Pediatric Urology

Editors

HILLARY L. COPP
ARMANDO J. LORENZO
ASEEM R. SHUKLA
ANTHONY A. CALDAMONE

UROLOGIC CLINICS
OF NORTH AMERICA

www.urologic.theclinics.com

Consulting Editor
SAMIR S. TANEJA

November 2018 • Volume 45 • Number 4

ELSEVIER

1600 John F. Kennedy Boulevard • Suite 1800 • Philadelphia, Pennsylvania, 19103-2899

http://www.theclinics.com

UROLOGIC CLINICS OF NORTH AMERICA Volume 45, Number 4
November 2018 ISSN 0094-0143, ISBN-13: 978-0-323-64314-6

Editor: Kerry Holland
Developmental Editor: Sara Watkins

Urologic Clinics of North America (ISSN 0094-0143) is published quarterly by Elsevier Inc., 360 Park Avenue South, New York, NY 10010-1710. Months of issue are February, May, August, and November. Business and Editorial Offices: 1600 John F. Kennedy Blvd., Suite 1800, Philadelphia, PA 19103-2899. Periodicals postage paid at New York, NY and additional mailing offices. Subscription prices are $374.00 per year (US individuals), $721.00 per year (US institutions), $100.00 per year (US students and residents), $431.00 per year (Canadian individuals), $901.00 per year (Canadian institutions), $515.00 per year (foreign individuals), $901.00 per year (foreign institutions), and $240.00 per year (Canadian and foreign students/residents). Foreign air speed delivery is included in all *Clinics* subscription prices. All prices are subject to change without notice. **POSTMASTER:** Send address changes to *Urologic Clinics of North America*, Elsevier Health Sciences Division, Subscription Customer Service, 3251 Riverport Lane, Maryland Heights, MO 63043. **Customer Service: 1-800-654-2452 (US). From outside the United States, call 1-314-447-8871. Fax: 1-314-447-8029. E-mail: JournalsCustomerServiceusa@elsevier.com (for print support) and JournalsOnlineSupport-usa@elsevier.com (for online support).**

Reprints. For copies of 100 or more, of articles in this publication, please contact the Commercial Reprints Department, Elsevier Inc., 360 Park Avenue South, New York, New York 10010-1710. Tel.: 212-633-3874; Fax: 212-633-3820; E-mail: reprints@ elsevier.com.

Urologic Clinics of North America is covered in MEDLINE/PubMed (*Index Medicus*), *Excerpta Medica, Current Contents/Clinical Medicine, Science Citation Index,* and *ISI/BIOMED.*

PROGRAM OBJECTIVE

The goal of *Urologic Clinics of North America* is to keep practicing urologists and urology residents up to date with current clinical practice in urology by providing timely articles reviewing the state of the art in patient care.

TARGET AUDIENCE

Practicing urologists, urology residents and other healthcare professionals practicing in the discipline of urology.

LEARNING OBJECTIVES

Upon completion of this activity, participants will be able to:
- Review epidemiology of, patient selection for, and psychological benefits of gender affirming surgery
- Discuss gender-affirming hormone therapy and surgical procedures
- Recognize long-term follow up and cancer screening for transgender patients

ACCREDITATION

The Elsevier Office of Continuing Medical Education (EOCME) is accredited by the Accreditation Council for Continuing Medical Education (ACCME) to provide continuing medical education for physicians.

The EOCME designates this enduring material for a maximum of 15 *AMA PRA Category 1 Credit*(s)™. Physicians should claim only the credit commensurate with the extent of their participation in the activity.

All other healthcare professionals requesting continuing education credit for this enduring material will be issued a certificate of participation.

DISCLOSURE OF CONFLICTS OF INTEREST

The EOCME assesses conflict of interest with its instructors, faculty, planners, and other individuals who are in a position to control the content of CME activities. All relevant conflicts of interest that are identified are thoroughly vetted by EOCME for fair balance, scientific objectivity, and patient care recommendations. EOCME is committed to providing its learners with CME activities that promote improvements or quality in healthcare and not a specific proprietary business or a commercial interest.

The planning committee, staff, authors and editors listed below have identified no financial relationships or relationships to products or devices they or their spouse/life partner have with commercial interest related to the content of this CME activity:

Liza M. Aguiar, MD; Andrea Balthazar, MD; Diana K. Bowen, MD; Luis H. Braga, MD, PhD; Megan A. Brockel, MD; Mark P. Cain, MD; Anthony A. Caldamone, MD, MMS, FAAP, FACS; Christopher S. Cooper, MD; Hillary L. Copp, MD, MS; Israel Franco, FAAP, FACS, MD; Daniela B. Gorduza, MD, FEAPU; C.D. Anthony Herndon, MD; Kerry Holland; Rakesh S. Joshi, MCh; Alison Kemp; Kathleen Kieran, MD, MS, MME; Robert Caleb Kovell, MD; Brad Kropp, MD; Armando J. Lorenzo, MD, MSc, FRCSC, FAAP, FACS; Pierre D.E. Mouriquand, MD, FRCS(Eng), FEAPU; Blake Palmer, MD; David M. Polanel, MD; Charmian A. Quigley, MBBS; Pramod P. Reddy, MD; Joshua D. Roth, MD; Kunj R. Sheth, MD; Margarett Shnorhavorian, MD, MPH; Aseem R. Shukla, MD; Alexander J. Skokan, MD; Arun K. Srinivasan, MD; Douglas W. Storm, MD; Samir Taneja, MD; Jason P. Van Batavia, MD; Vijaya M. Vemulakonda, MD, JD; Vignesh Viswanathan; Dan N. Wood, MD, PhD.

The planning committee, staff, authors and editors listed below have identified financial relationships or relationships to products or devices they or their spouse/life partner have with commercial interest related to the content of this CME activity:

Chester J. Koh, MD: participates on a speakers bureau and is a consultant/advisor for Intuitive Surgical.
Gregory E. Tasian, MD, MSc, MSCE: is a consultant/advisor for Allena Pharmaceuticals, Inc.

UNAPPROVED/OFF-LABEL USE DISCLOSURE

The EOCME requires CME faculty to disclose to the participants:
1. When products or procedures being discussed are off-label, unlabelled, experimental, and/or investigational (not US Food and Drug Administration [FDA] approved); and
2. Any limitations on the information presented, such as data that are preliminary or that represent ongoing research, interim analyses, and/or unsupported opinions. Faculty may discuss information about pharmaceutical agents that is outside of FDA-approved labelling. This information is intended solely for CME and is not intended to promote off-label use of these medications. If you have any questions, contact the medical affairs department of the manufacturer for the most recent prescribing information.

TO ENROLL

To enroll in the *Urologic Clinics of North America* Continuing Medical Education program, call customer service at 1-800-654-2452 or sign up online at http://www.theclinics.com/home/cme. The CME program is available to subscribers for an additional annual fee of USD $270.

METHOD OF PARTICIPATION

In order to claim credit, participants must complete the following:

1. Complete enrolment as indicated above.
2. Read the activity.
3. Complete the CME Test and Evaluation. Participants must achieve a score of 70% on the test. All CME Tests and Evaluations must be completed online.

CME INQUIRIES/SPECIAL NEEDS

For all CME inquiries or special needs, please contact elsevierCME@elsevier.com.

Contributors

CONSULTING EDITOR

SAMIR S. TANEJA, MD
The James M. Neissa and Janet Riha Neissa
Professor of Urologic Oncology, Professor of
Urology and Radiology, Director, Division of
Urologic Oncology, Vice Chair, Department
of Urology, NYU Langone Medical Center,
New York, New York

EDITORS

HILLARY L. COPP, MD, MS
Attending Pediatric Urology, UCSF Benioff
Children's Hospitals, San Francisco and
Oakland, Co-Director, UCSF Transitional
Urology Clinic, Associate Professor of
Urology, University of California, San Francisco
School of Medicine, San Francisco, California,
USA

**ARMANDO J. LORENZO, MD, MSc, FRCSC,
FAAP, FACS**
Staff Paediatric Urologist, Department of
Surgery, Division of Urology, Hospital for Sick
Children, Associate Professor, Department of
Surgery, Division of Urology, Associate
Scientist, Research Institute, Child Health
Evaluative Sciences, University of Toronto,
Toronto, Ontario, Canada

ASEEM R. SHUKLA, MD, FAAP
Attending Pediatric Urologist, Director,
Minimally Invasive Surgery, Endowed Chair in
Minimally Invasive Surgery, Associate
Professor of Surgery in Urology, Perelman
School of Medicine, University of
Pennsylvania, The Children's Hospital of
Philadelphia, Philadelphia, Pennsylvania, USA

**ANTHONY A. CALDAMONE, MD, MMS,
FAAP, FACS**
Professor of Surgery (Urology) and Pediatrics,
Hasbro Children's Hospital, The Warren Alpert
Medical School of Brown University, Division of
Pediatric Urology, Providence Rhode Island,
USA

AUTHORS

LIZA M. AGUIAR, MD
Assistant Professor of Surgery (Urology) and
Pediatrics, The Warren Alpert Medical School
of Brown University, Providence, Rhode Island,
USA

ANDREA BALTHAZAR, MD
Division of Urology, Resident in Urology,
Department of Surgery, Virginia
Commonwealth University School of Medicine,
VCU Medical Center, Richmond, Virginia, USA

DIANA K. BOWEN, MD
Fellow, Division of Urology, Perelman School of
Medicine, University of Pennsylvania, The
Children's Hospital of Philadelphia,
Philadelphia, Pennsylvania, USA

LUIS H. BRAGA, MD, PhD
Associate Professor, Department of Surgery,
Division of Urology, McMaster University,
Pediatric Urologist, McMaster Children's
Hospital, Hamilton, Ontario, Canada

MEGAN A. BROCKEL, MD
Assistant Professor, Department of
Anesthesiology, University of Colorado,
Children's Hospital Colorado, Aurora,
Colorado, USA

MARK P. CAIN, MD
Riley Hospital for Children at Indiana University
Health, Indianapolis, Indiana, USA

**ANTHONY A. CALDAMONE, MD, MMS,
FAAP, FACS**
Professor of Surgery (Urology) and Pediatrics,
Hasbro Children's Hospital, The Warren Alpert
Medical School of Brown University, Division of
Pediatric Urology, Providence Rhode Island,
USA

CHRISTOPHER S. COOPER, MD
Professor, Vice-Chair, Department of Urology,
University of Iowa, Carver College of Medicine,
Iowa City, Iowa, USA

ISRAEL FRANCO, FAAP, FACS, MD
Professor of Clinical Urology, Yale New Haven
Children's Hospital, New Haven, Connecticut,
USA

DANIELA B. GORDUZA, MD, FEAPU
Paediatric Urologist, Hospices Civils de Lyon,
Centre National de Référence Maladies Rares
sur le Développement Génital, Lyon, France

C.D. ANTHONY HERNDON, MD
Division Chief, Pediatric Urology, Division of
Urology, Department of Surgery, Co-Surgeon-
in-Chief, Children's Hospital of Richmond,
Virginia Commonwealth University School of
Medicine, VCU Medical Center, Richmond,
Virginia, USA

RAKESH S. JOSHI, MCh
Division of Paediatric Surgery, B.J. Medical
College and Civil Hospital, Ahmedabad,
Gujarat, India

KATHLEEN KIERAN, MD, MS, MME
Associate Professor, Division of Urology,
Seattle Children's Hospital, University of
Washington, Seattle, Washington, USA

CHESTER J. KOH, MD
Pediatric Urology, Baylor College of Medicine,
Texas Children's Hospital, Houston, Texas,
USA

ROBERT C. KOVELL, MD
Division of Urology, Assistant Professor,
Department of Surgery, University of
Pennsylvania Health System, The Children's
Hospital of Philadelphia, Perelman Center for
Advanced Medicine, Philadelphia,
Pennsylvania, USA

BRAD KROPP, MD
Medical Director, Pediatric Urology, Cook
Children's Health Care System, Fort Worth,
Texas, USA

**PIERRE D.E. MOURIQUAND, MD,
FRCS(Eng), FEAPU**
Professor and Head of the Department
of Paediatric Urology, Université
Claude-Bernard, Hospices Civils de Lyon
Centre National de Référence Maladies
Rares sur le Développement Génital, Lyon,
France

BLAKE PALMER, MD
Surgical Director of Renal Transplant, Pediatric
Urology, Cook Children's Health Care System,
Fort Worth, Texas, USA

DAVID M. POLANER, MD
Professor, Department of Anesthesiology,
University of Colorado, Children's Hospital
Colorado, Aurora, Colorado, USA

CHARMIAN A. QUIGLEY, MBBS
Pediatric Endocrinologist, Sydney Children's
Hospital, Randwick, New South Wales,
Australia

PRAMOD P. REDDY, MD
Director, Division of Pediatric Urology,
Professor, Department of Pediatrics, Cincinnati
Children's, University of Cincinnati College of
Medicine, University of Cincinnati, Cincinnati,
Ohio, USA

JOSHUA D. ROTH, MD
Riley Hospital for Children at Indiana University
Health, Indianapolis, Indiana, USA

KUNJ R. SHETH, MD
Pediatric Urology, Baylor College of Medicine,
Texas Children's Hospital, Houston, Texas,
USA

MARGARETT SHNORHAVORIAN, MD, MPH
Associate Professor, Division of Urology,
Seattle Children's Hospital, University of
Washington, Seattle, Washington, USA

ASEEM R. SHUKLA, MD, FAAP
Attending Pediatric Urologist, Director,
Minimally Invasive Surgery, Endowed Chair in
Minimally Invasive Surgery, Associate
Professor of Surgery in Urology, Perelman
School of Medicine, University of
Pennsylvania, The Children's Hospital of
Philadelphia, Philadelphia, Pennsylvania, USA

ALEXANDER J. SKOKAN, MD
Division of Urology, Resident, Department of
Surgery, University of Pennsylvania Health
System, Perelman Center for Advanced
Medicine, Philadelphia, Pennsylvania, USA

ARUN K. SRINIVASAN, MD
Pediatric Urology, The Children's Hospital of
Philadelphia, Philadelphia, Pennsylvania, USA

DOUGLAS W. STORM, MD
Clinical Assistant Professor, Department of
Urology, University of Iowa, Carver College of
Medicine, Iowa City, Iowa, USA

GREGORY E. TASIAN, MD, MSc, MSCE
Assistant Professor of Urology and
Epidemiology, Senior Scholar, Division of
Urology, Center for Pediatric Clinical
Effectiveness, Center for Clinical Epidemiology
and Biostatistics, Perelman School of
Medicine, University of Pennsylvania, The
Children's Hospital of Philadelphia,
Philadelphia, Pennsylvania, USA

JASON P. VAN BATAVIA, MD
Clinical Instructor, Pediatric Urology,
Division of Urology, The Children's Hospital
of Philadelphia, Philadelphia, Pennsylvania,
USA

VIJAYA M. VEMULAKONDA, MD, JD
Associate Professor, Department of
Urology, University of Colorado, Children's
Hospital Colorado, Aurora, Colorado,
USA

DAN N. WOOD, MD, PhD
Consultant Urologist, University
College London Hospitals, London,
United Kingdom

Contents

Preface: Pediatric Urology   xiii

Hillary L. Copp, Armando J. Lorenzo, Aseem R. Shukla, and Anthony A. Caldamone

Continuous Antibiotic Prophylaxis in Pediatric Urology   525

Douglas W. Storm, Luis H. Braga, and Christopher S. Cooper

> Continuous antibiotic prophylaxis (CAP) for urinary tract infection prevention in children with vesicoureteral reflux, hydronephrosis, and hydroureteronephrosis is reviewed. A more selective use of CAP is advocated based on a review of known individual risk factors in each of these conditions that subsequently helps identify the children most likely to benefit from CAP. Both short-term and potential long-term side effects of CAP are reviewed, including the impact of prophylactic antibiotics on bacterial resistance and the microbiome. Alternatives to continuous antibiotic prophylaxis including Vaccinium macrocarpon (Cranberry), probiotics, and vaccines are reviewed.

Pediatric Stone Disease   539

Diana K. Bowen and Gregory E. Tasian

> Once considered rare, pediatric nephrolithiasis has become a critical field of study in the last decade because of the rapid increase in incidence. Understanding the changing epidemiology and lifelong implications of pediatric stone disease is critically important to effectively manage the individual patient as well as identify risk factors for childhood onset that could be modified. Determining the role of diagnostic imaging in children is a unique challenge as limiting radiation and imaging stewardship should be priorities. Approaches to management have also changed, as technology continues to evolve and both medical and surgical options expand.

Anesthesia in the Pediatric Patient   551

Megan A. Brockel, David M. Polaner, and Vijaya M. Vemulakonda

> Improvements in anesthetic drugs and monitoring techniques over the past several decades have significantly reduced the anesthetic risks for pediatric patients. Neonates and infants are at increased risk for cardiovascular and pulmonary complications, and recent reports have led to concern that these young patients may be at risk for long-term detrimental neurodevelopmental effects as well. Although studies are currently under way to answer the question of anesthetic neurotoxicity in children, surgeons and anesthesiologists must work with parents to determine the best course of action for these vulnerable patients.

Urologic Evaluation and Management of Pediatric Kidney Transplant Patients   561

Blake Palmer and Brad Kropp

> Urologic causes of end-stage renal disease are estimated between 25% and 40% of causes. The goal of renal transplant in patients with chronic kidney disease is to provide renal replacement therapy with less morbidity, better quality of life, and improved overall survival compared with dialysis. A patient's urologic history can be a significant source of problems related to infections, recurrence of disease, and surgical complications. Many of the urologic risks are modifiable. Proper evaluation and

management can mitigate the potential problems after transplant, and these patients with complex urologic problems are seen to have similar graft function outcomes.

Neuropathic Bladder and Augmentation Cystoplasty

Joshua D. Roth and Mark P. Cain

571

Surgical indications for individuals with neuropathic bladder include unsafe urinary storage pressures, progressive upper tract deterioration, and continued urinary incontinence that is recalcitrant to oral pharmacologic or intradetrusor injection therapy and intermittent catheterization. Bladder augmentation is currently the gold standard surgical procedure used to increase bladder capacity and reduce storage pressures but has significant long-term risks. The medical and surgical management of neuropathic bladder, as well as long-term consequences of bladder augmentation, are reviewed.

Fertility Issues in Pediatric Urology

Kathleen Kieran and Margarett Shnorhavorian

587

Improved understanding of the pathogenesis and natural history of many urologic disorders, as well as advances in fertility preservation techniques, has increased the awareness of and options for management of fertility threats in pediatric patients. In children, fertility may be altered by oncologic conditions, by differences in sexual differentiation, by gonadotoxic drugs and other side effects of treatment for nonurologic disorders, and by urologic conditions, such as varicocele and cryptorchidism. Although fertility concerns are best addressed in a multidisciplinary setting, pediatric urologists should be aware of the underlying pathophysiology and management options to properly counsel and advocate for patients.

Transitional Urology

Robert C. Kovell, Alexander J. Skokan, and Dan N. Wood

601

The field of transitional urology has taken on an increasing importance in recent years as more individuals with congenital urologic issues are living and thriving into adulthood. This article reviews the transitional process itself, including barriers to successful transition and the consequences of failing to properly transition. Also provided is a broad overview of the urologic issues faced by patients who may benefit from lifelong care and the providers who will be helping them with transition and assuming their care.

Minimally Invasive Surgery in Pediatric Urology: Adaptations and New Frontiers

Kunj R. Sheth, Jason P. Van Batavia, Diana K. Bowen, Chester J. Koh, and Arun K. Srinivasan

611

As the frontiers of minimally invasive surgery (MIS) continue to expand, the availability and implementation of new technology in pediatric urology are increasing. MIS is already an integral part of pediatric urology, but there is still much more potential change to come as both recent and upcoming advances in laparoscopic and robotic surgery are surveyed.

Pediatric Urology and Global Health: Why Now and How to Build a Successful Global Outreach Program

Jason P. Van Batavia, Aseem R. Shukla, Rakesh S. Joshi, and Pramod P. Reddy

623

Global health programs in pediatric surgical fields are needed more than ever to ease the global burden of congenital anomalies. Pediatric urology is an ideal field for global health programs because genitourinary diseases account for a large proportion of congenital diseases and access to surgical subspecialists is lacking in most low- and middle-income countries. By following several key guidelines with particular emphasis on team building, visiting and local team collaboration, long-term commitment, and surgical training, global health partnerships can lead to a sustainable model for increasing surgical capacity.

Bladder Bowel Dysfunction

633

Liza M. Aguiar and Israel Franco

Bladder bowel dysfunction (BBD) describes a spectrum of lower urinary tract symptoms associated with bowel complaints. The true incidence of BBD is unknown; however, BBD symptoms represent approximately 40% of pediatric urology consultations. Given the close interaction between the bladder and bowel owing to their common innervation as well as associated pelvic floor muscles, patients often present with bowel complaints as well. Increasing awareness of BBD over the past 30 years has led to better diagnostic criteria and treatment methods. In this article, the authors review the clinical presentation, diagnostic approach, pathophysiology, and treatment options for children with BBD.

Prenatal Urinary Tract Dilatation

641

Andrea Balthazar and C.D. Anthony Herndon

Urinary tract dilatation (UTD) is the most common congenital anomaly detected on prenatal ultrasonography (US), affecting 1% to 3% of all pregnancies. This article focuses on the prenatal detection of UTD and the postnatal evaluation and management based on the UTD grading system risk assessment. Prophylactic antibiotics and postnatal imaging are discussed. The recent management trend is for a more conservative approach to minimize unnecessary testing and exposures to the fetus and neonate while detecting those who may have clinically significant disorder. The renal bladder US remains a critical part of the evaluation and helps guide further investigations.

Surgery of Anomalies of Gonadal and Genital Development in the "Post-Truth Era"

659

Daniela B. Gorduza, Charmian A. Quigley, Anthony A. Caldamone, and Pierre D.E. Mouriquand

This article aims to examine the current issues of debate concerning the management of atypical gonadal and genital development (AGD). Understanding this complex subject begins with defining the distinct AGD conditions, the aims and nature of surgical treatments, and the perceptions of affected individuals and their families. The evolving societal and medical contexts in this field are confronting facts and opinions, leading to a significant change in attitudes and approaches.

UROLOGIC CLINICS OF NORTH AMERICA

FORTHCOMING ISSUES

February 2019
**Surgical Advances in Female Pelvic
Reconstruction**
Craig V. Comiter, *Editor*

May 2019
**Emerging Technologies in Renal Stone
Management**
Ojas Shah and Briana Matlaga, *Editors*

August 2019
Modern Management of Testicular Cancer
Sia Daneshmand, *Editor*

RECENT ISSUES

August 2018
Advances in Urologic Imaging
Samir S. Taneja, *Editor*

May 2018
**Current Management of Invasive Bladder
and Upper Tract Urothelial Cancer**
Jeffrey M. Holzbeierlein, *Editor*

February 2018
**Contemporary Approaches to Urinary
Diversion and Reconstruction**
Michael S. Cookson, *Editor*

THE CLINICS ARE AVAILABLE ONLINE!
Access your subscription at:
www.theclinics.com

Preface
Pediatric Urology

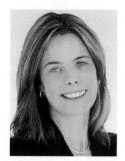 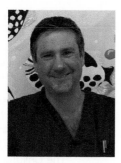 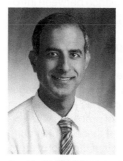 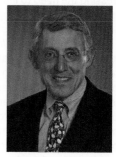

Hillary L. Copp, MD, MS   Armando J. Lorenzo, MD, MSc, FRCSC, FAAP, FACS   Aseem R. Shukla, MD, FAAP   Anthony A. Caldamone, MD, MMS, FAAP, FACS

Editors

Even if you are on the right track, you'll get run over if you just sit there.
—Will Rogers, quoted in the Sandusky –Register, The Week, May 2, 2016

Pediatric urology is a relatively young subspecialty, having received its accreditation as a subspecialty in the United States in 2007. Over the course of the last 30 years or so, there have been dramatic changes in our understanding of common pediatric urologic problems, which has influenced our management. One example is our understanding and management of vesicoureteral reflux and urinary tract infections in children. Reflux in particular is considered to be the anomaly that defined the subspecialty of pediatric urology. We had a very aggressive approach to its identification, as well as its management, as every child with reflux was either maintained on chronic antibiotic prophylaxis or surgically corrected. Today, we have a better understanding of its natural history, as well as stratification of the risk of reflux in individuals.

Similarly, when hydronephrosis was first discovered prenatally, we had a very aggressive approach to its management and were driven by the concept that, "Here we have a way to discover anomalies with the potential for renal injury before acquired renal damage ensues." Therefore, we felt that if these children were not intervened upon, preventable loss of renal function would result. We have since learned that it is the minority of this population that requires an intervention. And so it goes, on and on in pediatric urology. As we gain better understanding of a condition, we can refine management and become more selective with interventions. Thus, conservative management is becoming the rule rather than the exception for many of the pathologies we treat. Many challenges remain, as we have not yet adopted a universal classification system to allow us to rigorously study various evaluation and management protocols.

As our subspecialty matures, new problems have come into view. For example, we are becoming increasingly worried about long-term fertility issues related to conditions that we treat or treatments that we offer. Many centers in North America and Europe have developed fertility preservation teams to better study this complex issue and maximize future fertility potential. We have also broadened the scope of our counseling for surgical interventions early in life, including

Urol Clin N Am 45 (2018) xiii–xiv
https://doi.org/10.1016/j.ucl.2018.08.001

a more in-depth discussion of the potential neuro-cognitive risks of general anesthesia. Minimally invasive interventions are gaining popularity, changing the way we do many procedures, and stressing the need to find a balance between intro-duction of new technologies, morbidity, evidence-based practice, and costs.

In this issue of the *Urologic Clinics*, we tackle many of these topics and have selected certain areas of pediatric urology that we feel have under-gone significant changes in concept or manage-ment. Each of the authors has focused on updating our approach to these problems with sci-entific evidence. While many of these remain quite controversial, let us remember that the goal of argu-ment is not to win or lose but to make progress.

We would like to thank all the authors for their hard work in developing excellent articles for this issue. We would also like to thank our families for understanding the time that we put into our aca-demic pursuits.

Hillary L. Copp, MD, MS
UCSF Benioff Children's Hospitals
San Francisco and Oakland
UCSF Transitional Urology Clinic
University of California
San Francisco School of Medicine
550 16th Street, 5th Floor
San Francisco, CA 94158, USA

Armando J. Lorenzo, MD, MSc, FRCSC, FAAP, FACS
Department of Surgery
Division of Urology
Research Institute
Child Health Evaluative Sciences
University of Toronto
Hospital for Sick Children
555 University Avenue, Room M299
Toronto, Ontario M5G 1X8, Canada

Aseem R. Shukla, MD, FAAP
Minimally Invasive Surgery
Perelman School of Medicine at
the University of Pennsylvania
The Children's Hospital of Philadelphia
3401 Civic Center Boulevard
Philadelphia, PA 19104-4399, USA

Anthony A. Caldamone, MD, MMS, FAAP, FACS
Hasbro Children's Hospital
Warren Alpert Medical School of Brown University
Division of Pediatric Urology
2 Dudley Street, Suite 174
Providence, RI 02905, USA

E-mail addresses:
Hillary.Copp@ucsf.edu (H.L. Copp)
armando.lorenzo@sickkids.ca (A.J. Lorenzo)
ShuklaA@email.chop.edu (A.R. Shukla)
Anthony_Caldamone@brown.edu
(A.A. Caldamone)

Continuous Antibiotic Prophylaxis in Pediatric Urology

Douglas W. Storm, MD[a], Luis H. Braga, MD, PhD[b],
Christopher S. Cooper, MD[a],*

KEYWORDS

- Antibiotic prophylaxis • Vesicoureteral reflux • Prenatal hydronephrosis • Antibiotic resistance
- Microbiota • Megaureter • Side effects

KEY POINTS

- The use of antibiotic prophylaxis for pediatric urologic conditions has proven benefits and proven harms.
- The indiscriminate use of antibiotic prophylaxis for all children with vesicoureteral reflux and for those with all grades of hydronephrosis and hydroureteronephrosis is at best unnecessary and at worst harmful.
- Identification of risk factors for urinary tract infection, renal injury, and its long-term sequelae permits a more individualized and selective use of continuous antibiotic prophylaxis.
- Antibiotics affect the normal human microbiota, which is necessary for normal body functions and development.
- The full impact of prophylactic antibiotics, for better or worse, on the developing and aging body is unknown.

INTRODUCTION

The word prophylaxis from the Greek means to guard or prevent beforehand. Antibiotic prophylaxis in the context of Pediatric Urology is the attempt to prevent urinary tract infections (UTIs) in children who are at a higher risk, such as those with vesicoureteral reflux (VUR) and hydroureteronephrosis.

Evidence for or against the following statements regarding the use of antibiotic prophylaxis will be discussed in this article:

- The use of antibiotic prophylaxis for pediatric urologic conditions has proven benefit and proven harm.
- Nonselective or indiscriminate use of antibiotic prophylaxis for all children with VUR and for those with all grades of hydronephrosis (HN) and hydroureteronephrosis is at best unnecessary and at worst harmful.
- The full impact of prophylactic antibiotics, for better or worse, on the developing and aging body is unknown.

Over the last 2 decades, increased awareness of the truth of the previous statements by physicians and the public is leading to an increasingly selective approach to the use of prophylactic antibiotics. Although previously it was thought that most children with conditions such as VUR or hydronephrosis conferred a high risk of UTI and therefore they would benefit from continuous antibiotic prophylaxis (CAP), information from multiple

Disclosure Statement: None.
[a] Department of Urology, University of Iowa, Carver College of Medicine, 200 Hawkins Drive, 3RCP, Iowa City, IA 5224, USA; [b] Department of Surgery, Division of Urology, Mcmaster University, McMaster Children's Hospital, 1200 Main Street West, Hamilton, Ontario L8N 3Z5, Canada
* Corresponding author.
E-mail address: christopher-cooper@uiowa.edu

Urol Clin N Am 45 (2018) 525–538
https://doi.org/10.1016/j.ucl.2018.06.001

urologic.theclinics.com

studies now permit better identification of children most likely to benefit from antibiotic prophylaxis and thereby facilitate a more selective and individualized approach to health care. This article reviews the benefits and risks of antibiotic prophylaxis in the context of several common pediatric urologic conditions, including VUR, prenatally detected HN, and hydroureter. For each condition, patient characteristics that place the child at increased risk of UTI and its sequelae are noted. The impact of prophylactic antibiotics on bacterial resistance, the microbiome, and potential long-term side effects are reviewed. The article concludes with a discussion on the evolving field of alternatives to continuous antibiotic prophylaxis including prebiotics and probiotics.

VESICOURETERAL REFLUX

The greatest controversy regarding CAP in pediatric urology stems from their use in children with VUR. Without question, there is agreement that antibiotics kill bacteria and prevent UTIs. The reduction in UTIs in those children receiving CAP has been confirmed by the Randomized Intervention for Vesicoureteral Reflux (RIVUR) and Swedish Reflux trials.[1,2] What remains questioned is the practice of placing every child with VUR on CAP. In addition, controversy continues regarding the need to obtain a voiding cystourethrogram and diagnose VUR in children following their first febrile UTI.[3,4]

Over the last 2 decades, there has been increased recognition that many children with VUR do not benefit from either diagnosis or treatment of their condition.[5,6] The presence of reflux in many children is self-limited and innocuous; however, a subset of children with VUR benefit from both diagnosis and treatment with either CAP or operative intervention. The benefit comes in terms of prevention of recurrent UTIs and their associated morbidity as well as a reduction in kidney damage and its potential long-term sequelae. Many children with abnormal kidneys, including those with scars or a history of pyelonephritis, are at increased risk for end-stage renal disease later in life.[7] Identification of which children constitute the subset that benefit from antibiotics and/or surgical intervention continues to remain the greatest challenge to the advancement of VUR management.

Risk Factors

Multiple risk factors associated with recurrent UTI, persistent VUR, pyelonephritis, and renal scars have now been identified and when considered together help to better identify which children are most likely to benefit from antibiotic prophylaxis, and conversely, which children are unlikely to benefit. The severity or grade of VUR has been used as a primary factor in determining the likelihood of spontaneous reflux resolution and risk of pyelonephritis and renal injury. Higher grades of reflux are associated with decreased resolution rates and increased prevalence of renal scars.[8,9] In addition, VUR occurring earlier during bladder filling has been demonstrated to be a risk factor for breakthrough UTIs independent of grade.[10] In addition to grade and bladder volume at the onset of reflux, other factors predictive of reflux resolution, UTI, and/or the risk of renal injury include gender, age, race, laterality, bladder pressure at the onset of reflux, presence of renal scars, presence of bowel and bladder dysfunction, and a history of recurrent UTIs.[1,11–17] Knowledge of these factors may be used in a variety of available computer programs (ie, http://godot.urol.uic.edu/urocomp/svm_vur.html; https://www.choc.org/programs-services/urology/ireflux-risk-calculator/; https://uticalc.pitt.edu) to help predict the likelihood and timing of resolution or UTIs. These predictions may guide parents and clinicians in determining if the patient would benefit from earlier operative intervention as opposed to prolonged CAP.[14,18,19]

In addition, clinical efforts should be made at reducing a child's risk factors for UTI, such as correction of bladder or bowel dysfunction or consideration of circumcision in boys at high risk for UTI.

Bladder and Bowel Dysfunction

Bladder and bowel dysfunction (BBD) constitute the largest assessable risk factors for the development of UTI in children. Even on CAP, children with VUR and bowel and/or bladder dysfunction are at particularly high risk for developing recurrent pyelonephritis.[20–22] Recurrent UTIs are estimated to occur in about 45% to 56% of these children as opposed to 15% to 25% without BBD.[22,23] In addition, children with BBD also have a higher incidence of renal scarring, a lower spontaneous resolution rate, and a higher failure rate following antireflux surgery.[22,24] Treatment of a child's bladder dysfunction reduces recurrent UTIs and improves VUR resolution, and treatment of constipation significantly reduces recurrent UTIs and improves bladder function.[25,26] BBD alone is a risk factor for recurrent UTI but a child with BBD and any grade of VUR is at highest risk for recurrent UTI.[22]

Continuous Prophylactic Antibiotics with Vesicoureteral Reflux

Following an initial UTI, approximately 10% to 30% of children will develop at least one recurrent

UTI.[23,27–29] The recurrence rate is highest within the first 3 to 6 months following a UTI, and the more frequent and more recurrent a child's UTI is, the more likely he or she is to experience a subsequent UTI.[30–32] Neither the American Academy of Pediatrics (AAP) guidelines nor the National Institute of Health and Care Excellence guidelines recommend routinely prescribing prophylactic antibiotics to infants and children following their first UTI. Before the RIVUR trial and the Swedish reflux trials, the efficacy of prophylaxis in children with VUR was questioned by several relatively small randomized trials including children with low grades of VUR.[33–36] The RIVUR trial compared trimethoprim-sulfamethoxazole (TMP-SMX) prophylaxis with placebo in 607 children with grade I–IV VUR following UTI. The risk of febrile of symptomatic UTI recurrences was reduced by half in children receiving prophylaxis as compared with those receiving prophylaxis (25.5% vs 37.4%; relative risk, 0.68; 95% confidence interval [CI], 0.53–0.87), and this difference between the 2 treatment groups widened over time (**Fig. 1**).

Despite the findings noted earlier from the RIVUR trial, further review of the data revealed that 8 children would need to be treated with antibiotic prophylaxis for 2 years to prevent 1 case of febrile or symptomatic UTI. In addition, outcome renal scans (at the 2-year visit or 3–4 months after the child met treatment failure criteria) showed no significant difference between groups in the incidence of renal scarring (11.9% in the prophylaxis group and 10.2% in the placebo group; $P = .55$). The risk reduction for recurrent UTI was greatest in those children with BBD at baseline, a history of febrile UTI, or higher grades of VUR.[1]

As might be expected, the benefit of prophylactic antibiotics is more easily demonstrated when used in specific populations known to be at high risk for recurrent UTI such as girls with dilating VUR (ie, $\geq$ grade III).[19,37] The following risk factors associated with a low risk of recurrent UTI make it more difficult to demonstrate any benefit of prophylactic antibiotics: circumcised boys, no BBD, no recent history of UTI, normal renal ultrasound or DMSA scan, a lack of anatomic abnormalities, and nondilating VUR.[23] Knowledge of these risk factors is useful in identifying children with VUR most likely, and least likely, to benefit from continuous prophylactic antibiotics. Several recent studies have combined some of the previously identified risk factors in computational neural networks to better identify children with VUR at risk for breakthrough UTIs.[38,39]

A meta-analysis by de Bessa and colleagues[40] was conducted after the publication of the AAP 2011 recommendations. After initial analysis of the trials, CAP was determined to be beneficial only in children with high-grade VUR (Grade III/IV). However, with the addition of the data from the 2014 RIVUR study, the new pooled estimate supported the use of CAP in all children with VUR to prevent recurrent UTI, regardless of reflux grade. This benefit was further shown by the most recent systematic review and meta-analysis on the topic.[41] Wang and colleagues identified 1547 studies, of which 8 randomized controlled trials (RCTs) were selected to be included in their analysis. Pooled results demonstrated that CAP significantly reduced the risk of recurrent febrile or symptomatic UTI (pooled odds ratio [OR] 0.63). However, if UTIs occurred, there was an increased risk of antibiotic-resistant organisms (pooled OR 8.75). This meta-analysis also showed that a reduction in the number of new renal scars was not associated with CAP use.

As is the case with any systematic review, the applicability of these 2 meta-analyses heavily depends on the quality, validity, and heterogeneity of the included studies. Furthermore, although RCTs provide the best available evidence, they do not always reflect our clinical patient population. Therefore, these results must be interpreted with caution. Although it is tempting to simply extrapolate results of each RCT or systematic review beyond the study population to all children with VUR, this is risky. Each of the 8 RCTs had different patient cohorts, likely reflecting the differences in observed outcomes. The decision to use CAP is multifactorial, based on variables such as age, gender, clinical presentation, grade, presence of BBD, and circumcision status. Although risk calculators could be used to simplify clinical decision-making, a health care practitioner would ideally identify specific patient groups and

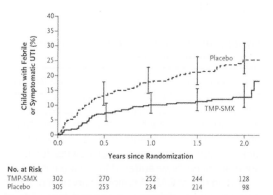

No. at Risk

TMP-SMX	302	270	252	244	128
Placebo	305	253	234	214	98

Fig. 1. Time to first recurrent febrile or symptomatic UTI. (*From* RIVUR Trial Investigators, Hoberman A, Greenfield SP, Mattoo TK, et al. Antimicrobial prophylaxis for children with vesicoureteral reflux. N Engl J Med 2014;370:2373; with permission.)

determine which RCT inclusion criteria best capture his or her child's clinical characteristics and apply the results accordingly instead of generalizing outcomes of systematic reviews to all children with VUR.

Reflux nephropathy/renal scarring

Although some studies have shown a small benefit in the use of antibiotic prophylaxis in preventing symptomatic and febrile UTIs, the prevention of renal scarring had not been established, mostly because of underpowering of studies. Hewitt[42] and coworkers performed a meta-analysis of 1427 subjects aged 18 years or younger looking at the effect of antibiotic prophylaxis in preventing UTI-mediated renal scarring. Their analysis revealed no influence of antibiotic prophylaxis in preventing renal scarring (pooled risk ratio, 0.83; 95% CI, 0.55–1.26). They performed a subgroup analysis, restricted to individuals with VUR, and again found no benefit of the use of antibiotic prophylaxis in preventing renal scarring (pooled risk ratio, 0.79, CI, 0.51–1.24).[42] Despite limitations to this study, which include the small number of studies, short duration of follow-up, and insufficient children with high-grade VUR, these results highlight the need to identify children at greatest risk of scarring in whom antibiotic prophylaxis is more likely to be beneficial. In addition, a lack of an identified area of renal damage or new scar by nuclear renal scan does not rule out the probability that a smaller degree of permanent renal injury is produced with each episode of pyelonephritis.

Children at risk for renal injury include those at risk for recurrent or breakthrough UTIs because renal scarring increases with an increasing number of febrile UTIs.[43] In addition, children with reflux and UTIs are at increased risk for renal scarring compared with children with UTIs and no reflux. Up to one-third of all patients with VUR have renal scars and in the International Reflux Study, 50% of children with grades III or IV reflux had scars at entry.[44] Of note, many "scars" identified on the initial renal imaging in children with VUR may actually be regions of congenital renal cortical dysplasia. Multiple studies demonstrate a direct correlation between increased prevalence of renal scarring and higher grades of reflux.[45] Renal scarring develops less often in nondilating forms of reflux.[46,47] A retrospective study of 120 patients demonstrated a significantly higher chance of developing a breakthrough UTI in children with grades III to V reflux and an abnormality on baseline DMSA scan compared with those without an abnormality (60% vs 6%, respectively).[48] In addition, renal scars are a negative predictor of reflux resolution independent of reflux grade.[12] Children with renal scars are also more likely to develop additional scars than children without renal scars.[47,49,50]

The presence of scars implies regions of renal damage and increases the risk for long-term adverse sequelae.[7] In one study with a mean follow-up of 12 years after an antireflux operation, children with unilateral renal scars had an 11% chance of developing hypertension and an 18.5% chance if they had bilateral renal scars.[51] Others have suggested the incidence of hypertension in children with bilateral renal scars is about 20%.[51] Children with severe bilateral renal scars are significantly more likely to develop proteinuria, chronic renal insufficiency, and failure than those with unilateral scars or unscarred kidneys.[7,52,53] These data strongly suggest that children with renal scars are at increased risk for further development of UTIs and scars and long-term clinical sequelae. These increased risks associated with renal scars needs to be considered along with the previously described risk factors for UTI and renal injury when selecting the subset of children most likely to benefit from prophylactic antibiotics.

Prompt antimicrobial treatment decreases the chance of permanent renal damage, as does the elimination of any subsequent episode of pyelonephritis.[54] If the social situation is such that a child may not be promptly diagnosed and treated for a febrile UTI, this child may be more likely to benefit from prophylactic antibiotics because a delay in treatment is associated with increased risk of renal injury and scar. One review noted that for every hour antimicrobial therapy was delayed in treating a febrile UTI, the odds of new renal scarring increased by 0.8%.[55] Others have shown that the odds of developing a renal scar double if antibiotics are begun after 72 hours from the start of a febrile UTI compared with children begun on antibiotics within 48 hours.[56]

Continuous Antibiotic Prophylaxis with Prenatal Hydronephrosis

CAP has been empirically recommended for newborns with prenatal HN to prevent UTI during the first 2 years of life. However, the quality of evidence to support such practice has been based on low levels of evidence.[57–59] Because of this lack of high-quality studies, guidelines for management of HN have suffered from inconsistencies regarding use of CAP. A national survey of practice patterns and antibiotic use showed that 56% of general pediatricians would routinely prescribe CAP for infants with prenatal HN.[60] Another survey revealed that pediatric nephrologists and urologists seem to agree on the perceived lack of

CAP benefit in children with unilateral low-grade HN; however, important discrepancies for bilateral and high grades of HN were noted.[61] Finally, an international survey has identified that pediatric urologists from the United States prescribed CAP at birth more often compared with their European colleagues (77% vs 40%, respectively; P<.001). However, similar proportions of pediatric urologists in the United States and in Europe (65%–70%) prescribe CAP for high-grade HN.[59]

In 2009, the Canadian Urological Association (CUA) guidelines on prenatal HN provided Grade D recommendation for CAP use in this population.[62] In 2010, the Society For Fetal Urology (SFU) consensus statement on HN recommended CAP only for infants with high-grade HN and for those with VUR.[63] On the other hand, the 2010 American Urological Association (AUA) guidelines on VUR suggested that CAP might not be necessary for children with asymptomatic VUR grades I and II (ie, without previous history of UTI).[23] Finally, the updated 2017 CUA-Pediatric Urologists of Canada (PUC) guidelines stated that the role of CAP initiated at birth is controversial but may be of greater benefit in infants with SFU grades III/IV HN and in cases with dilated ureters or bladder abnormalities. It was also suggested that women and uncircumcised men with prenatal HN may benefit more from prophylaxis than circumcised boys (Level 3 Evidence: Grade C Recommendation).[64]

Given these discrepancies within the literature, a systematic review, including data of nearly 4000 patients from 21 studies, was conducted in 2013 to summarize the latest evidence regarding CAP use in children with prenatal HN.[61] According to this review, overall pooled UTI rates were 4 times higher for patients with high-grade HN versus those with low-grade HN, as reported by others.[65] When HN grade was stratified according to CAP use, UTI rates were equivalent in children with low-grade HN, regardless of their CAP status (2.2% vs 2.8% with and without CAP, respectively). In patients with high-grade HN, UTI rates were significantly lower in those on versus not on CAP (14.6% vs. 28.9%). The number needed to treat was 7, meaning that 7 patients with high-grade HN needed to be on CAP in order to prevent one UTI.[61] Despite the heterogeneity of the included studies, an update of the previous systematic review confirmed the perceived value in providing CAP to infants with high-grade HN.[66] On the contrary, the European Association of Urology/European Society for Paediatric Urology Guidelines Panel recently released their statement saying that the benefits of CAP in a heterogeneous group of children with prenatal HN involving different causes remain unproven. However, that panel acknowledged that data from observational studies have shown that CAP reduces febrile UTI in particular subgroups, such as women, uncircumcised men, and those with hydroureteronephrosis.[67]

CAP in Primary Nonrefluxing Megaureters (Hydroureteronephrosis)

Evidence also suggests that the presence of hydroureter or ureterocele carries a significantly higher risk of UTI when compared with infants with isolated HN.[68] Patients with primary nonrefluxing megaureters (hydroureteronephrosis) have been studied in greater detail and found to have a much higher febrile UTI rate than those with isolated HN (19/59 [32%] versus 12/218 [6%]).[69] In a cohort study of 80 patients with primary megaureter with a mean follow-up of 26 months, febrile UTI developed in 34% of those infants within the first 6 months of life, leading the investigators to recommend CAP to this population.[70] In contrast, another study examined 47 children with 58 primary nonrefluxing megaureters and found an overall rate of febrile UTI of only 15%, with most of the events developing after 6 months of age,[71] which is contradictory to the current literature.[70,72,73] The British Association of Paediatric Urologists (BAPU) consensus on primary megaureter states that CAP is advisable for the first 6 to 12 months of life.[74] Circumcision and CAP use were the only factors associated with a reduction of UTI rates in infants with primary megaureters.[70,75] Furthermore, observational studies have shown that women and uncircumcised men with prenatal HN represent a high-risk group for development of UTI and are more likely to benefit from CAP to reduce that risk.[58,69,70,75,76]

Although it is thought that CAP may prevent UTI in children with prenatal HN, it is yet to be proved. An RCT comparing trimethoprim with placebo in infants with SFU grades III to IV HN is currently underway in order to answer this question.[77] Therefore, some investigators suggest institution of CAP at birth, whereas others, instead, recommend a low threshold for investigation and treatment of a suspected UTI.

Antibiotic resistance

Antibiotics are the primary treatment of bacterial infections. Since the original discovery of penicillin by Sir Alexander Fleming in 1928, antibiotic use has saved millions of lives. Unfortunately, an unintended side effect of antibiotics use has been the development of antibiotic resistance. Over time, the overuse of antibiotics and the lack of new antibacterial agents entering the market have resulted in a global crisis secondary to antibiotic resistance. In 2001, the World Health Organization (WHO) declared antibiotic resistance as a global public health problem, launching a global health strategy for containment of antimicrobial resistance.[78] In subsequent global action plans to curb antimicrobial resistance, the WHO declared that "Antibiotic resistance threatens the very core of modern medicine" and "without harmonized and immediate action on a global scale, the world is headed toward a post-antibiotic era in which common infections could once again kill."[79]

The overuse of antibiotics in the realm of pediatric urology, particularly with the use of prophylactic antibiotics (CAP), contributes to antibiotic resistance. CAP for UTIs has been associated with a 24-fold increased risk of resistant *Escherichia coli* to TMP-SMX.[80] Other studies have demonstrated the emergence of bacteria aside from *E coli* with high rates of resistance in children receiving prophylactic antibiotics.[81] Furthermore, Costelloe et al.[82] identified that antibiotic treatment resulted in a pooled OR for development of a UTI with antimicrobial resistance as 2.5 within 2 months of original treatment, falling to 1.3 within 12 months of treatment and that longer antibiotic treatment, such as through the use of CAP, was associated with a higher risk of antibiotic resistance.[82]

Over the last 10 years, numerous studies have evaluated the utility of prophylactic antibiotics in preventing recurrent infections in children with HN, VUR, and recurrent UTIs, with varied results. Despite differing conclusions, one apparent outcome is that CAP use does result in antibiotic resistance. A Cochrane Review in 2010 evaluated the effectiveness and risks associated with prophylactic antibiotic use in children to prevent recurrent UTIs. This review, which included 12 studies, concluded that the overall risk reduction of UTI recurrence in children placed on prophylactic antibiotics was modest at 8%, corresponding to the need to treat 12 to 13 children for 12 months to prevent a single UTI.[83] They noted that this benefit did not occur without risk. Namely, using the data from 2 studies,[19,34] they identified that breakthrough UTIs in children placed on prophylactic antibiotics are commonly resistant to their daily antimicrobial treatment. In the Montini and PRIVENT studies, 53% and 28% of the breakthrough infections, respectively, in the active treatment arms, were resistant to the active treatment drug.[19,84] This lead the investigators of the Cochrane Review to conclude that the small benefit of long-term prophylactic antibiotic use should be carefully weighed against the increased likelihood of bacterial resistance in subsequent infections.

These findings regarding antibiotic resistance secondary to CAP use are a common theme in other similar studies. The RIVUR study demonstrated those experiencing a breakthrough UTI with a statistically significant ($P<.001$) increased rate of resistance to TMP-SMX within the CAP cohort. Within the treatment group, 63.3% of all breakthrough UTIs from *E coli* were resistant to TMP-SMX compared with a 19.3% resistance rate to TMP-SMX within the placebo group. This study obtained rectal swabs at baseline, after treatment failure and at the end of the study, evaluating for TMP-SMX resistance. Although stool colonization with resistant *E coli* was more common in the prophylaxis group (27.6%) than in the placebo group (19.5%), the difference was not significant.

Breakthrough UTIs in children receiving antibiotic prophylaxis are not just singularly resistant to the prophylactic antimicrobial. Instead CAP use may lead to multidrug-resistant infections, resulting in serious and difficult to treat UTIs. An analysis by Selekman and colleagues[85] reviewed 1299 patients with recurrent UTIs from multiple different studies, in which co-trimoxazole was the most common drug used for prophylaxis (85%), and found that CAP children were more likely to have a multidrug-resistant infection (33% vs 6%, $P<.01$) and were more likely to receive broad spectrum antibiotics in treating their infection (68% vs 49%, $P = .004$). Therefore, CAP use significantly increases the acquired risk of coresistance and multidrug resistance. These multidrug-resistant infections may also contribute to an increased need for hospitalizations to treat pyelonephritis. Copp et al. identified that in California, pediatric hospitalizations for pyelonephritis increased 80% between 1985 and 2006, despite increasing support for outpatient treatment of such infections.[86] During this time, there was a 5-fold increase in resistant uropathogens. Although there are a multitude of factors that contributed to this higher hospitalization rate, increased uropathogen resistance may have played some role.

Antibiotic treatment may not only affect bacterial resistance within the patient taking the medication but may also result in resistant bacterial spread throughout a household. In a study by Samore at al., antibiotic therapy, particularly macrolides, increased the rate of ampicillin-resistant bacteria that was not limited to the patient but was found throughout individuals within the household who were not treated with antibiotics.[87] These findings demonstrate the far-reaching effects that antibiotics have both within the treated individual and the surrounding community.

Despite these pessimistic results, there are some opportunities for improvement and indications that improved antibiotic stewardship can improve antibiotic resistance. Studies by Nasrin and Gottesman demonstrated that by limiting the use of antibiotics such as B-lactam antibiotics and ciprofloxacin, there was a significant decrease in bacteria resistant to these antibiotics.[88] Unfortunately, this improvement in resistance was reversed immediately on reuse of these antibiotics. Pediatric urologists may assist in decreasing antibiotic resistance by being more selective in prescribing patterns regarding CAP based on consideration of individual risk factors as noted earlier in the sections on VUR, HN, and hydroureter.

In addition to limiting the situations in which CAP is prescribed, ensuring that only children with documented UTIs are treated with antibiotics will also limit antimicrobial use and lower antibiotic resistance. A recent study noted that nearly one-third of children younger than 2 years did not undergo either a urinalysis or a urine culture, before being treated with antibiotics for presumed UTI symptoms.[89] This is a clear contradiction to the recent AAP guidelines for UTI management, where obtaining a urine specimen for urinalysis and urine culture is recommended in a febrile infant without an apparent source for their fever.[90] Furthermore, treatment with proper antibiotics, even in an empirical fashion, could be helpful in decreasing antibiotic resistance. Previously, the Infectious Diseases Society of America and the European Society for Microbiology and Infectious Disease published guidelines for the treatment of uncomplicated UTIs.[91] They recommended that TMP-SMX not be used empirically if local resistance rates exceed 20%. However, in a recent study by Copp and colleagues,[92] they identified that 50% of children in the United States were prescribed TMP-SMX after developing a UTI, despite most regions having resistance rates exceeding the recommended 20%. In addition, they identified that 32% of these children were also prescribed a broad-spectrum antibiotic, which in turn has been shown to contribute to increased patient morbidity and cost, by prolonging antibiotic treatment, increasing the likelihood of office and emergency room visits, and increasing hospital admissions.[93] In addition, unnecessary exposure to these broad-spectrum antibiotics is in turn increasing resistance to these antimicrobials. To help reduce this, empirical prescribing of antibiotics based on a local antibiogram is recommended. Recent studies looking at UTI resistance patterns demonstrate that most UTIs are sensitive to narrow-spectrum antibiotics, including first-generation cephalosporins and nitrofurantoin.[94] The utilization of such infrequently used classes of antibiotics are commonly sufficient to treat an uncomplicated UTI, resulting in less exposure to broad-spectrum antibiotics, which may help reduce antibiotic resistance. In addition, these underutilized antibiotics have demonstrated continued low-resistance rates over time.

Antibiotic Impact on the Microbiota

Microbiota is the collection of bacteria, archaea, fungi, protozoa, and viruses that inhabit parts of a host. In humans, there is an incredibly large number of microbials that colonize the oral and nasal cavities, the skin surface, and the gastrointestinal tracts. In fact, it is estimated that microbial cells outnumber human cells 10 to 1, and the colon is the most heavily colonized site. Health care providers are now beginning to understand that microbiota plays a critical role in normal body function and that a normal functioning microbiome plays an important role in host immunity, metabolism, and resistance to pathogens. In addition, shifts in the "normal" microbiota may lead to disease states.[95]

One way in which our normal microbiota is adversely affected is through the use of antibiotics. In general, the practitioner's goal when administering an antibiotic consists of targeting specific bacteria that may reside at an exact niche, resulting in infection. Unfortunately, antibiotics are not well targeted and their administration may result in undesired consequences by killing bacteria at other "noninfected" sites. Therefore, although antibiotics are designed to target pathogenic organisms, unrelated members of various microbiota are also affected, especially within the gut microbiota.[96,97] These effects may be long lasting, even after treatment with the antibiotic has been completed. Studies have shown that antibiotic treatment is followed by a decrease in microbiota diversity, but generally within days to weeks after treatment, most of the microbiota returns, resembling the pretreatment state.[97–99] However, some original members of the microbiota are lost indefinitely, which may exert short-term and long-term effects on patient health. In addition, repeated treatment with antibiotics generates larger short-term and long-term changes in the composition of the gastrointestinal microbiota.[100]

Health care–associated infections provide examples of consequences secondary to shifts in the human microbiota as a result of antibiotic treatment. Antimicrobial therapy is probably the biggest risk factor of development of *Clostridium difficile*–associated diarrhea.[101] In certain healthy individuals, *C difficile* is naturally present within the gastrointestinal microbiota. Antibiotic therapy leads to dysbiosis within the gastrointestinal tract, leading to a *C difficile* infection. As the *C difficile* transitions from its colonization state, to an infectious state, it then becomes a toxin-producing pathogen that may then cause pseudomembranous colitis. Similarly, antibiotics also increase human susceptibility to salmonellosis. Adler and colleagues[102] demonstrated that antibiotic-treated infants, as compared with antibiotic naive infants, were more likely to be infected by Salmonella.

Potential Long-Term Side Effects of Prophylactic Antibiotics

Antibiotics affect the microbiota of the gastrointestinal tract, which plays a multifunctional role involving enhancement of host digestion, energy turnover, metabolism, absorption of nutrients, barrier against pathogens, and development of the immune and nervous systems.[103] In addition to development of bacterial antibiotic resistance, early-life antibiotic exposure has been associated with increased adiposity in animal models, and observational studies in children have reported associations between antibiotic exposure and increased body mass.[104–107] Antibiotics affect the gut microbiota, and the link between altered gut microbiota and human metabolism is becoming increasingly apparent.[108] In addition, alterations to the gut microbiota have been noted to affectt and impair bone growth and development.[109–111]

The impact of oral antibiotics on animal growth has been well established for decades, with greater increases in weight noted when antibiotics are administered earlier in life.[105,106] The impact of the microbiota on weight and adiposity is demonstrated in rats undergoing alteration of their microbiota via fecal transplant from obese and lean human donors. These rats all received identical diets and caloric intake yet developed different body mass phenotypes, which matched the obese or lean human fecal donors' phenotype.[112] More recently, studies have addressed the association between antibiotics and obesity in children. Ajslev and colleagues[113] reported that exposure to antibiotics in the first 6 months of life was associated with a subsequent risk of being overweight in childhood. The impact of early exposure to antibiotics on body mass was also confirmed by Trasande and colleagues.[114] Other studies reported reversible, persistent, or progressive effects of antibiotic use on children's body mass index trajectories, with different effects by age, suggesting that antibiotic use influenced weight gain throughout childhood.[107,115] An electronic health record review of 64,580 children at the Children's Hospital of Philadelphia demonstrated an increased risk of developing childhood obesity associated with both broad-spectrum antibiotics and cumulative exposure for those receiving 4 or more antibiotic courses.[116] However, a recent retrospective, longitudinal study of more than 38,000 children did not find a statistically significant association between short-term antibiotic use within the first 6 months of life and weight gain.[107] In addition, a secondary analysis of data from a randomized clinical trial of 300 children on prophylactic antibiotics failed to show any significant difference in weight gain compared with controls.[117] The data from the studies mentioned earlier suggest that higher cumulative antibiotic dosage exposure and broader spectrum antibiotic exposure may have greater impact on the gut microbiota with a subsequent increased chance of long-term side effects including obesity.

Investigators have begun to identify other possible associations between shifts in the microbiome and subsequent development of diseases. In addition, our understanding of microbiome development, which begins in infancy and early childhood, has also increased. Just as there are milestones in child maturity, there seems to be developmental milestones for the human microbiome and disruptions in this growth, at times because of antibiotic exposure, may result in lifelong consequences in the composition and function of the gut ecosystem.[118,119] Several recent studies suggest an association between childhood asthma and neonatal antibiotic exposure.[120,121] Other studies demonstrate an association between pediatric antibiotic exposure and subsequent inflammatory bowel disease and celiac disease, as well as rheumatoid arthritis and type 1 diabetes.[95,122] The full impact of antimicrobials through alterations in the gut microbiota on metabolism, growth, as well as other potential side effects on the immune, digestive, and nervous system remain to be defined.[104]

Alternatives to Prophylactic Antibiotics

After reviewing the possible side effects associated with CAP, it would be ideal if there were safer effective alternatives to using antibiotics for prophylaxis. In this section potential alternatives to CAP are reviewed.

Vaccinium macrocarpon (cranberry)

The cranberry subgenus, Vaccinium macrocarpon, is one of the most common agents used to try to prevent UTIs in adult women. It has also been tried in children, in whom its compliance has been shown to be better than oral antibiotics without associated side effects.[19,123] Cranberry's mechanism of action resides in the action of its proanthocyanidin on mannose-resistant P-fimbriated E coli strains. The proanthocyanidin prevents adhesion of fimbriae to a specific receptor on the uroepithelial cell. This effect can occur at concentrations as low as 75 ug/mL.[124,125]

Most studies evaluating the effectiveness of cranberry in preventing UTIs have been performed in adults. To date, the data are incomplete but encouraging. In postmenopausal women, although cranberry juice did not significantly reduce the number of UTIs as compared with placebo, it did reduce the number of infections caused by P-fimbriated E coli.[126] In addition, a recent Cochrane review, which included 10 studies and over 1000 women, identified that cranberry juice did decrease the number of symptomatic UTIs over a 12-month period.[127] The evidence of cranberry efficacy in children is less clear. A double-blind randomized placebo-controlled study involving 225 children demonstrated no significant reduction in UTI recurrence for children taking cranberry juice. However, it did demonstrate a reduction in the actual number of recurrences and the need for antibiotic use.[128]

Probiotics

Probiotics are live organisms that when administered in adequate amounts confer a health benefit to the host. In the past, probiotics have been predominantly used to restore or improve dysbiotic gastrointestinal microbiota. As such, they have most commonly been prescribed to treat problems such as antibiotic-associated diarrhea or infectious diarrhea. The concept behind the use of probiotics to prevent UTI development is known as the competitive theory, in which disruption of the natural flora (through antibiotic use or disease development) renders patients prone to severe infection with pathogenic microorganisms. A strategy to restore a host-supportive bacterial flora and a microenvironment resistant to infection involves the use of probiotics.

To date, most of the studies investigating the use of probiotics to prevent UTIs have focused on adult women. Women with reduced lactobacilli within their vaginal flora have been shown to be more prone to recurrent UTIs. Therefore, studies have focused on restoring Lactobacilli within the vaginal microbiome. Stapleton and colleagues[129] performed a double-blind placebo-controlled study in which a Lactobacillus crispatus intravaginal suppository probiotic or placebo was instilled in 100 women for 10 weeks. After a 10-week follow-up, they noted a reduced risk of recurrent UTI development within the treatment arm. When evaluating the use of probiotics in children, there currently are limited studies. Previously, Darouiche and colleagues[130] tested the topical use of probiotics in patients with neurogenic bladder. After instillation of a benign E coli strain into the bladder of these patients, they found decreased rates of recurrent UTIs, especially in those in whom the bladder was successfully colonized with the benign E coli.

Other probiotic studies using advances in genetic engineering have focused on augmenting the gut microbiota with engineered bacterial strains. In vitro studies using engineered Lactococcus lactis to express and deliver antimicrobial peptides against Escherichia faecium have shown reduction of pathogen counts by 10,000-fold.[131] In addition, "sense and destroy" probiotics have been formulated that encode sensors for pathogenic bacterial strains. On detection of a pathogen, these probiotics activate a genetic program to kill the target bacteria.[132]

Bacterial interference from probiotic use has also been studied. Darouiche and colleagues[133,134] performed 2 studies in which patients with a neurogenic bladder after a spinal cord injury are intentionally colonized with a nonpathogenic strain of E coli (E coli 83972 and E coli HU21117). These pilot studies demonstrated safety after bladder instillation as well as a reduced risk of symptomatic UTI development with pathogenic E coli in these patients.

Vaccine therapy

Current vaccinology approaches have focused on targeting certain virulence factors, such as FimH or type 1 fimbriae on uropathogenic E coli, which is the most common bacteria causing UTIs. Although no current vaccine is available in the United States, a few products are available in other countries. Uro-Vaxom is currently available in Europe and Canada. Studies to date, which have been limited to adults, have only demonstrated modest protection against UTI development.[135] Although no current vaccine exists within the United States and the data surrounding vaccine development are preliminary, this is an exciting endeavor and may be a breakthrough treatment alternative for patients suffering from recurrent UTIs in the future.

SUMMARY

The common and widespread practice of relatively nonselective use of CAP for children with VUR, HN, and hydroureteronephrosis is beginning to change. Better identification of individual risk factors for UTI and subsequent renal injury and its sequelae now permit a more selective and beneficial use of CAP. Both the short and potential long-term side effects of antibiotics demand such a selective use of CAP by health care providers. A reduction in the use of antibiotics will help decrease the development of bacterial resistance on both an individual and community basis. In addition, limited use of antibiotics will decrease the impact on a child's microbiota, which is increasingly being recognized to play a major role in normal body functions and development. The pediatric urologist must also continue to reduce correctable risk factors for UTIs on an individual basis so that the need and use of CAP in these children may be decreased. A strong need for proven viable alternatives to CAP continues to exist with ample opportunity for further scientific exploration in the areas of prebiotics, probiotics, and vaccines. Current practice patterns affect and shape the future for each of our patients as well as the treatment options that will subsequently be available for health care providers. The known negative impact of these current practice patterns dictates the need to change our practice now.

REFERENCES

1. Hoberman A, Greenfield SP, Mattoo TK, et al. Antimicrobial prophylaxis for children with vesicoureteral reflux. N Engl J Med 2014;370(25):2367–76.
2. Brandstrom P, Esbjorner E, Herthelius M, et al. The Swedish reflux trial in children: I. Study design and study population characteristics. J Urol 2010; 184(1):274–9.
3. Reaffirmation of AAP Clinical Practice Guideline. The diagnosis and management of the initial urinary tract infection in febrile infants and young children 2-24 months of age. Pediatrics 2016;138(6) [pii:e20163026].
4. Wan J, Skoog SJ, Hulbert WC, et al. Section on Urology response to new Guidelines for the diagnosis and management of UTI. Pediatrics 2012; 129(4):e1051–3.
5. Cooper CS, Chung BI, Kirsch AJ, et al. The outcome of stopping prophylactic antibiotics in older children with vesicoureteral reflux. J Urol 2000;163(1):269–72 [discussion: 272–3].
6. Cooper CS, Austin JC. Vesicoureteral reflux: who benefits from surgery? Urol Clin North Am 2004; 31(3):535–41, x.
7. Calderon-Margalit R, Golan E, Twig G, et al. History of childhood kidney disease and risk of adult end-stage renal disease. N Engl J Med 2018;378(5): 428–38.

8. Elder JS, Peters CA, Arant BS Jr, et al. Pediatric vesicoureteral reflux guidelines panel summary report on the management of primary vesicoureteral reflux in children. J Urol 1997;157(5):1846–51.
9. Tiihonen K, Ouwehand AC, Rautonen N. Human intestinal microbiota and healthy ageing. Ageing Res Rev 2010;9(2):107–16.
10. Alexander SE, Arlen AM, Storm DW, et al. Bladder volume at onset of vesicoureteral reflux is an independent risk factor for breakthrough febrile urinary tract infection. J Urol 2015;193(4): 1342–6.
11. McMillan ZM, Austin JC, Knudson MJ, et al. Bladder volume at onset of reflux on initial cystogram predicts spontaneous resolution. J Urol 2006;176(4 Pt 2):1838–41.
12. Nepple KJ, Knudson MJ, Austin JC, et al. Abnormal renal scans and decreased early resolution of low grade vesicoureteral reflux. J Urol 2008; 180(4 Suppl):1643–7 [discussion: 1647].
13. Nepple KG, Knudson MJ, Austin JC, et al. Adding renal scan data improves the accuracy of a computational model to predict vesicoureteral reflux resolution. J Urol 2008;180(4 Suppl):1648–52 [discussion: 1652].
14. Knudson MJ, Austin JC, Wald M, et al. Computational model for predicting the chance of early resolution in children with vesicoureteral reflux. J Urol 2007;178(4 Pt 2):1824–7.
15. Knudson MJ, Austin JC, McMillan ZM, et al. Predictive factors of early spontaneous resolution in children with primary vesicoureteral reflux. J Urol 2007; 178(4 Pt 2):1684–8.
16. Van Arendonk KJ, Madsen MT, Austin JC, et al. Nuclear cystometrogram-determined bladder pressure at onset of vesicoureteral reflux predicts spontaneous resolution. Urology 2007;69(4): 767–70.
17. Cooper CS, Madsen MT, Austin JC, et al. Bladder pressure at the onset of vesicoureteral reflux determined by nuclear cystometrogram. J Urol 2003; 170(4 Pt 2):1537–40 [discussion: 1540].
18. Shaikh N, Hoberman A, Hum SW, et al. Development and validation of a calculator for estimating the probability of urinary tract infection in young febrile children. JAMA Pediatr 2018;172(6):550–6.
19. Craig JC, Simpson JM, Williams GJ, et al. Antibiotic prophylaxis and recurrent urinary tract infection in children. N Engl J Med 2009;361(18):1748–59.
20. Leslie B, Moore K, Salle JL, et al. Outcome of antibiotic prophylaxis discontinuation in patients with persistent vesicoureteral reflux initially presenting with febrile urinary tract infection: time to event analysis. J Urol 2010;184(3):1093–8.
21. Sillen U, Brandstrom P, Jodal U, et al. The Swedish reflux trial in children: v. Bladder dysfunction. J Urol 2010;184(1):298–304.

22. Keren R, Shaikh N, Pohl H, et al. Risk factors for recurrent urinary tract infection and renal scarring. Pediatrics 2015;136(1):e13–21.

23. Peters CA, Skoog SJ, Arant BS Jr, et al. Summary of the AUA guideline on management of primary vesicoureteral reflux in children. J Urol 2010; 184(3):1134–44.

24. Chesney RW, Carpenter MA, Moxey-Mims M, et al. Randomized Intervention for Children With Vesicoureteral Reflux (RIVUR): background commentary of RIVUR investigators. Pediatrics 2008; 122(Suppl 5):S233–9.

25. Loening-Baucke V. Urinary incontinence and urinary tract infection and their resolution with treatment of chronic constipation of childhood. Pediatrics 1997;100(2 Pt 1):228–32.

26. Erickson BA, Austin JC, Cooper CS, et al. Polyethylene glycol 3350 for constipation in children with dysfunctional elimination. J Urol 2003;170(4 Pt 2): 1518–20.

27. Winberg J, Bergstrom T, Jacobsson B. Morbidity, age and sex distribution, recurrences and renal scarring in symptomatic urinary tract infection in childhood. Kidney Int Suppl 1975;4:S101–6.

28. Nuutinen M, Uhari M. Recurrence and follow-up after urinary tract infection under the age of 1 year. Pediatr Nephrol 2001;16(1):69–72.

29. Shaikh N, Morone NE, Bost JE, et al. Prevalence of urinary tract infection in childhood: a meta-analysis. Pediatr Infect Dis J 2008;27(4):302–8.

30. Winberg J, Andersen HJ, Bergstrom T, et al. Epidemiology of symptomatic urinary tract infection in childhood. Acta Paediatr Scand Suppl 1974;(252):1–20.

31. Kasanen A, Sundquist H, Elo J, et al. Secondary prevention of urinary tract infections. The role of trimethoprim alone. Ann Clin Res 1983;15(Suppl 36):1–36.

32. McCracken GH Jr. Recurrent urinary tract infections in children. Pediatr Infect Dis 1984;3(3 Suppl):S28–30.

33. Garin EH, Olavarria F, Garcia Nieto V, et al. Clinical significance of primary vesicoureteral reflux and urinary antibiotic prophylaxis after acute pyelonephritis: a multicenter, randomized, controlled study. Pediatrics 2006;117(3):626–32.

34. Montini G, Rigon L, Zucchetta P, et al. Prophylaxis after first febrile urinary tract infection in children? A multicenter, randomized, controlled, noninferiority trial. Pediatrics 2008;122(5):1064–71.

35. Pennesi M, Travan L, Peratoner L, et al. Is antibiotic prophylaxis in children with vesicoureteral reflux effective in preventing pyelonephritis and renal scars? A randomized, controlled trial. Pediatrics 2008;121(6):e1489–94.

36. Roussey-Kesler G, Gadjos V, Idres N, et al. Antibiotic prophylaxis for the prevention of recurrent urinary tract infection in children with low grade vesicoureteral reflux: results from a prospective randomized study. J Urol 2008;179(2):674–9 [discussion: 679].

37. Brandstrom P, Esbjorner E, Herthelius M, et al. The Swedish reflux trial in children: III. Urinary tract infection pattern. J Urol 2010;184(1):286–91.

38. Hidas G, Billimek J, Nam A, et al. Predicting the risk of breakthrough urinary tract infections: primary vesicoureteral reflux. J Urol 2015;194(5):1396–401.

39. Arlen AM, Alexander SE, Wald M, et al. Computer model predicting breakthrough febrile urinary tract infection in children with primary vesicoureteral reflux. J Pediatr Urol 2016;12(5):288.e1-5.

40. de Bessa J Jr, de Carvalho Mrad FC, Mendes EF, et al. Antibiotic prophylaxis for prevention of febrile urinary tract infections in children with vesicoureteral reflux: a meta-analysis of randomized, controlled trials comparing dilated to nondilated vesicoureteral reflux. J Urol 2015;193(5 Suppl): 1772–7.

41. Wang ZT, Wehbi E, Alam Y, et al. A reanalysis of the RIVUR trial using a risk classification system. J Urol 2018;199(6):1608–14.

42. Hewitt IK, Pennesi M, Morello W, et al. Antibiotic prophylaxis for urinary tract infection-related renal scarring: a systematic review. Pediatr 2017;139(5) [pii:e20163145].

43. Jodal U. The natural history of bacteriuria in childhood. Infect Dis Clin North Am 1987;1(4):713–29.

44. Weiss R, Duckett J, Spitzer A. Results of a randomized clinical trial of medical versus surgical management of infants and children with grades III and IV primary vesicoureteral reflux (United States). The international reflux study in children. J Urol 1992;148(5 Pt 2):1667–73.

45. Hoberman A, Charron M, Hickey RW, et al. Imaging studies after a first febrile urinary tract infection in young children. N Engl J Med 2003;348(3): 195–202.

46. Bailey RR, Lynn KL, Smith AH. Long-term followup of infants with gross vesicoureteral reflux. J Urol 1992;148(5 Pt 2):1709–11.

47. Ylinen E, Ala-Houhala M, Wikstrom S. Risk of renal scarring in vesicoureteral reflux detected either antenatally or during the neonatal period. Urology 2003;61(6):1238–42 [discussion: 1242–3].

48. Mingin GC, Nguyen HT, Baskin LS, et al. Abnormal dimercapto-succinic acid scans predict an increased risk of breakthrough infection in children with vesicoureteral reflux. J Urol 2004;172(3):1075–7 [discussion: 1077].

49. Lenaghan D, Whitaker JG, Jensen F, et al. The natural history of reflux and long-term effects of reflux on the kidney. J Urol 1976;115(6):728–30.

50. Olbing H, Claesson I, Ebel KD, et al. Renal scars and parenchymal thinning in children with

vesicoureteral reflux: a 5-year report of the International Reflux Study in Children (European branch). J Urol 1992;148(5 Pt 2):1653–6.

51. Wallace DM, Rothwell DL, Williams DI. The long-term follow-up of surgically treated vesicoureteric reflux. Br J Urol 1978;50(7):479–84.

52. Jodal U, Lindberg U. Guidelines for management of children with urinary tract infection and vesicoureteric reflux. Recommendations from a Swedish state-of-the-art conference. Swedish Medical Research Council. Acta Paediatr Suppl 1999; 88(431):87–9.

53. Mor Y, Leibovitch I, Zalts R, et al. Analysis of the long-term outcome of surgically corrected vesicoureteric reflux. BJU Int 2003;92(1):97–100.

54. Oh MM, Kim JW, Park MG, et al. The impact of therapeutic delay time on acute scintigraphic lesion and ultimate scar formation in children with first febrile UTI. Eur J Pediatr 2012;171(3):565–70.

55. Shaikh N, Mattoo TK, Keren R, et al. Early antibiotic treatment for pediatric febrile urinary tract infection and renal scarring. JAMA Pediatr 2016;170(9): 848–54.

56. Karavanaki KA, Soldatou A, Koufadaki AM, et al. Delayed treatment of the first febrile urinary tract infection in early childhood increased the risk of renal scarring. Acta Paediatr 2017;106(1):149–54.

57. Walsh TJ, Hsieh S, Grady R, et al. Antenatal hydronephrosis and the risk of pyelonephritis hospitalization during the first year of life. Urology 2007;69(5): 970–4.

58. Zareba P, Lorenzo AJ, Braga LH. Risk factors for febrile urinary tract infection in infants with prenatal hydronephrosis: comprehensive single center analysis. J Urol 2014;191(5 Suppl):1614–8.

59. Merguerian PA, Herz D, McQuiston L, et al. Variation among pediatric urologists and across 2 continents in antibiotic prophylaxis and evaluation for prenatally detected hydronephrosis: a survey of American and European pediatric urologists. J Urol 2010;184(4 Suppl):1710–5.

60. Yiee JH, Tasian GE, Copp HL. Management trends in prenatally detected hydronephrosis: national survey of pediatrician practice patterns and antibiotic use. Urology 2011;78(4):895–901.

61. Braga LH, Mijovic H, Farrokhyar F, et al. Antibiotic prophylaxis for urinary tract infections in antenatal hydronephrosis. Pediatrics 2013;131(1):e251–61.

62. Psooy K, Pike J. Investigation and management of antenatally detected hydronephrosis. Can Urol Assoc J 2009;3(1):69–72.

63. Nguyen HT, Herndon CD, Cooper C, et al. The Society for Fetal Urology consensus statement on the evaluation and management of antenatal hydronephrosis. J Pediatr Urol 2010;6(3):212–31.

64. Capolicchio JP, Braga LH, Szymanski KM. Canadian Urological Association/Pediatric Urologists of Canada guidelines on the investigation and management of antenatally detected hydronephrosis. Can Urol Assoc J 2018;12(4):85–92.

65. Szymanski KM, Al-Said AN, Pippi Salle JL, et al. Do infants with mild prenatal hydronephrosis benefit from screening for vesicoureteral reflux? J Urol 2012;188(2):576–81.

66. Easterbrook B, Capolicchio JP, Braga LH. Antibiotic prophylaxis for prevention of urinary tract infections in prenatal hydronephrosis: an updated systematic review. Can Urol Assoc J 2017;11(1–2Suppl1):S3–11.

67. Silay MS, Undre S, Nambiar AK, et al. Role of antibiotic prophylaxis in antenatal hydronephrosis: a systematic review from the European Association of Urology/European Society for Paediatric Urology Guidelines Panel. J Pediatr Urol 2017;13(3): 306–15.

68. Lee NG, Marchalik D, Lipsky A, et al. Risk factors for catheter associated urinary tract infections in a pediatric institution. J Urol 2016;195(4 Pt 2): 1306–11.

69. Braga LH, Farrokhyar F, D'Cruz J, et al. Risk factors for febrile urinary tract infection in children with prenatal hydronephrosis: a prospective study. J Urol 2015;193(5 Suppl):1766–71.

70. Braga LH, D'Cruz J, Rickard M, et al. The fate of primary nonrefluxing megaureter: a prospective outcome analysis of the rate of urinary tract infections, surgical indications and time to resolution. J Urol 2016;195(4 Pt 2):1300–5.

71. DiRenzo D, Persico A, DiNicola M, et al. Conservative management of primary non-refluxing megaureter during the first year of life: a longitudinal observational study. J Pediatr Urol 2015;11(4): 226.e1-6.

72. Gimpel C, Masioniene L, Djakovic N, et al. Complications and long-term outcome of primary obstructive megaureter in childhood. Pediatr Nephrol 2010;25(9):1679–86.

73. Song SH, Lee SB, Park YS, et al. Is antibiotic prophylaxis necessary in infants with obstructive hydronephrosis? J Urol 2007;177(3):1098–101 [discussion: 1101].

74. Farrugia MK, Hitchcock R, Radford A, et al. British Association of Paediatric Urologists consensus statement on the management of the primary obstructive megaureter. J Pediatr Urol 2014;10(1): 26–33.

75. Herz D, Merguerian P, McQuiston L. Continuous antibiotic prophylaxis reduces the risk of febrile UTI in children with asymptomatic antenatal hydronephrosis with either ureteral dilation, high-grade vesicoureteral reflux, or ureterovesical junction obstruction. J Pediatr Urol 2014;10(4):650–4.

76. Zee RS, Herbst KW, Kim C, et al. Urinary tract infections in children with prenatal hydronephrosis:

a risk assessment from the Society for Fetal Urology Hydronephrosis Registry. J Pediatr Urol 2016; 12(4):261.e1-7.

77. Braga LH, Ruzhynsky V, Pemberton J, et al. Evaluating practice patterns in postnatal management of antenatal hydronephrosis: a national survey of Canadian pediatric urologists and nephrologists. Urology 2014;83(4):909–14.

78. World Health Organization. WHO global strategy for containment of antimicrobial resistance, vol. 2013. Geneva (Switzerland): WHO; 2001.

79. World Health Organization. Global action plan on antimicrobial resistance. Geneva (Switzerland): WHO; 2015.

80. Allen UD, MacDonald N, Fuite L, et al. Risk factors for resistance to "first-line" antimicrobials among urinary tract isolates of Escherichia coli in children. CMAJ 1999;160(10):1436–40.

81. Cheng CH, Tsai MH, Huang YC, et al. Antibiotic resistance patterns of community-acquired urinary tract infections in children with vesicoureteral reflux receiving prophylactic antibiotic therapy. Pediatrics 2008;122(6):1212–7.

82. Costelloe C, Metcalfe C, Lovering A, et al. Effect of antibiotic prescribing in primary care on antimicrobial resistance in individual patients: systematic review and meta-analysis. BMJ 2010;340:c2096.

83. Williams G, Craig JC. Long-term antibiotics for preventing recurrent urinary tract infection in children. Cochrane Database Syst Rev 2011;(3):CD001534.

84. Montini G, Toffolo A, Zucchetta P, et al. Antibiotic treatment for pyelonephritis in children: multicentre randomised controlled non-inferiority trial. BMJ 2007;335(7616):386.

85. Selekman RS, Shapiro DJ, Copp HL. Antimicrobial exposure and uropathogen resistance: an analysis of individual patient data from RCTs on antibiotic prophylaxis and prevention of UTI. American Urology Association Annual Meeting. New Orleans, LA, May 15–19, 2015.

86. Copp HL, Halpern MS, Maldonado Y, et al. Trends in hospitalization for pediatric pyelonephritis: a population based study of California from 1985 to 2006. J Urol 2011;186(3):1028–34.

87. Samore MH, Tonnerre C, Hannah EL, et al. Impact of outpatient antibiotic use on carriage of ampicillin-resistant Escherichia coli. Antimicrob Agents Chemother 2011;55(3):1135–41.

88. Nasrin D, Collignon PJ, Roberts L, et al. Effect of beta lactam antibiotic use in children on pneumococcal resistance to penicillin: prospective cohort study. BMJ 2002;324(7328):28–30.

89. Copp HL, Yiee JH, Smith A, et al. Use of urine testing in outpatients treated for urinary tract infection. Pediatrics 2013;132(3):437–44.

90. Subcommittee on Urinary Tract Infections, Steering Committee on Quality Improvement and Management, Roberts KB. Urinary tract infection: clinical practice guideline for the diagnosis and management of the initial UTI in febrile infants and children 2 to 24 months. Pediatrics 2011; 128(3):595–610.

91. Gupta K, Hooton TM, Naber KG, et al. International clinical practice guidelines for the treatment of acute uncomplicated cystitis and pyelonephritis in women: a 2010 update by the Infectious Diseases Society of America and the European Society for Microbiology and Infectious Diseases. Clin Infect Dis 2011;52(5):e103–20.

92. Copp HL, Shapiro DJ, Hersh AL. National ambulatory antibiotic prescribing patterns for pediatric urinary tract infection, 1998-2007. Pediatrics 2011; 127(6):1027–33.

93. Yen ZS, Davis MA, Chen SC, et al. A cost-effectiveness analysis of treatment strategies for acute uncomplicated pyelonephritis in women. Acad Emerg Med 2003;10(4):309–14.

94. Edlin RS, Shapiro DJ, Hersh AL, et al. Antibiotic resistance patterns of outpatient pediatric urinary tract infections. J Urol 2013;190(1):222–7.

95. Keeney KM, Yurist-Doutsch S, Arrieta MC, et al. Effects of antibiotics on human microbiota and subsequent disease. Annu Rev Microbiol 2014;68:217–35.

96. Jakobsson HE, Jernberg C, Andersson AF, et al. Short-term antibiotic treatment has differing long-term impacts on the human throat and gut microbiome. PLoS One 2010;5(3):e9836.

97. Jernberg C, Lofmark S, Edlund C, et al. Long-term ecological impacts of antibiotic administration on the human intestinal microbiota. ISME J 2007; 1(1):56–66.

98. Dethlefsen L, Huse S, Sogin ML, et al. The pervasive effects of an antibiotic on the human gut microbiota, as revealed by deep 16S rRNA sequencing. PLoS Biol 2008;6(11):e280.

99. De La Cochetiere MF, Durand T, Lepage P, et al. Resilience of the dominant human fecal microbiota upon short-course antibiotic challenge. J Clin Microbiol 2005;43(11):5588–92.

100. Dethlefsen L, Relman DA. Incomplete recovery and individualized responses of the human distal gut microbiota to repeated antibiotic perturbation. Proc Natl Acad Sci U S A 2011;108(Suppl 1):4554–61.

101. Kelly CP, Pothoulakis C, LaMont JT. Clostridium difficile colitis. N Engl J Med 1994;330(4):257–62.

102. Adler JL, Anderson RL, Boring JR, et al. A protracted hospital-associated outbreak of salmonellosis due to a multiple-antibiotic-resistant strain of Salmonella indiana. J Pediatr 1970;77(6):970–5.

103. Cox LM, Blaser MJ. Antibiotics in early life and obesity. Nat Rev Endocrinol 2015;11(3):182–90.

104. Cooper CS. Fat, demented and stupid: an unrecognized legacy of pediatric urology? J Pediatr Urol 2017;13(4):341–4.

105. Luckey TD, Moore PR, Elvehjem CA, et al. The activity of synthetic folic acid in purified rations for the chick. Science 1946;103(2684):682–4.

106. Jukes TH. Antibiotics in animal feeds and animal production. BioScience 1972;22(9):526–34.

107. Schwartz BS, Pollak J, Bailey-Davis L, et al. Antibiotic use and childhood body mass index trajectory. Int J Obes (Lond) 2016;40(4):615–21.

108. Tremaroli V, Backhed F. Functional interactions between the gut microbiota and host metabolism. Nature 2012;489(7415):242–9.

109. Guss JD, Horsfield MW, Fontenele FF, et al. Alterations to the gut microbiome impair bone strength and tissue material properties. J Bone Miner Res 2017;32(6):1343–53.

110. Sjogren K, Engdahl C, Henning P, et al. The gut microbiota regulates bone mass in mice. J Bone Miner Res 2012;27(6):1357–67.

111. Yan J, Herzog JW, Tsang K, et al. Gut microbiota induce IGF-1 and promote bone formation and growth. Proc Natl Acad Sci U S A 2016;113(47):E7554–63.

112. Ellekilde M, Selfjord E, Larsen CS, et al. Transfer of gut microbiota from lean and obese mice to antibiotic-treated mice. Sci Rep 2014;4:5922.

113. Ajslev TA, Andersen CS, Gamborg M, et al. Childhood overweight after establishment of the gut microbiota: the role of delivery mode, pre-pregnancy weight and early administration of antibiotics. Int J Obes (Lond) 2011;35(4):522–9.

114. Trasande L, Blustein J, Liu M, et al. Infant antibiotic exposures and early-life body mass. Int J Obes (Lond) 2013;37(1):16–23.

115. Saari A, Virta LJ, Sankilampi U, et al. Antibiotic exposure in infancy and risk of being overweight in the first 24 months of life. Pediatrics 2015;135(4):617–26.

116. Bailey LC, Forrest CB, Zhang P, et al. Association of antibiotics in infancy with early childhood obesity. JAMA Pediatr 2014;168(11):1063–9.

117. Edmonson MB, Eickhoff JC. Weight gain and obesity in infants and young children exposed to prolonged antibiotic prophylaxis. JAMA Pediatr 2017;171(2):150–6.

118. Smith MI, Yatsunenko T, Manary MJ, et al. Gut microbiomes of Malawian twin pairs discordant for kwashiorkor. Science 2013;339(6119):548–54.

119. Stefka AT, Feehley T, Tripathi P, et al. Commensal bacteria protect against food allergen sensitization. Proc Natl Acad Sci U S A 2014;111(36):13145–50.

120. Murk W, Risnes KR, Bracken MB. Prenatal or early-life exposure to antibiotics and risk of childhood asthma: a systematic review. Pediatrics 2011;127(6):1125–38.

121. Ortqvist AK, Lundholm C, Kieler H, et al. Antibiotics in fetal and early life and subsequent childhood asthma: nationwide population based study with sibling analysis. BMJ 2014;349:g6979.

122. Hviid A, Svanstrom H, Frisch M. Antibiotic use and inflammatory bowel diseases in childhood. Gut 2011;60(1):49–54.

123. Uhari M, Nuutinen M, Turtinen J. Adverse reactions in children during long-term antimicrobial therapy. Pediatr Infect Dis J 1996;15(5):404–8.

124. Foo LY, Lu Y, Howell AB, et al. The structure of cranberry proanthocyanidins which inhibit adherence of uropathogenic P-fimbriated Escherichia coli in vitro. Phytochemistry 2000;54(2):173–81.

125. Howell AB, Reed JD, Krueger CG, et al. A-type cranberry proanthocyanidins and uropathogenic bacterial anti-adhesion activity. Phytochemistry 2005;66(18):2281–91.

126. Stapleton AE, Dziura J, Hooton TM, et al. Recurrent urinary tract infection and urinary Escherichia coli in women ingesting cranberry juice daily: a randomized controlled trial. Mayo Clin Proc 2012;87(2):143–50.

127. Goldman RD. Cranberry juice for urinary tract infection in children. Can Fam Physician 2012;58(4):398–401.

128. Salo J, Uhari M, Helminen M, et al. Cranberry juice for the prevention of recurrences of urinary tract infections in children: a randomized placebo-controlled trial. Clin Infect Dis 2012;54(3):340–6.

129. Stapleton AE, Au-Yeung M, Hooton TM, et al. Randomized, placebo-controlled phase 2 trial of a Lactobacillus crispatus probiotic given intravaginally for prevention of recurrent urinary tract infection. Clin Infect Dis 2011;52(10):1212–7.

130. Darouiche RO, Thornby JI, Cerra-Stewart C, et al. Bacterial interference for prevention of urinary tract infection: a prospective, randomized, placebo-controlled, double-blind pilot trial. Clin Infect Dis 2005;41(10):1531–4.

131. Geldart K, Borrero J, Kaznessis YN. Chloride-inducible expression vector for delivery of antimicrobial peptides targeting antibiotic-resistant enterococcus faecium. Appl Environ Microbiol 2015;81(11):3889–97.

132. Hwang IY, Tan MH, Koh E, et al. Reprogramming microbes to be pathogen-seeking killers. ACS Synth Biol 2014;3(4):228–37.

133. Darouiche RO, Hull RA. Bacterial interference for prevention of urinary tract infection: an overview. J Spinal Cord Med 2000;23(2):136–41.

134. Darouiche RO, Green BG, Donovan WH, et al. Multicenter randomized controlled trial of bacterial interference for prevention of urinary tract infection in patients with neurogenic bladder. Urology 2011;78(2):341–6.

135. Bauer HW, Rahlfs VW, Lauener PA, et al. Prevention of recurrent urinary tract infections with immunoactive E. coli fractions: a meta-analysis of five placebo-controlled double-blind studies. Int J Antimicrob Agents 2002;19(6):451–6.

Pediatric Stone Disease

Diana K. Bowen, MD[a],*, Gregory E. Tasian, MD, MSc, MSCE[b]

KEYWORDS

- Pediatrics • Urology • Nephrolithiasis • Diagnostic imaging • Medical management

KEY POINTS

- The greatest increases in the incidence of nephrolithiasis are among adolescents.
- Ultrasound should be the initial diagnostic imaging study obtained for pediatric patients with suspected kidney or ureteral stones.
- A complete metabolic evaluation, including a 24-hour urine collection, should be obtained for patients who begin forming stones during childhood.
- Surgical management should be informed by the size and location of the stone as well as the preferences of the patient and family after counseling about stone clearance probabilities and effects of treatment.

EPIDEMIOLOGY

The incidence of pediatric nephrolithiasis has increased by estimates of 4% to 10% annually over the last 2 decades.[1–4] The greatest increase has been seen in older children, with the 12- to 17-year-old age group driving this overall increase in one 25-year retrospective study.[3] In addition to the adolescent age group, women and African Americans showed the greatest increase in incidence within a 20-year population-based study conducted in South Carolina.[5] Female adolescents appear to have the highest rates of nephrolithiasis in several studies for unclear reasons, which is in contrast to the adult population.[1,5]

Geographically, adult kidney stones are more common in the Southeastern United States, which is often referred to as the "stone belt."[6,7] Within the Pediatric Health Information System from 1999 to 2008, hospitals in the Midwest (45%) and South (35%) indeed had the highest prevalence of pediatric stone disease encounters.[2] More recently, a study using the Nationwide Inpatient Sample and Nationwide Emergency Department Sample

(NEDS) databases echoed this, demonstrating the Southern region of the United States had the highest prevalence of pediatric stone disease, although overall regional variation was not statistically significant.[8]

Stone Composition

Stone composition is a critical piece of understanding the cause and different patterns of stone disease in children as well as informing secondary prevention strategies. The overall population distribution of stone composition is similar between adults and children, with calcium oxalate comprising the majority, although calcium phosphate is slightly more common in children (9% vs 5%).[9] Any stone passed by a patient or obtained during surgery should be sent for analysis to help guide diagnosis and treatment.

Metabolic Abnormalities

Metabolic abnormalities that increase the risk of nephrolithiasis can be identified in 75% to 84% of children, with hypercalciuria and hypocitraturia

Disclosures: D.K. Bowen has no commercial or financial conflicts of interest to disclose. G.E. Tasian is a consultant for Allena Pharmaceuticals.
^a Division of Urology, Department of Surgery, University of Pennsylvania Perelman School of Medicine and The Children's Hospital of Philadelphia, 3rd Floor, Wood Building, 3401 Civic Center Boulevard, Philadelphia, PA 19104, USA; ^b Division of Urology, Center for Pediatric Clinical Effectiveness, Center for Clinical Epidemiology and Biostatistics, University of Pennsylvania Perelman School of Medicine, The Children's Hospital of Philadelphia, 3rd Floor, Wood Building, 3401 Civic Center Boulevard, Philadelphia, PA 19104, USA
* Corresponding author.
E-mail address: dkbowen@gmail.com

being the most commonly reported.[10,11] Although estimates differ in the literature, 34% to 50% of pediatric stone-formers will have hypercalciuria and up to 68% will have hypocitraturia.[12–14] Most commonly, hypercalciuria (Ca excretion >4 mg/kg/d in children older than 2 years) is idiopathic.[15] Low urine volume is another common finding on urine analysis and metabolic workup and should not be forgotten. Occasionally metabolic abnormalities can aid in the diagnosis of certain conditions due to a unique combination of urinary abnormalities combined with patient factors, such as in distal renal tubular acidosis (RTA). Other specific disorders are beyond the scope of this article.

Environmental Exposures

Many theories exist to explain the recent increase in nephrolithiasis; however, no all-encompassing cause has been identified. Increasingly, risk for stone disease is viewed as a composite of multiple factors rather than just one exposure or genetic abnormality. This "exposome," the accumulation of environmental exposures during an individual's lifetime that affects risk of stone disease, is then viewed through the lens of a person's genetic and intrinsic metabolic predisposition.[16]

The role of diet is inherently connected to metabolic abnormalities, and there are many dietary factors that may be contributing to increased stone formation during childhood. Both well-known risk factors for nephrolithiasis, children in the United States are drinking less water and taking in greater daily amounts of sodium than is recommended.[17–19] To this end, a 2-year randomized controlled trial (RCT; PUSH: Prevention of Urinary Stones with Hydration) is currently underway to assess the impact of increased fluid intake on the recurrence rate of nephrolithiasis in both adults and children (12–18 year old).[20] Consumption of sugary drinks, especially those with fructose, may also be a contributing factor, although this has not been studied. Excessive animal protein and sodium intake are each independent risk factors for hypercalciuria, with the latter also decreasing urinary citrate.[10] The role of dietary oxalate is less clear, and the evidence especially for children is low for a cause-and-effect relationship of diet modification.

Although diet plays a role, likely more complex interactions between multiple variables are responsible in the end. For example, because the full relationship of dietary intake, absorption, and extraction is complicated, other minerals are being studied for their potential role, for example, zinc. Based on prior in vitro studies suggesting zinc affects calcium metabolism and thus kidney stone formation, a recent case-control trial of 12- to 18-year-old stone-formers and controls matched for age, sex, and race examined the relationship between dietary zinc intake and urinary zinc excretion.[21] The investigators found an association between insufficient dietary zinc intake and increased odds of stone formation in the adolescent population.

The current epidemic of childhood obesity and adult literature linking diet/lifestyle factors to stone disease have prompted several investigations assessing the role of body mass index (BMI) and obesity rates in pediatric nephrolithiasis. This body of literature has conflicting results on whether a relationship exists, including a 25-year series that found no link between kidney stones and BMI.[3,22,23] Most recently, a large population-based study investigated this idea within a cohort of Jewish Israeli adolescents who underwent a mandatory medical assessment before army enlistment at 17 years of age. Over a 30-year period, the reported prevalence of stone disease increased starting in 1995 to 2012 at a rate of 6% annually, with a concurrent trend of increasing BMI among male candidates. Higher BMI was found in stone-formers versus controls, with an odds ratio (OR) for nephrolithiasis of 1.7 in BMI of 30 or greater.[4] Expounding further on this possible link, Cambareri and associates[24] studied 206 otherwise healthy pediatric stone-formers across 4 institutions and 24-hour urinary parameters as influenced by BMI. The investigators found that overweight or obese pediatric stone-formers have lower urinary volume and elevated uric acid compared with their normal-weight peers.

A link between the environment and nephrolithiasis has been shown by demonstrating the temperature dependence of kidney stone presentations.[25] However, no studies have identified one temperature metric as the best predictor for vulnerable populations, and almost all use "dry-bulb" temperature metrics without taking into account the complex relationship between temperature and humidity. Recently, Ross and colleagues[26] performed a time series analysis to estimate differences between predicted and observed stone presentations for different daily temperature metrics and relative humidity in the South Carolina claims database over a period of almost 20 years. They found the combination of temperature and relative humidity best determines the risk of kidney stone presentation, suggesting that moist temperature metrics (wet-bulb temperatures and heat index) are more appropriate to use in studies than dry-bulb temperature metrics, particularly in the summer.[26]

Medical Disorders, Anatomic Abnormalities, and Medications

Anatomic or structural abnormalities, such as ureteropelvic junction obstruction, posterior urethral valves, duplicated system, bladder exstrophy, or prior lower urinary tract diversion, predisposes a patient to stone formation due to functional or anatomic obstruction with stasis of urine. Although anatomic abnormalities are diagnosed often in known pediatric stone-formers, most patients with these abnormalities (95%–99%) will not form stones, suggesting a multifactorial process.[27] Medical conditions, such as inflammatory bowel disease, cystic fibrosis, nephrocalcinosis, renal dysplasia, and nonambulatory patients with cerebral palsy, are all associated with stone formation. Topiramate, a medication frequently used to treat patients with seizures and migraine headaches, is a carbonic anhydrase inhibitor that causes a mixed RTA resulting in decreased citrate excretion and increased urine pH and is associated with calcium phosphate stones. Other carbonic anhydrase inhibitors, such as zonisamide and acetazolamide, are associated with nephrolithiasis. Further complicating the picture for patients with epilepsy, a ketogenic diet is an effective nonpharmacologic treatment but is associated with an increased prevalence of kidney stones ranging from 3% to 6% incidence over a 2-year diet duration.[28] Other medication exposures associated with increased risk of stone formation are calcitriol, steroids, antiretrovirals, and vitamin C or D use. Finally, neonates found to have nephrocalcinosis will commonly have a history of furosemide or loop diuretics, promoting hypercalciuria.

Genetics

Pediatric patients are more likely to have a monogenic cause of stone disease than adults, although this is still rare overall. Monogenic causes of nephrolithiasis include cystinuria, hypoxanthine guanine phosphoribosyltransferase mutations, primary xanthinuria, and primary hyperoxaluria. Cystinuria accounts for 5% to 10% of pediatric nephrolithiasis and at least 2 genes are known to be causative of this autosomal recessive defect in amino acid transport.[29]

In prior studies, up to 50% of nephrolithiasis/nephrocalcinosis has been attributed to heritability.[30,31] In an international cohort of 143 individuals less than 18 years old who had either one episode of nephrolithiasis or ultrasound (US) diagnosis of nephrocalcinosis, patients were examined for the presence of mutations in 30 genes that are known to cause these conditions if mutated.[32] Mutations were detected in 14 genes, with those patients diagnosed at a younger age more likely to have autosomal recessive conditions. This study identified a causative mutation in 17% of all patients, which is consistent with prior studies showing 1 in 5 pediatric patients will harbor a monogenic mutation.[31,32] The same laboratory more recently performed whole exome sequencing (WES) for the same 30 genes within 51 families in whom a member presented less than 25 years of age with a stone or nephrocalcinosis. Twenty-two patients and 15 families (30%) were found with a mutation, with most presenting at <10 years of age and autosomal recessive mutations being the most common (80%).[33] Whether there is a role for WES in the future in children to help establish a diagnosis or possibly guide treatment remains to be seen.[34]

ECONOMIC IMPACT

The overall economic burden of nephrolithiasis is tremendous and has increased from estimates of $2.1 billion annually in 2000 to now exceed $10 billion annually.[7,35] The cost of pediatric nephrolithiasis is just beginning to be elucidated. A longitudinal study of South Carolina emergency departments (ED) from 1996 to 2007 demonstrated that not only did the incidence of nephrolithiasis encounters in the ED increase 4-fold from 7.9 to 18.5 per 100,000 over the 12-year period but also the total adjusted charges increased from $3.4 million to $12.6 million.[1] Using the 2009 NEDS and Kids' Inpatient Database, 2 databases managed by the Healthcare Cost and Utilization Project (HCUP) with a 20% stratified sample of US hospitals, an estimate of median charges for the year 2009 was $13,922 for inpatient admission and $3991 for ED charges, with weighted annual totals of $229 million and $149 million, respectively.[36]

More recently, Young and colleagues[8] analyzed HCUP databases from 2006 to 2012 to determine a longitudinal economic burden of pediatric nephrolithiasis. The investigators found that, although the number of encounters was not significantly different, the mean charges for both emergency department (ED) visits and inpatient admissions increased significantly from 2006 to 2012 (by 60% and 102%, respectively). Total annual charges for ER and inpatient encounters increased from $230 million in 2006 to $395 million in 2012; these were unadjusted for inflation, but the investigators note that this increase outpaced inflation. In the adult literature, inpatient care and ambulatory surgery seem to be key drivers of cost.[35] Although the specific drivers for increased costs in pediatrics have yet to be delineated, partly because of the difficulty in assessing true costs from hospital charges and natural limitations of nationally representative databases, the charges in Young's study were higher in encounters associated with an operation. To date, there has been no robust direct comparison of costs in pediatric surgical treatment.

DIAGNOSIS

Diagnosis of nephrolithiasis in pediatrics relies on clinical acumen in combination with imaging and selective laboratory testing. Common presenting signs and symptoms include abdominal or flank pain, dysuria, nausea or vomiting, as well as hematuria. In younger children, the symptoms are often vague and poorly localized; thus, a high level of suspicion is important with the aid of diagnostic tests, including a urinalysis. Specifically seeking out a prior stone history or family history of nephrolithiasis is important. Additional laboratory tests, including a chemistry panel, complete blood count, and urine culture, are sent as indicated.

Stones may often be discovered incidentally on imaging or when nephrolithiasis had not been considered, due to the presentation of many children with nonspecific pain or vomiting.[37] Marzuillo and colleagues[38] reviewed the current evidence on "occult" pediatric nephrolithiasis (stones not seen on US) and found half or more of the children with nephrolithiasis could present with abdominal/flank pain and no specific urinary symptoms and thus required a high degree of suspicion for diagnosis especially if less than 8 years old.

US imaging is considered the first-line diagnostic imaging study in children with suspected ureteral or kidney stones.[37] A renal and bladder US is ideal for children given their relative lack of body fat for image quality, the lack of ionizing radiation, and the relatively low cost.[11] It is known that US is less sensitive (70%) than computed tomography (CT); however, US is an adequate screening tool to diagnose most clinically significant stones.[39] Johnson and colleagues[40] found that although US did miss some stones, it was sufficient for diagnosis of 89% of stones that ultimately needed surgical intervention. Imaging characteristics of urinary tract stones are discrete echogenic foci that produce posterior acoustic shadowing; however, small stones and modern USs with harmonic or spatial compounding imaging may not cast an acoustic shadow. A confirmatory finding is twinkle artifact, a color Doppler phenomenon that appears as a rapid change of color immediately behind a stationary object, which must be performed at the maximum pulse repetition frequency for the US machine.[11]

Despite the recommended use of US as the first diagnostic imaging study obtained for children with suspected ureteral or kidney stones, there is widespread use of CT as a first-line study likely given its wide availability and near 100% sensitivity and specificity. A cross-sectional study of 9228 children with nephrolithiasis from 2003 to 2011 using the Marketscan commercial insurance claims database found that 63% of children underwent an initial CT study, whereas only 24% had an US first. Substantial regional variation exists in CT utilization; in one study, children in the southeastern United States had the highest odds of initial CT (OR 1.27).[41] More recently, low-dose CT studies that use scanning sequences (ie, stone protocol) have been introduced because they dramatically reduce total radiation exposure to <3 mSv but maintain a diagnostic sensitivity of 96.6% for nephrolithiasis.[11] The accuracy of low-dose CT specifically for pediatric nephrolithiasis, however, has not been confirmed. Outside of US and CT, plain abdominal radiograph is another option for evaluation, as combining x-ray with US can increase sensitivity for ureteral stones, however is not used routinely for children in clinical practice.[39]

Currently, US is the first-line imaging method, with low-dose CT reserved for indeterminate cases or if further clarification is necessary (ie, special cases of surgical planning).[37,42] The authors' institution provides a clinical pathway for nephrolithiasis presenting in the ED to help facilitate this decision making (**Fig. 1**). Future studies to identify barriers to the use of US as the primary modality at all hospitals are needed.

ACUTE STONE EPISODE MANAGEMENT
Medical Expulsive Therapy

In a stable child with a ureteral stone, conservative management is indicated. The 2016 American Urological Association (AUA) and Endourological Society guidelines recommend medical expulsive therapy (MET) using alpha-blockers for pediatric patients with uncomplicated ureteral stones <10 mm.[43] Alpha-adrenergic antagonists block receptors in the ureter involved in smooth muscle contraction, thereby leading to dilation and easier passage of a stone. In the adult literature, randomized trials have demonstrated that both tamsulosin and nifedipine (a calcium channel blocker) increase stone passage, whereas alpha-antagonists also decrease time to stone passage, reduce pain requirements, and are cost-effective.[44–46] Recent studies in adults suggest that the greatest benefit of MET is for distal stones >5 mm among adults.[46,47]

ED Pathway for Evaluation and Treatment of Children with Suspected Nephrolithiasis

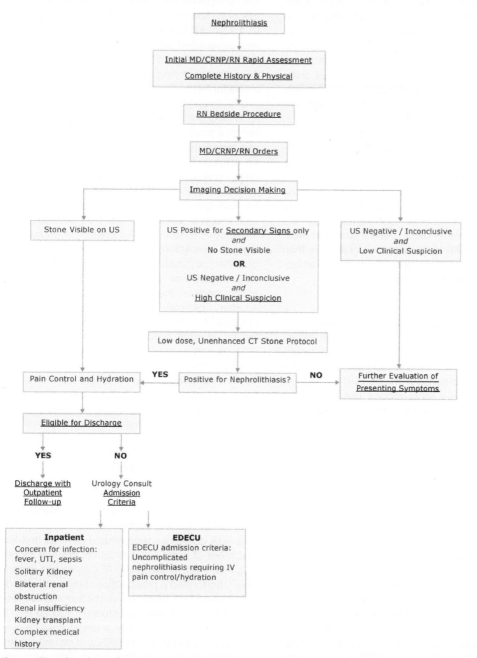

Fig. 1. Clinical pathway for acute nephrolithiasis presentations at the Children's Hospital of Philadelphia (CHOP). EDECU, Emergency Department Extended Care Unit; IV, intravenous; MD/CRNP/RN, doctor/certified registered nurse practitioner/registered nurse; UTI, urinary tract infection. (*From* Children's Hospital of Philadelphia (CHOP). ED Pathway for Evaluation and Treatment of Children with Suspected Nephrolithiasis. Published April 2018. Available at: http://www.chop.edu/clinical-pathway/nephrolithiasis-suspected-emergent-care-clinical-pathway. CHOP Clinical Pathways Program: G. Tasian, MD, MSc, MSCE; L. Copelovitch, MD; N. Plachter, CRNP; K. Ashcroft, CRNP; S. Schneider, PA-C. Accessed April 1, 2018; with permission.)

Thus far, there have been 4 small randomized clinical trials and 2 retrospective studies addressing MET in pediatric patients.[48,49] Tasian and colleagues[49] showed a higher stone expulsion rate with tamsulosin versus analgesics alone for stones less than 10 mm in a multi-institutional cohort. A 2016 meta-analysis and systematic review of the pediatric literature identified only 5 studies of sufficient quality, 3 RCTs, and 2 retrospective cohorts, with pooled results (465 patients) demonstrating that MET significantly increased the odds of spontaneous stone passage (OR 2.21, 95% confidence interval [CI] 1.4–3.5), although concerns about biases affecting published outcomes given the various study designs should be noted.[50] Interestingly, Tian and associates[48] published a systematic review shortly thereafter including 5 studies in which 4 were blinded RCTs. They found higher stone expulsion rates and no significant adverse effects with both of the adrenergic alpha-antagonists (doxazosin and tamsulosin). In their analysis, tamsulosin significantly decreased the time to stone expulsion but doxazosin did not. The investigators conclude that adrenergic alpha-antagonists are effective and safe for distal ureteral stones in pediatric patients with distal ureteral stones less than 10 mm. Of note, none of the RCTs in children examined calcium channel blockers.[48]

Surgery

Operative intervention in children is necessary when ureteral stones fail to pass spontaneously or renal stones become symptomatic. Up to 22% of acute stone episodes in children will require surgery.[2] Lower pole renal stones pose a unique problem because they often present incidentally, but the need for intervention in children is unknown. Dos Santos and colleagues[51] retrospectively evaluated 224 children with lower pole stones and found that 53.5% spontaneously passed the stone, 25% remained asymptomatic and the stone did not grow, and intervention was performed in 21.4%; these stones tended to be larger or grew with time.

As in adults, the main modalities are shockwave lithotripsy (SWL), ureteroscopy (URS), and percutaneous nephrolithotomy (PCNL). SWL had previously been the gold standard for pediatric stone disease; however, recent procedure trends at children's hospitals suggest URS is being used more within the last decade.[52,53] In fact, Wang and colleagues[52] found in their analysis of pediatric hospitals from 2000 to 2008 that URS became more common in later years as well as if there was a ureteral stone code as opposed to a renal stone code alone. Hospital variation was the single most important identifiable factor driving choice between SWL and URS in this study.

Concerns have been raised regarding the deleterious long-term effects of SWL on the pediatric kidney with respect to hypertension (HTN). A population-based retrospective study of 11,570 adult patients with incident nephrolithiasis, including 1319 who underwent SWL and 919 who underwent URS, found a significant increased risk of HTN with SWL (hazard ratio [HR] 1.34, 95% CI 1.15, 1.57) but not URS.[54] Nephrolithiasis itself was associated with a significant risk for chronic kidney disease (HR 1.82, 95% CI 1.67, 1.98), thus compounding the effects of SWL for a stone-former.

URS in children, however, carries its own technical risks and challenges, ranging from manipulation of a smaller ureter in young children to access of a reconstructed urinary tract in complex cases. An attempt to limit the number of anesthetics a child receives is an important benchmark; thus, studies of both stone clearance and re-treatment for each type of procedure are important. Despite technological advances, such as semirigid ureteroscopes as small as 4.5 French, ureteral stenting is sometimes required before definitive treatment of passive dilation of the ureter and subsequent ureteral access if the ureter will not accommodate the ureteroscope, thus adding another general anesthetic to one stone episode.[53,55] Ellison and colleagues[53] recently looked at total procedure volume of URS and SWL as well as 90-day re-treatment for pediatric nephrolithiasis in the Pediatric Health Information System database. The investigators found that SWL and age less than 5 years were associated with re-treatment. Interestingly, patients who underwent both prestenting and a stent at the time of URS or SWL had greatly reduced odds of re-treatment (66%) versus those with stenting at only one of those time points.

The location and size of the stone play obvious and important roles in stone clearance and thus selection of procedure, and this data are unfortunately often not available in claims database reviews. Current AUA guidelines recommend SWL as first-line treatment of kidney and proximal ureteral stones less than 2 cm in children.[43] Mokhless and associates[56] performed a prospective comparative study of URS and SWL in 60 young children with a mean age of 2.4 ± 1.3 years for stones 10 to 20 mm in size. Stone clearance after a single session was 70% in SWL and 86.6% in URS, and no major complications occurred in either group. Follow-up was 3 months with US and plain radiograph, at which time the overall stone clearance was 93.3% and 96.6%, respectively.[56]

In an older group with mean age of 10 years, Featherstone and colleagues[57] reviewed URS for large stones >1 cm in which most stones were located in the kidney. Eighteen patients underwent 35 procedures with a mean of 1.8 procedures per patient (range 1–4); only 6 patients achieved stone-free status after the first URS, but overall stone clearance was 89% at a follow-up of

2.7 years. A ureteral access sheath of 9.5 French was used in almost half of the procedures (49%) and a postoperative stent in 60%.[57] Access sheaths of 9.5 through 14 French have been described in series with good success as defined by stone-free rates and rare postoperative ureteral strictures.[58,59] It is the authors' opinion that active dilation should not be undertaken, and that the risks and benefits of prestenting for passive dilation be carefully considered.

The 2016 AUA guidelines state that both PCNL and SWL are acceptable if the stone burden is greater than 20 mm.[43] However, there is a paucity of data regarding SWL in pediatric patients with large stone burden, and with the possible long-term risks of SWL combined with the likelihood for repeat surgical interventions, the authors implore caution with this approach. PCNL is reasonable for these patients despite a higher risk of complications, and an important technique for the subset of pediatric patients with reconstructed lower urinary tracts. Technical advances in equipment have not only enabled PCNL to be used in pediatric patients, but also have contributed to the advent of mini- and micro-PCNL to decrease morbidity. Mini-PCNL refers to access tracts of less than 20 to 24 French, whereas micro-PCNL utilizes tracts less than 10 French.[60] Published experience with PCNL in children is still limited, with most reports limited to retrospective series demonstrating feasibility and safety.[61,62] Last, an important factor in surgical management should be the inherent radiation exposure involved. One study reported their median fluoroscopy time of URS (1.6 minutes unilateral and 2.5 minutes bilateral) and PCNL (11.7 minutes) and calculated its radiation exposure equivalent to be 3 mSv for URS and 16.8 mSv for PCNL.[63] Given that current guidelines recommend a maximum dose of less than 20 mSv/y over a 5-year period, and that each stone episode comes with additional diagnostic radiation, every attempt should be made to limit the cumulative amount of radiation.[64] To mitigate this factor, intraoperative US has now been described in several feasibility studies for SWL, URS, and PCNL.[65–67]

LONG-TERM MANAGEMENT AND PREVENTION OF RECURRENCE
Recurrence

After acute management of any pediatric stone episode, focus must shift to further diagnostic workup for prevention of recurrence and long-term management. It was previously thought that recurrence rates in pediatric nephrolithiasis were lower than adults at 16% to 19% versus 50% (within 5–10 years), respectively; however, these likely are not representative of the current population because they were performed when the incidence was much lower and the follow-up times were drastically different.[68,69]

To answer this, Tasian and colleagues[70] performed a contemporary (2008–2014) retrospective cohort study of 285 healthy patients aged 3 to 18 years old to determine recurrence rates as defined by a new stone on imaging associated with symptoms (pain and/or vomiting). Using survival analysis, among patients who presented with their first kidney stone during childhood, there was a 50% probability of recurrence within 3 years of the index stone. The risk of lifelong stone formation, identifiable abnormalities commonly found on metabolic workup, and the high risk of recurrence are the rationale for a thorough metabolic evaluation that includes 24-hour urine analysis and serum chemistries (including basic metabolic panel, magnesium, phosphorus, and uric acid) for any patient that forms a stone in childhood.

Metabolic Evaluation

Interestingly, there is a lack of consensus regarding metabolic workup and methods to decrease recurrence, because there are no published guidelines specific to pediatric stone-formers. The current AUA guidelines do not specifically address pediatric patients, whereas the EAU does recommend analyzing 24-hour urine collections in high-risk patients in order to decrease recurrence.[42,71] In addition to demonstrating higher rates of recurrence in children and adolescents, the study by Tasian and colleagues[70] was powered to detect differences in recurrence rates stratified by those who obtained a 24-hour urine analysis. The investigators demonstrated a 60% reduction in risk of recurrence in patients who completed at least one 24-hour analysis, preliminary evidence that completing a 24-hour urine analysis does make a difference. As a test, 24-hour urine collection appears to be a reliable tool in children; however, the importance of a single versus repeated collection is unclear. In a study of more than 700 children, Ellison and colleagues[72] demonstrated concordance in the excretion of two 24-hour urinary samples collected closely together, with modestly good agreement in excretions of calcium, oxalate, and citrate. However, the investigators found that the risk of recurrence may be misclassified in up to 25% of pediatric stone-formers if only a single 24-hour urine analysis is used, arguing for the importance of a second collection before initiating therapy.[72]

Metabolic analysis ideally helps to stratify those children who may benefit from medical intervention after their first stone episode, and defining normal values within the pediatric population is important to this end. Reference values are provided in **Table 1**. Aside from accepted independent risk factors such as hypercalciuria, Defoor and colleagues[73] assessed whether a calcium-to-citrate ratio might improve stratification in a retrospective review. A total of 73 solitary stone-formers and 92 recurrent stone-formers were included, matched for age (12.7 and 13.3 years, respectively), gender, and BMI, then compared with a smaller control group (n = 29) that was slightly younger (9.6 years). The investigators found that in their cohort, the mean calcium-to-citrate ratio was significantly higher in recurrent stone-formers (0.64) than in controls (0.33) and solitary stone-formers (0.41); the difference between controls and solitary stone-formers did not reach significance.[73] Whether the sensitivity and accuracy of this test will elevate it to have a role in predicting recurrence remains to be seen.

Some investigators have argued that a full metabolic evaluation may not be needed in all pediatric patients. Given that the metabolic evaluation of their modern pediatric stone population resembled the adult population with predominantly low urine volume and hypocitraturia, Bevill and colleagues[12] argue that more selective testing based on stone composition or spot urine tests could be entertained. However, a cutoff of 250 mg/d as opposed to a weight-based formula (>4 mg/kg/d) was used and resulted in a very low incidence (11%). Their results are incongruent with several other series and would need to be confirmed in larger studies; therefore, caution should be exercised. Furthermore, urinary parameters change significantly with age, and thus, management strategies will likely be different for younger versus older children.[74] Many clinicians will obtain a spot urinary calcium-to-creatinine ratio as an initial assessment of hypercalciuria; however, this is inherently limited in diagnostic scope and is perhaps most useful for children who are not yet toilet trained, with or without other random urinary metabolites (uric acid, citrate, oxalate).[15,27] At the authors' institution, patients undergo a serum basic metabolic profile, magnesium, phosphorus, and uric acid; a 24-hour urine analysis if toilet trained or a urinalysis and spot urine for calcium, creatinine, oxalate, and citrate if not toilet trained. It is important to remember that 24-hour urine chemistries must be indexed to the patient's

Table 1
Metabolic evaluation: normal urinary solute values and reference ranges

Metabolite	Age	Random[a]	24 h[b]	Litholink Total Excretion Reference Ranges (Adult)
Calcium	0–6 mo	<0.8 mg/mg	<4 mg/kg/d	Male: <250 mg/d
	7–12 mo	<0.6 mg/mg		Female: <200 mg/d
	>24 mo	<0.21 mg/mg		
Oxalate	0–6 mo	<0.26 mg/mg	<40 mg/1.73 m²	20–40 mg/d
	7–24 mo	<0.11 mg/mg		
	2–5 y	<0.08 mg/mg		
	5–14 y	<0.06 mg/mg		
	>16 y	<0.03 mg/mg		
Citrate	0–17 y	>0.2–0.42 mg/mg	Males: >130 mg/g	Male: >450 mg/d Female: >550 mg/d
			Females: >300 mg/g	
	>18 y		Males: >450 mg/g	
			Females: >550 mg/g	
Uric acid	>2 y	0.56 mg/dL GFR[c]	<815 mg/1.73 m²	Male: <0.8 g/d
				Female: <0.75 g/d
Cystine	>6 mo	<0.075 mg/mg	<50 mg/1.73 m²	

Abbreviation: GFR, glomerular filtration rate.
  [a] Random samples are a ratio of the urine metabolite (mg) to urine creatinine (mg).
  [b] Twenty-four-hour samples: urine oxalate, uric acid, and cystine measurement corrected for body surface area (m²); urine citrate (mg) measured as ratio to urine creatinine (g).
  [c] Random sample urine uric acid (mg/dL) × plasma creatinine (mg/dL)/urine creatinine (mg/dL).
  Adapted from Copelovitch L. Urolithiasis in children: medical approach. Pediatr Clin North Am 2012;59:885; with permission.

creatinine, body weight, or body surface area for smaller children (see **Table 1**).

Dietary Interventions and Targeted Therapy

As in adult stone management, a cornerstone first-line treatment of all stone-formers regardless of underlying cause is increased fluid intake. Specific dietary modifications can be made to target 24-hour urine results, such as decreased sodium intake to combat hypercalciuria. Importantly, calcium restriction is not recommended for stone-formers given the increased risk of incident stone formation and osteoporosis.[15] Similarly, children should not restrict their animal protein intake and aim for 100% of the daily recommended allowance, due to the need for protein to sustain growth.

Further therapy may become necessary if dietary changes alone are insufficient, or if a known genetic/metabolic condition is identified. **Table 2** lists specific metabolic abnormalities and the corresponding dietary and medical targeted therapy. Alkali agents such as potassium citrate or potassium-magnesium citrate may be used, preferentially to sodium citrate given the associated increased sodium delivery to the nephron. Special circumstances require very thoughtful use of medications, such as patients who are on a ketogenic diet for epilepsy. Potassium citrate may be used because these patients have hypercalciuria as well as hypocitraturia and urine acidification. In a cohort of 313 patients on a ketogenic diet from Johns Hopkins, 198 children were started on oral potassium citrate either empirically (106) or "preventively" due to the presence of hypercalciuria (92), versus 105 who were not started on medication.[28] Between the 2 groups, preventative use of oral potassium citrate was associated with a decreased incidence of kidney stones (2.0% vs 10.5%; $P = .003$). Furthermore, empiric administration resulted in stone incidence of 0.9% versus 6.7% in the preventive group ($P = .02$).[28] Other specific pharmacologic interventions are listed in **Table 2**.

Follow-up Imaging and Surveillance

After dietary or pharmacologic interventions have been instituted, a follow-up urinary metabolic analysis should be repeated several months after. Patients taking medications with a side-effect profile must be followed closely. The optimal timing of follow-up and diagnostic

Table 2
Recommended dietary intake and targeted therapies for specific metabolic abnormalities

Metabolic Abnormality	Dietary Recommendation	Medication
Low urine volume	Fluid intake sufficient to maintain urine output >2.5 L for adults and >30 mL/kg/d for younger patients (weak evidence)	
Hypocitraturia	Increase potassium-rich fruits and vegetables Citrate supplementation	Potassium citrate 2–4 mEq/kg/d Sodium citrate
Hypercalciuria	Maintain normal dietary calcium intake, low salt diet <2 g/d	Thiazide diuretic (eg, hydrochlorothiazide 1–2 mg/kg/d) up to 25–50 mg daily
Hyperoxaluria	Limit dietary oxalate Discontinue vitamin C supplements due to increased risk of CaOx stone if hyperoxaluria Maintain high Ca intake	
Hyperuricosuria	Urinary alkalinization Decrease nondairy protein and Sodium Intake Increase fluid intake	Allopurinol 4–10 mg/kg/d Potassium citrate
Cystinuria	Higher fluid intake than general dietary recommendations: 1.5-2 L/m^2 Decrease sodium intake	Tiopronin (alpha-mercaptopropionylglycine) D-Pencillamine Potassium citrate

Abbreviation: CaOx, calcium oxalate.

testing is undefined, although should be guided in some part by the risk status of the patient's diagnosis, with high-risk or recurrent stone-formers being seen in joint nephrology/urology clinic if possible. At the authors' institution currently, pediatric patients are seen every 6 months with a renal bladder US for the first 2 years after the initial stone and until 24-hour urinary analysis returns to normal.

FUTURE DIRECTIONS

Pediatric stone disease is a rapidly evolving field of study and should continue on that trajectory as we begin to more fully understand the drivers behind its rising incidence. Further refining risk categories and necessary evaluations may offer more tailored treatment regimens based on patient characteristics. Could a genetic approach be useful? Langman[34] points to WES in the follow-up study of 51 families examining the same 30 genes as the Braun study. WES identified 22 patients within 15 families with a mutation; the majority (80%) was autosomal recessive.[34] He suggests a step-wise approach to look intensively for genetic causes in children who are less than 5 year old, especially with a history of consanguinity or nephrocalcinosis.

Equally important as defining patient risk for evaluation and treatment is defining and studying these outcomes from a patient perspective. A disease-specific instrument for nephrolithiasis was released only in 2013, and earlier studies used a generic short form-36 that encompasses 8 health domains.[75] As pediatric stone disease is comparatively understudied, it is not surprising that there is even less known about pediatric patient-reported outcomes.

REFERENCES

1. Sas DJ, Hulsey TC, Shatat IF, et al. Increasing incidence of kidney stones in children evaluated in the emergency department. J Pediatr 2010;157(1):132–7.
2. Routh JC, Graham DA, Nelson CP. Epidemiological trends in pediatric urolithiasis at United States free-standing pediatric hospitals. J Urol 2010;184(3):1100–4.
3. Dwyer ME, Krambeck AE, Bergstralh EJ, et al. Temporal trends in incidence of kidney stones among children: a 25-year population based study. J Urol 2012;188(1):247–52.
4. Alfandary H, Haskin O, Davidovits M, et al. Increasing prevalence of nephrolithiasis in association with increased body mass index in children: a population based study. J Urol 2018;199(4):1044–9.
5. Tasian GE, Ross ME, Song L, et al. Annual incidence of nephrolithiasis among children and adults in South Carolina from 1997 to 2012. Clin J Am Soc Nephrol 2016;11(3):488–96.
6. Soucie JM, Thun MJ, Coates RJ, et al. Demographic and geographic variability of kidney stones in the United States. Kidney Int 1994;46(3):893–9.
7. Pearle MS, Calhoun EA, Curhan GC, Urologic Diseases of America Project. Urologic diseases in America project: urolithiasis. J Urol 2005;173(3):848–57.
8. Young BJ, Tejwani R, Wang HH, et al. Is the economic impact and utilization of imaging studies for pediatric urolithiasis across the United States increasing? Urology 2016;94:208–13.
9. Kirejczyk JK, Porowski T, Filonowicz R, et al. An association between kidney stone composition and urinary metabolic disturbances in children. J Pediatr Urol 2014;10(1):130–5.
10. Tasian GE, Copelovitch L. Evaluation and medical management of kidney stones in children. J Urol 2014;192(5):1329–36.
11. Colleran GC, Callahan MJ, Paltiel HJ, et al. Imaging in the diagnosis of pediatric urolithiasis. Pediatr Radiol 2017;47(1):5–16.
12. Bevill M, Kattula A, Cooper CS, et al. The modern metabolic stone evaluation in children. Urology 2017;101:15–20.
13. Kovacevic L, Wolfe-Christensen C, Edwards L, et al. From hypercalciuria to hypocitraturia - a shifting trend in pediatric urolithiasis. J Urol 2012;188:1623–7.
14. Penido MG, Srivastava T, Alon US. Pediatric primary urolithiasis: 12-year experience at a Midwestern Children's Hospital. J Urol 2013;189(4):1493–7.
15. Copelovitch L. Urolithiasis in children: medical approach. Pediatr Clin North Am 2012;59(4):881–96.
16. Scales CD Jr, Tasian GE, Schwaderer AL, et al. Urinary stone disease: advancing knowledge, patient care, and population health. Clin J Am Soc Nephrol 2016;11(7):1305–12.
17. Kant AK, Graubard BI. Contributors of water intake in US children and adolescents: associations with dietary and meal characteristics–National Health and Nutrition Examination Survey 2005-2006. Am J Clin Nutr 2010;92(4):887–96.
18. Cogswell ME, Yuan K, Gunn JP, et al. Vital signs: sodium intake among U.S. School-aged children - 2009-2010. MMWR Morb Mortal Wkly Rep 2014;63(36):789–97.
19. Clark MA, Fox MK. Nutritional quality of the diets of US public school children and the role of the school meal programs. J Am Diet Assoc 2009;109(2 Suppl):S44–56.
20. Prevention of Urinary Stones with Hydration (PUSH) Trial. NIDDK. Available at: www.clinicaltrials.gov. Accessed April 14, 2018.

21. Tasian GE, Ross ME, Song L, et al. Dietary zinc and incident calcium kidney stones in adolescence. J Urol 2017;197(5):1342–8.

22. Kokorowski PJ, Routh JC, Hubert KC, et al. Association of urolithiasis with systemic conditions among pediatric patients at children's hospitals. J Urol 2012;188(4 Suppl):1618–22.

23. Kim SS, Luan X, Canning DA, et al. Association between body mass index and urolithiasis in children. J Urol 2011;186(4 Suppl):1734–9.

24. Cambareri GM, Giel DW, Bayne AP, et al. Do overweight and obese pediatric stone formers have differences in metabolic abnormalities compared with normal-weight stone formers? Urology 2017;101: 26–30.

25. Tasian GE, Pulido JE, Gasparrini A, et al. Daily mean temperature and clinical kidney stone presentation in five U.S. metropolitan areas: a time-series analysis. Environ Health Perspect 2014;122(10):1081–7.

26. Ross ME, Vicedo-Cabrera AM, Kopp RE, et al. Assessment of the combination of temperature and relative humidity on kidney stone presentations. Environ Res 2018;162:97–105.

27. McKay CP. Renal stone disease. Pediatr Rev 2010; 31(5):179–88.

28. McNally MA, Pyzik PL, Rubenstein JE, et al. Empiric use of potassium citrate reduces kidney-stone incidence with the ketogenic diet. Pediatrics 2009; 124(2):e300–4.

29. Shekarriz B, Stoller ML. Cystinuria and other noncalcareous calculi. Endocrinol Metab Clin North Am 2002;31:951–77.

30. Goldfarb DS, Fischer ME, Keich Y, et al. A twin study of genetic and dietary influences on nephrolithiasis: a report from the Vietnam Era Twin (VET) Registry. Kidney Int 2005;67(3):1053–61.

31. Halbritter J, Baum M, Hynes AM, et al. Fourteen monogenic genes account for 15% of nephrolithiasis/nephrocalcinosis. J Am Soc Nephrol 2015; 26(3):543–51.

32. Braun DA, Lawson JA, Gee HY, et al. Prevalence of monogenic causes in pediatric patients with nephrolithiasis or nephrocalcinosis. Clin J Am Soc Nephrol 2016;11(4):664–72.

33. Daga A, Majmundar AJ, Braun DA, et al. Whole exome sequencing frequently detects a monogenic cause in early onset nephrolithiasis and nephrocalcinosis. Kidney Int 2018;93(1):204–13.

34. Langman CB. A rational approach to the use of sophisticated genetic analyses of pediatric stone disease. Kidney Int 2018;93(1):15–8.

35. Litwin MS, Saigal CS. Urologic Diseases in America. US Department of Health and Human Services, Public Health Service, National Institutes of Health, National Institute of Diabetes and Digestive and Kidney Diseases. Washington, DC: US Government Printing Office; 2012. p. 314–45.

36. Wang HH, Wiener JS, Lipkin ME, et al. Estimating the nationwide, hospital based economic impact of pediatric urolithiasis. J Urol 2015;193(5 Suppl): 1855–9.

37. Riccabona M, Avni FE, Blickman JG, et al. Imaging recommendations in paediatric uroradiology. Minutes of the ESPR uroradiology task force session on childhood obstructive uropathy, high-grade fetal hydronephrosis, childhood haematuria, and urolithiasis in childhood. ESPR Annual Congress, Edinburgh, UK, June 2008. Pediatr Radiol 2009;39(8): 891–8.

38. Marzuillo P, Guarino S, Apicella A, et al. Why we need a higher suspicion index of urolithiasis in children. J Pediatr Urol 2017;13(2):164–71.

39. Passerotti C, Chow JS, Silva A, et al. Ultrasound versus computerized tomography for evaluating urolithiasis. J Urol 2009;182(4 Suppl):1829–34.

40. Johnson EK, Faerber GJ, Roberts WW, et al. Are stone protocol computed tomography scans mandatory for children with suspected urinary calculi? Urology 2011;78(3):662–6.

41. Tasian GE, Pulido JE, Keren R, et al. Use of and regional variation in initial CT imaging for kidney stones. Pediatrics 2014;134(5):909–15.

42. Turk C, Petrik A, Sarica K, et al. EAU guidelines on diagnosis and conservative management of urolithiasis. Eur Urol 2016;69(3):468–74.

43. Assimos D, Krambeck A, Miller NL, et al. Surgical management of stones: American Urological Association/Endourological Society Guideline, PART I. J Urol 2016;196(4):1153–60.

44. Pickard R, Starr K, MacLennan G, et al. Medical expulsive therapy in adults with ureteric colic: a multicentre, randomised, placebo-controlled trial. Lancet 2015;386(9991):341–9.

45. Hollingsworth JM, Rogers MA, Kaufman SR, et al. Medical therapy to facilitate urinary stone passage: a meta-analysis. Lancet 2006;368(9542):1171–9.

46. Ye Z, Zeng G, Yang H, et al. Efficacy and safety of tamsulosin in medical expulsive therapy for distal ureteral stones with renal colic: a multicenter, randomized, double-blind, placebo-controlled trial. Eur Urol 2017. https://doi.org/10.1016/j.eururo. 2017.10.033.

47. Dahm P, Sukumar S, Hollingsworth J. Medical expulsive therapy for distal ureteral stones: the verdict is in. Eur Urol 2018;73:392–3.

48. Tian D, Li N, Huang W, et al. The efficacy and safety of adrenergic alpha-antagonists in treatment of distal ureteral stones in pediatric patients: a systematic review and meta-analysis. J Pediatr Surg 2017; 52(2):360–5.

49. Tasian GE, Cost NG, Granberg CF, et al. Tamsulosin and spontaneous passage of ureteral stones in children: a multi-institutional cohort study. J Urol 2014; 192(2):506–11.

50. Velazquez N, Zapata D, Wang HH, et al. Medical expulsive therapy for pediatric urolithiasis: Systematic review and meta-analysis. J Pediatr Urol 2015; 11(6):321–7.

51. Dos Santos J, Lopes RI, Veloso AO, et al. Outcome analysis of asymptomatic lower pole stones in children. J Urol 2016;195(4 Pt 2):1289–93.

52. Wang HH, Huang L, Routh JC, et al. Shock wave lithotripsy vs ureteroscopy: variation in surgical management of kidney stones at freestanding children's hospitals. J Urol 2012;187(4):1402–7.

53. Ellison JS, Shnorhavorian M, Oron A, et al. Risk factors for repeat surgical intervention in pediatric nephrolithiasis: a pediatric health information system database study. J Pediatr Urol 2018;14(3): 245.e1–6.

54. Denburg MR, Jemielita TO, Tasian GE, et al. Assessing the risk of incident hypertension and chronic kidney disease after exposure to shock wave lithotripsy and ureteroscopy. Kidney Int 2016;89(1):185–92.

55. Kim S, Kolon T, Canter D, et al. Pediatric flexible ureteroscopic lithotripsy: the Children's Hospital of Philadelphia. J Urol 2008;180(6):2616–9.

56. Mokhless IA, Abdeldaeim HM, Saad A, et al. Retrograde intrarenal surgery monotherapy versus shock wave lithotripsy for stones 10 to 20 mm in preschool children: a prospective, randomized study. J Urol 2014;191(5 Suppl):1496–9.

57. Featherstone NC, Somani BK, Griffin SJ. Ureteroscopy and laser stone fragmentation (URSL) for large (>/=1 cm) paediatric stones: outcomes from a university teaching hospital. J Pediatr Urol 2017; 13(2):202.e1–7.

58. Smaldone MC, Cannon GM Jr, Wu HY, et al. Is ureteroscopy first line treatment for pediatric stone disease? J Urol 2007;178(5):2128–31 [discussion: 31].

59. Singh A, Shah G, Young J, et al. Ureteral access sheath for the management of pediatric renal and ureteral stones: a single center experience. J Urol 2006;175(3):1080–2.

60. Bonzo JR, Tasian GE. The emergence of kidney stone disease during childhood-impact on adults. Curr Urol Rep 2017;18(6):44.

61. Yadav SS, Aggarwal SP, Mathur R, et al. Pediatric percutaneous nephrolithotomy-experience of a tertiary care center. J Endourol 2017;31(3):246–54.

62. Silay MS, Tepeler A, Atis G, et al. Initial report of microperc in the treatment of pediatric nephrolithiasis. J Pediatr Surg 2013;48(7):1578–83.

63. Ristau BT, Dudley AG, Casella DP, et al. Tracking of radiation exposure in pediatric stone patients: the time is now. J Pediatr Urol 2015;11(6):339.e1-5.

64. Wrixon AD. New ICRP Recommendations. J Radiol Prot 2008;28(2):161–8.

65. Goren MR, Goren V, Ozer C. Ultrasound-guided shockwave lithotripsy reduces radiation exposure and has better outcomes for pediatric cystine stones. Urol Intl 2016;98(4):429–35.

66. Desai M, Ridhorkar V, Patel S, et al. Pediatric percutaneous nephrolithotomy: assessing impact of technical innovations on safety and efficacy. J Endourol 1999;13(5):359–64.

67. Morrison JC, Kawal T, Van Batavia JP, et al. Use of ultrasound in pediatric renal stone diagnosis and surgery. Curr Urol Rep 2017;18(3):22.

68. Pietrow PKPJ, Adams MC, Shyr Y, et al. Clinical outcome of pediatric stone disease. J Urol 2002; 167:670–3.

69. Diamond DA, Menon M, Lee P, et al. Etiological factors in pediatric stone recurrence. J Urol 1989;142(2 Pt 2):606–8.

70. Tasian GE, Kabarriti AE, Kalmus A, et al. Kidney stone recurrence among children and adolescents. J Urol 2017;197(1):246–52.

71. Pearle MS, Goldfarb DS, Assimos DG, et al. Medical management of kidney stones: AUA guideline. J Urol 2014;192(2):316–24.

72. Ellison JS, Hollingsworth JM, Langman CB, et al. Analyte variations in consecutive 24-hour urine collections in children. J Pediatr Urol 2017;13(6):632.e1-7.

73. DeFoor W, Jackson E, Schulte M, et al. Calcium-to-citrate ratio distinguishes solitary and recurrent urinary stone forming children. J Urol 2017;198(2): 416–21.

74. Cambareri GM, Kovacevic L, Bayne AP, et al. National multi-insitutional cooperative on urolithiasis in children: age is a significant predictor of urine abnormalities. J Pediatr Urol 2015;11(4):218–23.

75. Ellison JS, Williams M, Keeley FX Jr. Patient-reported outcomes in nephrolithiasis: can we do better? J Endourol 2018;32(1):10–20.

Anesthesia in the Pediatric Patient

Megan A. Brockel, MD[a],*, David M. Polaner, MD[a], Vijaya M. Vemulakonda, MD, JD[b]

KEYWORDS

- Pediatric anesthesia • Regional anesthesia • Neurotoxicity • ERAS • Surgical decision making

KEY POINTS

- General anesthesia has a low rate of serious complications in children.
- Neonates and infants generally have a higher risk of cardiovascular and pulmonary morbidity and mortality when compared with older children and adults.
- Concerns about neurotoxicity appear strongest in infants with longer or repeated anesthetic exposures, but adverse findings in animal models have not clearly translated into humans.
- Regional anesthesia may help to reduce the need for, or moderate, the exposure to intraoperative general anesthetic agents and may improve postoperative outcomes.

INTRODUCTION

Unlike in the adult population, where regional anesthesia may be used as an alternative to general anesthesia, surgery in the pediatric patient relies on use of general anesthesia for most cases. Although general anesthesia is often supplemented with regional anesthesia to reduce perioperative pain and stress, anesthesia in children is not without risk, which may vary based on the age of the child. These risks have been highlighted in recent years, with studies suggesting that prolonged or repetitive anesthetic exposure in early childhood may adversely affect brain development. Due to these potential risks, the Food and Drug Administration issued a warning cautioning about the risks of prolonged anesthetic exposure in children younger than 3 years and suggesting the potential benefit of delaying elective surgery when medically appropriate.[1] The purpose of this article is to discuss the evolution of current pediatric anesthetic practice, the potential risks of general anesthesia in young children, and possible alternatives to, or techniques of moderating, exposure to general anesthesia. We also offer our approach to making decisions with families about the optimal timing of and anesthetic approach to nonemergent urologic surgery in children.

SURGICAL STRESS AND BENEFIT OF ANESTHESIA IN CHILDREN

More than 30 years ago, it was common practice for newborns to undergo surgical procedures with only intermittent nitrous oxide or no anesthesia at all. This practice stemmed from widely held beliefs that neonates did not sense pain and that anesthetic techniques available at the time were too high risk. In 1987, Anand and colleagues[2] performed a randomized controlled trial in which preterm infants undergoing ligation of a patent ductus arteriosus received either nitrous oxide and muscle relaxant or nitrous oxide and muscle relaxant plus fentanyl. Major hormonal responses to surgical stress were significantly greater in the nonfentanyl than in the fentanyl group. Beyond this, infants in the nonfentanyl group were more likely to require an increase in ventilatory support after surgery and to experience circulatory and metabolic complications postoperatively. This

Disclosure Statement: The authors have nothing to disclose.
[a] Department of Anesthesiology, University of Colorado, Children's Hospital Colorado, Anschutz Medical Campus, 13123 East 16th Avenue, Aurora, CO 80045, USA; [b] Department of Urology, University of Colorado, Children's Hospital Colorado, Anschutz Medical Campus, 13123 East 16th Avenue, Aurora, CO 80045, USA
* Corresponding author.
E-mail address: Megan.brockel@childrenscolorado.org

and other studies sparked interest in neonatal pain, the associated stress response, and short-term and long-term outcomes of untreated pain in the neonatal period. A decade later, Taddio and colleagues[3] found that circumcised infants showed a stronger response to the pain associated with a subsequent vaccination than uncircumcised infants. Among the circumcised infants, those who had preoperative treatment with a eutectic mixture of local anesthetics (EMLA) had an attenuated pain response to subsequent vaccination.

These studies, along with others, mounted a strong argument that pain in the neonatal period is physiologically disruptive and developmentally detrimental in both the short-term and the long-term. This evidence combined with the development of newer, safer anesthetic medications and monitoring capability led to widespread acceptance of administration of anesthesia and treatment of pain in neonates undergoing painful procedures as standard of care.

RISKS OF GENERAL ANESTHESIA

It is widely recognized and well-documented that the risk of both significant morbidity and mortality associated with surgical procedures requiring anesthesia has decreased significantly over the past 50 years. Although it was previously assumed that pediatric mortality rates are greater than those for adults, recent data suggest that, with the exception of infants, rates for children and young adults are similar.[4] The mortality rates among children undergoing noncardiac surgery range from 0.4 to 1.6 per 10,000 anesthetics, although, among neonates and infants, mortality rates are much higher.[5]

The Pediatric Perioperative Cardiac Arrest (POCA) Registry was formed in 1994 in an effort to elucidate the factors and outcomes associated with cardiac arrest in anesthetized children. Institutions that provide anesthesia to children were offered an opportunity to voluntarily enroll in the registry. In the first 4 years (1994–1997), 63 institutions enrolled and submitted 289 cases of cardiac arrest (defined as the need for chest compressions or as death in anesthetized children 18 years of age or younger). Cardiac arrest related to anesthesia had an incidence of 1.4 ± 0.45 (mean ± standard deviation) per 10,000 instances of anesthesia and a mortality rate of 26%. Medication-related (37%) and cardiovascular (32%) causes of cardiac arrest were most common. Cardiac depression from halothane was responsible for two-thirds of all medication-related arrests. Infants younger than 1 year accounted for 55% of all anesthesia-related arrests. Patients with severe underlying disease and those having emergency surgery were most likely to have a fatal outcome.[6]

In an update from the POCA registry published in 2007, cases submitted to the registry in the 7 years since the original report (1998–2004) were analyzed.[7] In the interim, halothane use had declined in favor of sevoflurane and, with this, the proportion of medication-related arrests declined from 37% to 18% ($P<.05$). Cardiovascular causes of arrest, including hypovolemia due to blood loss and hyperkalemia due to blood transfusion, were proportionally more common. The most common cause of respiratory-related arrests was laryngospasm and the most common cause of equipment-related arrests was lung and vascular injury caused by insertion of central venous catheters.

Cardiovascular

Beyond cardiovascular complications associated with perioperative blood loss and transfusion, children (especially infants) are at risk of bradycardia under anesthesia. Cardiac output in infants and children is heart rate dependent, and a slowing of the heart rate is necessarily associated with a reduction in cardiac output. As such, bradycardia under anesthesia is associated with significant morbidity. In an epidemiologic study, Keenan and colleagues[8] found that the frequency of bradycardia (defined as heart rate <100 beats per minute) during anesthesia was 1.27% during the first year of life and decreased to 0.65% in the third and 0.16% in the fourth year. Causes included disease or surgery in 35%, inhalational agent in 35%, and hypoxemia in 22%. Morbidity included hypotension in 30%, asystole or ventricular fibrillation in 10%, and death in 8%. Treatment involved epinephrine in 30% and chest compressions in 25%. Associated factors included higher American Society of Anesthesiologists physical status and longer surgery.

Pulmonary

Laryngospasm, bronchospasm, and upper respiratory tract infections

Laryngospasm, defined as sustained reflex closure of the false and true vocal cords, is a potentially life-threatening emergency typically occurring in a light plane of anesthesia during induction or emergence from anesthesia. The incidence of laryngospasm varies dramatically among studies, with factors that increase the frequency of laryngospasm including young age, history of reactive airway disease, recent upper respiratory tract infection (URI), and second-hand smoke exposure. These same factors also increase the frequency of perioperative bronchospasm.

In addition to laryngospasm and broncho-spasm, recent URIs increase the risk of other peri-operative adverse events. For the perioperative risk to return to baseline, elective surgery should be postponed 4 to 6 weeks after a URI. As children may have as many as 10 URIs per year, many pe-diatric anesthesiologists use 2 to 4 weeks as a more reasonable timeframe for which to postpone elective surgery after a URI. Patient and proce-dural factors, such as patient comorbidities, URI duration and symptoms, airway management (facemask is associated with the least complica-tions in the setting of a URI, followed by a laryngeal mask, followed by an endotracheal tube), and type and duration of the operation are all factors that are considered in the decision-making process. Extra caution should be taken with children whose infections are associated with fever, mucopurulent secretions, signs of lower respiratory tract involve-ment (wheezing or rhonchi), and changes in behavior (eating, activity, sleep), as these findings significantly increase the risk of perioperative adverse events. Similarly, respiratory illness in children with associated underlying chronic respi-ratory disease should be a signal for increased caution.

Fasting and Aspiration

Preoperative fasting policies are universally imple-mented before elective procedures to reduce the likelihood of regurgitation and aspiration of gastric contents that can occur when protective airway re-flexes are lost under anesthesia. Although the inci-dence of aspiration is rare, reports on the outcomes following aspiration events are conflict-ing. Some investigators report that pulmonary aspiration is associated with nearly no mortality, whereas others associate aspiration events with significant morbidity and mortality.[9] The highest-risk time for an aspiration event is during induction, and patient factors associated with aspiration include full stomach, bowel obstruction, abdom-inal pain, diabetes, and trauma. Anesthetic factors include inadequate or light anesthesia and inap-propriate choice of airway management (eg, use of a laryngeal mask in a patient at high risk of aspi-ration). Some have voiced concerns that the cur-rent guidelines of 6 hours for solids, 4 hours for breast milk, and 2 hours for clear liquids may be unnecessarily restrictive, and patients often fast for much longer than is beneficial.[10] Prolonged fasting comes with its own set of detrimental metabolic and behavioral consequences in children, and some advocate for a revision of the current guidelines.[10] Until new research becomes available to elucidate the safety of liberalized fast-ing, clinicians must educate parents about both the importance of fasting and the unnecessariness of fasting for too long, while paying special atten-tion to patients who are at increased risk for aspi-ration events.

Apnea and Former Premature Infants

The first prospective study demonstrating the risk of apnea after anesthesia in former premature in-fants was published in 1983[11] and since that time, numerous studies have sought to identify risk factors and define the period of susceptibility. The cause is thought to be an inability of the imma-ture brainstem to control and regulate breathing after an anesthetic and it has been established that infants born before 36 weeks' conceptual age are at risk. A meta-analysis of 8 prospective studies of former premature infants undergoing inguinal herniorrhaphy reported that the postcon-ceptual age required to reduce the risk to less than 1% with 95% confidence was 54 weeks in in-fants born at 35 weeks' gestational age and 56 weeks in those born before 32 weeks' gesta-tion.[12] Some have suggested that the risk of apnea is less after a spinal anesthetic than it is after a general anesthetic; however, case reports of ap-nea after spinal anesthesia have been published and most pediatric anesthesiologists recommend monitoring of all premature infants for 24 hours af-ter an anesthetic regardless of the technique.[13]

Neurotoxicity

In 2003, Jevtovic-Todorovic et al[14] reported that commonly used anesthetic agents cause wide-spread neurodegeneration and persistent learning deficits in newborn rats. The investigators expressed concern that their findings may trans-late to humans with anesthetic agents causing apoptotic neuronal death in the developing human brain.[15] Although experts in the pediatric commu-nity voiced concern over the applicability of the an-imal data to human subjects,[16] they agreed that further investigation was certainly warranted.

The animal evidence that anesthetic exposure may produce adverse microstructural and neuro-developmental performance effects is both strong and consistent across species, ranging from ro-dents to nonhuman primates. Most of these studies, however, have used anesthetic exposures that are quite long, in excess of that which the vast majority of human infants receive. Many have also been criticized for experimental protocols in which the exposure is limited to an anesthetic, without the concomitant exposure to surgery that may moderate some of the neuroanatomic effects of anesthesia. Finally, the effects of a nurturing and robust salutary developmental environment, which can leverage the neuroplasticity of young brains, has not been replicated in many animal experimental protocols. The most recent primate studies have tried to address these criticisms, and still have pointed to adverse neurodevelopmental outcomes with long anesthetic exposures. Yet, the translation of these results to human studies has been both inconsistent and unclear at best.

With only one exception, all human studies have used retrospective methodologies, which leaves even the finest case-control and propensity-score adjusted investigations subject to unmeasured confounding. A series of retrospective analysis from the Mayo group looked at large cohorts of children exposed to no, 1, or multiple anesthetics before the age of 3 years. All, including the most recent and most sophisticated, found that children with single exposures were not different from controls, but multiple anesthetics were associated with diminished scholastic performance in later years. A very large retrospective cohort analysis from Canada found that although multiparameter scholastic testing showed statistically significant performance differences in children who received anesthetics in infancy, those differences were so small as to be clinically negligible. Several large twin studies from Europe, in which twin pairs were either concordant or discordant for anesthetic exposure, showed no differences. Finally, an ambidirectional study (in which exposure to anesthesia or not was retrospective, but follow-up with matched sibling controls was prospective) found no differences.

The reasons for such widely divergent outcomes of these clinical studies are not entirely clear, and might be due to unmeasured confounders and biases, differences in outcome metrics, or other methodological factors. There is only one prospective randomized clinical trial to date, the GAS (general anesthesia vs spinal) trial, in which more than 700 infants were randomized to receive either general anesthesia or spinal anesthesia for inguinal herniorrhaphy followed by neurodevelopmental testing 2 and 5 years after surgery. At this time, although the final results are pending, the 2-year examinations showed no differences between groups, suggesting that a short (1-hour) exposure to general anesthesia does not result in adverse developmental outcomes. The effect of longer exposures in humans remains uncertain. Anesthetic techniques that can mitigate or reduce exposure to agents suspected of causing adverse effects (all gamma-aminobutyric acid-*ergic* and

N-Methyl-D-aspartate [NMDA] receptor antagonists) may be considered in the putative at-risk population of infants 2 years of age and younger undergoing long (longer than 3 hours) anesthetics. These include regional anesthetics or analgesics, opioids, and possibly alpha agonists, such as dexmedetomidine, all of which can be combined with lower-dose general anesthetics.

At the present time, the data support that surgery without anesthesia has harmful short-term and long-term effects while providing anesthesia to neonates for surgery may or may not have harmful effects of its own. Until the effects of anesthesia on the developing brain are better understood, pediatric surgeons and anesthesiologists must navigate this time of relative uncertainty with the best interests of our young patients in mind. Techniques to mitigate the amount of exposure to anesthetic agents that have been implicated in nonhuman studies as adversely affecting neurodevelopment are discussed later in this article, and have additional benefits as well. The medical necessity for the operation and its most salutary timing for best outcome remains the primary consideration, whereas theoretic concerns regarding anesthetic neurotoxicity should take precedence only when the operation can be safely postponed without fear of adversely affecting the outcome.

ALTERNATIVES AND ADJUNCTS TO GENERAL ANESTHESIA

In recent years, much interest has developed surrounding the concept of multimodal analgesia as a strategy to optimize analgesia while minimizing side effects. With multimodal anesthesia and pain management, regional anesthesia, opioids, and adjuvants, including acetaminophen, nonsteroidal anti-inflammatory drugs, alpha agonists, NMDA receptor antagonists, and gabapentinoids are used in combination to reduce the concentration of volatile anesthetics that patients require during surgery and the amount of opioids used during the intraoperative and postoperative periods. Concerns over anesthetic neurotoxicity in neonates and the opioid crisis in the United States have heightened interest in multimodal strategies, whereas published data supporting the safety and efficacy of regional anesthesia in children[17] and the applicability of Enhanced Recovery after Surgery (ERAS) protocols in children[18,19] have contributed to their implementation.

Regional Anesthesia in Children

In the past 2 decades, there has been a tremendous surge in the use of pediatric regional anesthesia. The expansion of practice, from basic neuraxial techniques (caudal and epidural blocks) to spinal anesthesia and peripheral nerve and plexus blockade, has been fueled by several developments, including the widespread availability and use of ultrasound guidance, better understanding of drug toxicity, recognition of the benefits of these blocks, and increasingly high-quality and quantitative evidence about safety. Several large-scale projects to collect prospective multicenter data on safety and complications have been performed, all indicating very low rates of serious complications and sequelae. Two 1-year studies from the French Language Society for Pediatric Anesthesia (ADARPEF)[20,21] demonstrated a high degree of safety, as did a large study or epidural blocks in children from the Association of Pediatric Anaesthetists of the UK and Ireland.[22] The Pediatric Regional Anesthesia Network (PRAN) was begun in 2007 as a research network and registry to collect highly audited prospective data on regional anesthetics in children.[23] The database now contains more than 150,000 blocks, and is an ongoing project, so its data will continue to grow in power as more cases are accrued. Several important results from PRAN have been published, and because accurate denominator data are available, complication and adverse event incidences can be calculated. Notable findings include the following:

- The incidence of serious complications is extremely low, corroborating the results of the ADARPEF and APAGBI studies.[17,24–26]
- The risk of serious complications (nerve injury, local anesthetic systemic toxicity) when regional blocks in children are performed under general anesthesia is no greater, and may be significantly lower, than when performed in awake or sedated subjects.[27]
- The most common adverse event in all blocks was technical problems related to catheters (eg, accidental dislodgement, kinking), suggesting that a significant improvement in efficacy could be achieved with better fixation techniques.
- Subgroup analyses particularly pertinent to urology include the finding of no temporary or permanent sequelae following caudal block,[28] no serious complications related to transverse abdominis plane block,[26] and a high degree of safety with no long-term sequelae or complications of epidural blocks in neonates.

There is currently controversy regarding the relationship between caudal block and the incidence of urethrocutaneous fistula following hypospadias repair.[29–31] There is a strong possibility that the disparity in results is due to unmeasured confounding, sparse data bias, or collinearity in these retrospective studies,[32–34] and thus PRAN (among several other consortia) is currently carrying out a prospective randomized controlled trial of caudal versus penile block in hypospadias repair.

In pediatric urology specifically, regional techniques are being used both as the sole anesthetic and as adjuncts to general anesthesia for infants and children undergoing surgical procedures. Spinal anesthesia is a viable alternative to general anesthesia for infants undergoing lower abdominal surgery with reported success rates of more than 80%.[35,36] Successful use of continuous infusion of local anesthetic through caudal catheters for inguinal hernia repairs in infants both with and without supplemental intravenous sedation has also been reported.[37,38]

Although regional techniques can be used as an alternative to general anesthesia, in pediatric practice they are used more commonly as an adjunct to general anesthesia. Potential advantages of using neuraxial anesthesia in combination with general anesthesia in neonates and infants include a reduction in intraoperative requirements for volatile anesthetics, opioids, and neuromuscular blocking agents, mitigation of the surgical stress response, earlier tracheal extubation, improvement in postoperative analgesia, and reduction in hospital length of stay.[39]

Enhanced Recovery After Surgery in Children

ERAS is a multimodal, multidisciplinary approach to perioperative care that started in Europe in the 1990s. Over the past 20 years, ERAS protocols have been implemented and studied in adult surgical care and have resulted in reductions in length of hospital stay and complications of 30% to 50% while readmissions and costs are also reduced.[40] ERAS protocols typically consist of approximately 20 preoperative, intraoperative, and postoperative elements and include opioid-sparing analgesic strategies including regional analgesia and adjunctive pain medications. Although ERAS started mainly with colorectal surgery, it has been shown to improve outcomes in almost all major adult surgical specialties. Unfortunately, despite abundant evidence supporting improved outcomes with enhanced recovery protocols in adults, data in pediatric populations are relatively sparse. A 2016 systematic review found only 5 relevant studies on the use of pediatric enhanced recovery protocols.[41]

To address this disparity and evaluate the safety and efficacy of an ERAS protocol in a pediatric population, a pediatric ERAS protocol was implemented at the authors' institution for patients undergoing urologic reconstruction as a pilot study in 2014.[18] The protocol was adapted from adult ERAS protocols and included 16 preoperative, intraoperative, and postoperative elements (Table 1). Patients younger than 18 years undergoing an operation that involved a bowel anastomosis were eligible for inclusion. No other exclusion criteria were defined. Thirteen patients were included prospectively, and they were propensity matched in a 1:2 ratio to recent historical controls (2009–2014) with no differences seen in baseline variables. Length of stay decreased from 8 days historically to 5 days in the ERAS cohort. National

mean length of stay for the same procedures ranges from 7 to 10 days. The small pilot nature of the study was underpowered to show significant differences in length of stay. Emergency department visits, readmissions, and reoperations did not increase with ERAS. There was a significant decrease in overall 90-day complications from 2.1 per patient to 1.3 per patient ($P = .035$).

Short and colleagues[19] also implemented a similar protocol for pediatric patients undergoing colorectal surgery. A retrospective review was conducted including 43 patients in the pre-enhanced recovery protocol period and 36 patients in the post-enhanced recovery protocol period. The median length of stay decreased from 5 days to 3 days in the post-enhanced recovery protocol period ($P = .01$). The complication

Table 1
Elements appropriate for use in adolescent patients undergoing elective intestinal operations

Adult ERAS Protocol Elements for Colonic Surgery	Element Included in Pediatric ERAS Protocol for Intestinal Surgery?	Element Included in Pediatric ERAS Protocol for Urologic Reconstruction?
Preoperative education and counseling	Yes	Yes
Preoperative optimization	Yes	No
Avoidance of routine use of mechanical bowel preparation	No	Yes
Minimization of preoperative fasting	Yes	Yes
Avoidance of routine use of sedative premedication	Not mentioned	Yes
Thromboembolism prophylaxis	Yes	Yes
Antimicrobial prophylaxis	Yes	Yes
Anesthetic protocol	Yes	Yes
Minimally invasive technique	Yes	Yes
Maintenance of normothermia	Yes	Yes
Goal-directed fluid therapy	Yes	Yes
Avoidance of peritoneal drains	Yes	Yes
Avoidance of nasogastric tubes	Yes	Yes
Early removal of urinary catheters	Yes	Yes
Prevention of postoperative ileus	Yes	Yes
Nausea and vomiting prophylaxis	Yes	Yes
Opioid-sparing postoperative analgesia	Yes	Yes
Perioperative nutritional care	Yes	Yes
Postoperative glucose control	No	No
Early mobilization	Yes	Yes

Abbreviation: ERAS, enhanced recovery after surgery.
Data from Refs.[18,42,43]

rate and 30-day readmission rate were not significantly different in the pre-enhanced and post-enhanced recovery periods.

In an effort to adapt and apply well-studied adult ERAS protocols to pediatric populations, a multidisciplinary team used a modified Delphi process to develop a pediatric-specific ERAS protocol for use in adolescents undergoing elective intestinal procedures. The process included literature review, surveys, and expert panel discussion including author MAB. The multidisciplinary expert panel included surgeons, gastroenterologists, anesthesiologists, nurses, and patient and family representatives. The investigators defined a protocol composed of 19 elements appropriate for use in adolescent patients undergoing elective intestinal operations (see **Table 1**). Although early data supporting the use of ERAS protocols in children is promising, more work is needed to learn how to best develop and implement these care pathways for young patients.

SURGICAL COUNSELING AND DECISION MAKING IN THE PEDIATRIC PATIENT

Although the risks of surgery and associated anesthesia exposure in young children is not inconsequential, they must be weighed against the risks of not intervening. Risks of surgery in the young child include not only the neurodevelopmental and respiratory risks, but also potential emotional and psychological risks of separation anxiety, which may be significant between 15 and 24 months of age.[44] Additionally, studies have suggested an increased risk of night terrors or other emotional trauma in children undergoing surgery between ages 1 and 3 years.[44] These risks must be weighed against the risks of observation, including risk to fertility potential in the undescended testis,[45,46] risks of renal injury in the obstructed kidney,[47] and potential risk to self-image in children with hypospadias or other genital anomalies (**Table 2**).[44,48]

Our approach to counseling families about these risks includes both actively engaging families in the decision-making process and providing transparency regarding what is known and what is unknown about the risks of surgery (including anesthetic risks) versus observation in infants and young children. Although prior studies suggest that discussion of "worst case scenarios" may be anxiety-provoking, a comprehensive discussion that includes goals of treatment, medical indications/necessity for intervention, and potential alternatives/contingency plans may serve to increase parental trust and confidence in the decision and reduce parental decisional conflict.[49] When discussing elective surgery of relatively short duration (<2 hours) in an otherwise healthy child, such as orchiopexy or hypospadias, we

---

Table 2
Surgical counseling and decision making in the pediatric patient

Procedure	Age at Surgery	Anesthetic Approach	Special Considerations
Orchiopexy	6–12 mo	General with caudal block	Laryngospasm may occur with manipulation of the testis in the setting of light anesthesia with a laryngeal mask airway (LMA)
Hypospadias/Penile surgery	6–18 mo	General with penile, pudendal, or caudal block	
Inguinal herniorrhaphy	Neonatal or infant period	Spinal block, caudal block, or general with caudal block	
Pyeloplasty/ureteral surgery	Variable	General with caudal block or epidural catheter if open	Timing dependent on underlying risk of renal injury
Reconstruction	Variable	General with regional block (neuraxial or peripheral), optimize nonopioid adjuncts	Consider multidisciplinary care within an ERAS pathway

Abbreviation: ERAS, enhanced recovery after surgery.
Data from Refs.[44–48]

continue to recommend surgery in the first year of life due to the relatively low neurodevelopmental risk. In the setting of more complex surgical decision making, in which surgical times may be prolonged or in which the risk of multiple surgeries is higher, such as treatment of differences in sexual development, ongoing discussions over a series of clinical visits may facilitate the development of the surgeon-parent relationship and help the clinician better gauge and address parental priorities and concerns in developing a surgical plan. Finally, we recommend proactive anesthetic and surgical planning with the anesthesiology team in advance of surgical scheduling and highly encourage preoperative consultation with an anesthesiologist to discuss anesthetic risks whenever the potential risk of anesthetic exposure is heightened due to complexity of the procedure, underlying patient condition, or parent concern.

To mitigate the risks posed by general anesthesia in the neonate and young child, we recommend that anesthesia be administered under the supervision of a pediatric anesthesiologist with experience and understanding of the nuanced developmental changes in infancy and childhood. Use of adjuvant local and regional anesthesia should be considered to reduce exposure to inhaled agents and minimize the need for postoperative narcotics. Additionally, surgical teams should work to limit the number of anesthetic exposures in the first 3 years of life by working to combine procedures performed under a single anesthetic if this can be done without significantly increasing the duration of anesthetic exposure.[50]

Ultimately, the decision for surgery from an anesthetic risk perspective is similar to the decision for surgery more globally and should be tailored based on the anesthesiologist's assessment of risk of anesthetic exposure, the surgeon's assessment of risk of delayed intervention, and the parent's underlying goals and preferences. By actively engaging all parties in the decision-making process and ensuring that all necessary information is shared, we believe that we are able to optimize the care of our patients despite our current limited knowledge about the long-term risks of early anesthetic exposure.

SUMMARY

Over the past 30 years, the pendulum has swung from avoidance of anesthesia in neonates to routine administration of anesthesia in neonates and infants as standard of care. Although administration of anesthesia has become safer in terms of cardiovascular and pulmonary complications, recent concerns over the long-term effects of these agents on the neurodevelopment of young patients have given cause for pediatric anesthesiologists and surgeons to question current practice while actively seeking answers to this question with prospective, randomized controlled trials. Until more conclusive evidence is achieved, thoughtful conversations among surgeons, anesthesiologists, and parents to make decisions based on risks and benefits to our young patients are the best course of action. For those children who do require surgery and anesthesia at a young age, multimodal anesthesia and analgesia including regional techniques and adjuncts optimize analgesia, reduce the exposure to volatile anesthetics, and may reduce risks. Although one might consider postponing elective operations in these youngest patients until they are older, the current evidence suggests that the decision should be primarily based on the need and optimal timing of the operation.

REFERENCES

1. United States Food and Drug Administration. FDA drug safety communication: FDA review results in new warnings about using general anesthetics and sedation drugs in young children and pregnant women. 2016. Available at: https://www.fda.gov/Drugs/DrugSafety/ucm532356.htm. Accessed April 9, 2018.
2. Anand KJ, Sippell WG, Aynsley-Green A. Randomised trial of fentanyl anaesthesia in preterm babies undergoing surgery: effects on the stress response. Lancet 1987;1(8527):243–8.
3. Taddio A, Katz J, Ilersich AL, et al. Effect of neonatal circumcision on pain response during subsequent routine vaccination. Lancet 1997;349(9052):599–603.
4. Flick R. Clinical complications in pediatric anesthesia. In: Gregory G, Andropoulos D, editors. Gregory's pediatric anesthesia. 5th edition. West Sussex (England): Wiley-Blackwell; 2012. p. 1152–82.
5. Flick RP, Sprung J, Harrison TE, et al. Perioperative cardiac arrests in children between 1988 and 2005 at a tertiary referral center: a study of 92,881 patients. Anesthesiology 2007;106(2):226–37 [quiz: 413–4].
6. Morray JP, Geiduschek JM, Ramamoorthy C, et al. Anesthesia-related cardiac arrest in children: initial findings of the Pediatric Perioperative Cardiac Arrest (POCA) Registry. Anesthesiology 2000;93(1):6–14.
7. Bhananker SM, Ramamoorthy C, Geiduschek JM, et al. Anesthesia-related cardiac arrest in children: update from the Pediatric Perioperative Cardiac Arrest Registry. Anesth Analg 2007;105(2):344–50.

8. Keenan RL, Shapiro JH, Kane FR, et al. Bradycardia during anesthesia in infants. An epidemiologic study. Anesthesiology 1994;80(5):976–82.

9. Kelly CJ, Walker RW. Perioperative pulmonary aspiration is infrequent and low risk in pediatric anesthetic practice. Paediatr Anaesth 2015;25(1):36–43.

10. Frykholm P, Schindler E, Sumpelmann R, et al. Preoperative fasting in children: review of existing guidelines and recent developments. Br J Anaesth 2018;120(3):469–74.

11. Liu LM, Cote CJ, Goudsouzian NG, et al. Life-threatening apnea in infants recovering from anesthesia. Anesthesiology 1983;59(6):506–10.

12. Cote CJ, Zaslavsky A, Downes JJ, et al. Postoperative apnea in former preterm infants after inguinal herniorrhaphy. A combined analysis. Anesthesiology 1995;82(4):809–22.

13. Polaner D. Anesthesia for same-day surgical procedures. In: Davis P, Cladis F, Motoyama E, editors. Smith's anesthesia for infants and children. 8th edition. Philadelphia: Elsevier; 2011. p. 1058–76.

14. Jevtovic-Todorovic V, Hartman RE, Izumi Y, et al. Early exposure to common anesthetic agents causes widespread neurodegeneration in the developing rat brain and persistent learning deficits. J Neurosci 2003;23(3):876–82.

15. Ikonomidou C, Bittigau P, Koch C, et al. Neurotransmitters and apoptosis in the developing brain. Biochem Pharmacol 2001;62(4):401–5.

16. Anand KJ, Soriano SG. Anesthetic agents and the immature brain: are these toxic or therapeutic? Anesthesiology 2004;101(2):527–30.

17. Polaner DM, Taenzer AH, Walker BJ, et al. Pediatric Regional Anesthesia Network (PRAN): a multi-institutional study of the use and incidence of complications of pediatric regional anesthesia. Anesth Analg 2012;115(6):1353–64.

18. Rove KO, Brockel MA, Saltzman AF, et al. Prospective study of enhanced recovery after surgery protocol in children undergoing reconstructive operations. J Pediatr Urol 2018;14(3):252.e1–9.

19. Short HL, Heiss KF, Burch K, et al. Implementation of an enhanced recovery protocol in pediatric colorectal surgery. J Pediatr Surg 2018;53(4):688–92.

20. Ecoffey C, Lacroix F, Giaufre E, et al. Epidemiology and morbidity of regional anesthesia in children: a follow-up one-year prospective survey of the French-Language Society of Paediatric Anaesthesiologists (ADARPEF). Paediatr Anaesth 2010; 20(12):1061–9.

21. Giaufré E, Dalens B, Gombert A. Epidemiology and morbidity of regional anesthesia in children: a one-year prospective survey of the French-Language Society of Pediatric Anesthesiologists. Anesth Analg 1996;83(5):904–12.

22. Llewellyn N, Moriarty A. The national pediatric epidural audit. Paediatr Anaesth 2007;17(6):520–33.

23. Polaner DM, Martin LD, PRAN Investigators. Quality assurance and improvement: the Pediatric Regional Anesthesia Network. Paediatr Anaesth 2011;22(1): 115–9.

24. Suresh S, Schaldenbrand K, Wallis B, et al. Regional anaesthesia to improve pain outcomes in paediatric surgical patients: a qualitative systematic review of randomized controlled trials. Br J Anaesth 2014; 113(3):375–90.

25. Walker BJ, Long JB, De Oliveira GS, et al. Peripheral nerve catheters in children: an analysis of safety and practice patterns from the pediatric regional anesthesia network (PRAN). Br J Anaesth 2015;115(3): 457–62.

26. Long JB, Birmingham PK, De Oliveira GS Jr, et al. Transversus abdominis plane block in children: a multicenter safety analysis of 1994 cases from the PRAN (Pediatric Regional Anesthesia Network) database. Anesth Analg 2014;119(2):395–9.

27. Taenzer AH, Walker BJ, Bosenberg AT, et al. Asleep versus awake: does it matter? Pediatric regional block complications by patient state: a report from the Pediatric Regional Anesthesia Network. Reg Anesth Pain Med 2014;39(4):279–83.

28. Suresh S, Long J, Birmingham PK, et al. Are caudal blocks for pain control safe in children? An analysis of 18,650 caudal blocks from the Pediatric Regional Anesthesia Network (PRAN) database. Anesth Analg 2015;120(1):151–6.

29. Taicher BM, Routh JC, Eck JB, et al. The association between caudal anesthesia and increased risk of postoperative surgical complications in boys undergoing hypospadias repair. Paediatr Anaesth 2017; 27(7):688–94.

30. Kim MH, Im YJ, KIL HK, et al. Impact of caudal block on postoperative complications in children undergoing tubularised incised plate urethroplasty for hypospadias repair: a retrospective cohort study. Anaesthesia 2016;71(7):773–8.

31. Zaidi RH, Casanova NF, Haydar B, et al. Urethrocutaneous fistula following hypospadias repair: regional anesthesia and other factors. Paediatr Anaesth 2015;25(11):1144–50.

32. Braga LH, Jegatheeswaran K, McGrath M, et al. Cause and effect versus confounding—is there a true association between caudal blocks and tubularized incised plate repair complications? J Urol 2017; 197(3 Pt 2):845–51.

33. Ayubi E, Safiri S. The association between caudal anesthesia and increased risk of postoperative surgical complications in boys undergoing hypospadias repair: comment on data sparsity. Paediatr Anaesth 2017;27(9):974.

34. Polaner DM, Almenrader N, Vemulakonda V. Caudal analgesia, hypospadias, and urethrocutaneous fistula: does association mean causality? Paediatr Anaesth 2017;27(7):676–7.

35. Frawley G, Bell G, Disma N, et al. Predictors of failure of awake regional anesthesia for neonatal hernia repair: data from the general anesthesia compared to spinal anesthesia study–comparing apnea and neurodevelopmental outcomes. Anesthesiology 2015;123(1):55–65.

36. Whitaker EE, Wiemann BZ, DaJusta DG, et al. Spinal anesthesia for pediatric urological surgery: reducing the theoretic neurotoxic effects of general anesthesia. J Pediatr Urol 2017;13(4):396–400.

37. Waurick K, Sauerland C, Goeters C. Dexmedetomidine sedation combined with caudal anesthesia for lower abdominal and extremity surgery in expreterm and full-term infants. Paediatr Anaesth 2017;27(6):637–42.

38. Mueller CM, Sinclair TJ, Stevens M, et al. Regional block via continuous caudal infusion as sole anesthetic for inguinal hernia repair in conscious neonates. Pediatr Surg Int 2017;33(3):341–5.

39. Goeller JK, Bhalla T, Tobias JD. Combined use of neuraxial and general anesthesia during major abdominal procedures in neonates and infants. Paediatr Anaesth 2014;24(6):553–60.

40. Ljungqvist O, Scott M, Fearon KC. Enhanced recovery after surgery: a review. JAMA Surg 2017;152(3):292–8.

41. Shinnick JK, Short HL, Heiss KF, et al. Enhancing recovery in pediatric surgery: a review of the literature. J Surg Res 2016;202(1):165–76.

42. Gustafsson UO, Scott MJ, Schwenk W, et al. Guidelines for perioperative care in elective colonic surgery: Enhanced Recovery After Surgery (ERAS((R))) Society recommendations. World J Surg 2013;37(2):259–84.

43. Short HL, Taylor N, Piper K, et al. Appropriateness of a pediatric-specific enhanced recovery protocol using a modified Delphi process and multidisciplinary expert panel. J Pediatr Surg 2018;53(4):592–8.

44. Timing of elective surgery on the genitalia of male children with particular reference to the risks, benefits, and psychological effects of surgery and anesthesia. American Academy of Pediatrics. Pediatrics 1996;97(4):590–4.

45. Elder JS. Surgical management of the undescended testis: recent advances and controversies. Eur J Pediatr Surg 2016;26(5):418–26.

46. Kolon TF, Herndon CD, Baker LA, et al. Evaluation and treatment of cryptorchidism: AUA guideline. J Urol 2014;192(2):337–45.

47. Arora S, Yadav P, Kumar M, et al. Predictors for the need of surgery in antenatally detected hydronephrosis due to UPJ obstruction–a prospective multivariate analysis. J Pediatr Urol 2015;11(5):248.e1-5.

48. van der Horst HJ, de Wall LL. Hypospadias, all there is to know. Eur J Pediatr 2017;176(4):435–41.

49. Chotai PN, Nollan R, Huang EY, et al. Surgical informed consent in children: a systematic review. J Surg Res 2017;213:191–8.

50. Wall LB, Spitler J. Anesthesia in the pediatric patient. J Hand Surg 2014;39(1):146–8.

Urologic Evaluation and Management of Pediatric Kidney Transplant Patients

Blake Palmer, MD*, Brad Kropp, MD

KEYWORDS

- Kidney transplant • Pediatric urology • Renal transplant • Urology evaluation
- Transplant evaluation

KEY POINTS

- Pediatric urologists play an important role in the evaluation of patients with end-stage renal disease and the management of posttransplant patients.
- Patients with unmanaged lower urinary tract dysfunction will have higher rates of complications and increased graft dysfunction, but these can be normalized when appropriately managed by a pediatric urologist.
- Most studies indicated that posttransplantation patients with a history of lower urinary tract dysfunction and/or reconstruction will have a higher incidence of urinary tract infections, but not have worse graft function outcomes.

INTRODUCTION

The first successful kidney transplant occurred between identical twins in December 1954, and the first report of a successful renal transplant in a pediatric patient was in 1966.[1–3] Since that time, the goal of renal transplantation in patients with chronic kidney disease (CKD) has been to provide renal replacement therapy with less morbidity, better quality of life, and improved overall survival compared with dialysis across all ages, genders, races, and causes of end-stage renal disease (ESRD).[4–7] Secondary improvements after renal transplantation in children include improved growth, school attendance, and cognitive functioning. It has been shown to also be cost-effective compared with dialysis.[4,8]

Urologic causes of ESRD are estimated between 25% and 40% of causes. Classic United Network for Organ Sharing (UNOS) categories do not allow for identification of specific urologic causes nor distinct classification of all diseases (**Table 1**).

Renal transplantation should be considered another renal replacement therapy for ESRD but not a cure. It is generally considered the optimal form of therapy, but not all patients with CKD have similar risks and benefits from renal transplantation.[9] The goals of the evaluation process are to identify and mitigate risks and optimize benefits for these patients. It should be understood that not all CKD patients are candidates for transplantation, although most will ultimately be suitable. One goal of the evaluation process is to identify the appropriate timing of transplantation wherein a patient may not be ready for transplantation at the current time but may ultimately be a good candidate in the future due to growth or modifications of risk factors. Throughout the evaluation process, the underlying purpose to identify and optimize a potential transplant candidate should be kept in mind. Another goal is to identify transplantation surgical risks for the procedure in general and specifically regarding the key components of the procedure related to the vascular and

Disclosure Statement: None.
Pediatric Urology, Cook Children's Health Care System, 750 8th Avenue, 6th Floor, Fort Worth, TX 76104, USA
* Corresponding author.
E-mail address: blake.palmer@cookchildrens.org

Table 1	
Causes of end-stage renal disease in pediatric population	
Cause	**%**
Aplasia/hypoplasia/dysplasia	15.8
Obstructive uropathy	15.3
Focal segmental glomerulosclerosis	11.7
Reflux nephropathy	5.2
Polycystic disease	3.0
Chronic glomerulonephritis	3.2
Medullary cystic disease	2.7
Hemolytic uremic syndrome	2.6
Prune belly	2.5
Congenital nephrotic syndrome	2.6
Familial nephritis	2.3
Cystinosis	2.1
Pyelonephritis/interstitial nephritis	1.7

Data from North American Pediatric Renal Trials and Collaborative Studies. NAPRTCS 2010 Annual Transplant Report. NAPRTCS 2010. Available at: https://web.emmes.com/study/ped/annlrept/2010_Report.pdf.

urologic reconstruction that are integral to the procedure. It is also important during the evaluation process to understand the reasons that kidneys can fail after transplant and from where posttransplant morbidity is derived. These causes of graft dysfunction include recurrence of disease, immunologic rejection, acquired infections, medication side effects, and surgical complications. A patient's urologic history can be a significant source of problems related to infections, recurrence of disease, and surgical complications.[10,11] Many of the urologic risks are modifiable, and this is important in the preparation before transplantation.

Description of Evaluation Process

The renal transplant process is initiated when the primary nephrologist officially refers the patient to a transplant center. The referral is made when the progression of CKD to ESRD is inevitable, and long-term renal replacement therapy will be needed. The referral for transplant evaluation can be done before the initiation of dialysis. There are significant short- and long-term benefits to preemptive transplantation in appropriate situations. In the pediatrics population, preemptive transplants occurred 28.7% of the time during the 2010 to 2012 time period.[12] Typically this is done when the estimated creatinine clearance is less than 20 mL/min. In the pediatric population, this can be done at an earlier level for cases when the risks of CKD-associated sequelae are greater

than the risks of transplantation. Typically, this is in a case when growth impairment, electrolyte disturbances, uremia, persistent anemia, metabolic acidosis, and metabolic bone disease are profound and refractory to other management options.[13,14]

The evaluation process is comprehensive and requires a multidisciplinary team that includes a pediatric nephrologist, transplant surgeon, transplant coordinator, pediatric urologist, nurse, social worker, child psychologist or mental health provider, dietitian, pharmacist, and anesthesiologist. This team may include other medical specialty providers on an as-needed basis to provide comprehensive medical clearance and often can require but is not limited to specialists in infectious disease, cardiology, pulmonology, hematology, oncology, hepatology, gastroenterology, dermatology, otolaryngology, and so forth. The process starts with an intake contact with the parent/caregiver. Usually an education step occurs to ensure the family and patient are well versed on the steps of the process and ramifications of an organ transplant. The evaluation will include a thorough medical and surgical history, a comprehensive physical examination, and a psychosocial examination by a pertinent professional. This is to ensure the patient and support network are prepared for the transplant process. Compatibility testing is done with blood typing and histocompatibility testing. Other tests will include but are not limited to serum and urine testing, serology testing, chest radiograph, echocardiogram, electrocardiogram, and dental examination.

The role of the pediatric urologist is to prepare the patient from a urinary perspective for a new transplant and identify risks for complications after transplant (**Table 2**). A thorough urologic history and examination with special attention to the questions outlined in **Box 1** will provide the pediatric urologist with a framework for their pretransplant evaluation. The goals are to ensure that the patient has a normal functioning lower urinary tract system for the transplanted kidney. However, many of the patients undergoing the evaluation process will need specific urologic conditions addressed before clearance for transplantation to decrease potential complications and morbidity. Some of these specific issues are addressed here.

Need for Pretransplant Native Nephrectomy

It is estimated that of 10% to 20% of pediatric recipients may need a unilateral or bilateral native nephrectomy before transplantation.[15,16] It is important to consider the indications for pretransplant native nephrectomy (PTNN; **Box 2**)

Table 2 Causes of renal allograft failure in pediatric recipients	
Chronic rejection	40.5%
Acute rejection	10.5
Medication nonadherence	5.9
Graft thrombosis	6.9
Death with functioning graft	8.2
Disease recurrence	7.8
Focal segmental glomerulosclerosis	46.0
Membranoproliferative glomerulonephritis	8.9
Hemolytic-uremic syndrome	8.9
Oxalosis	5.0
Chronic glomerulonephritis	3.5
Others	27.7

Data from United States Organ Transplantation. OPTN and SRTR annual data report 2011. US Department Health and Human Services 2012. Available at: http://srtr.transplant.hrsa.gov/annual_reports/2011/pdf/00_intro_12.pdf.

Box 1
Questions for the pediatric urologist to answer during evaluation?

- Cause or renal disease? Is it a primary urologic disease process (ie, PUV) or did urologic disease contribute to renal failure (ie, recurrent pyelonephritis episodes)?
- Is this the first transplant? If they have had a prior transplant, did they have any urologic problems?
- What is their current native kidney status? Last renal ultrasound and images reviewed?
- What is their current bladder status and management? Last voiding study or urodynamics and results reviewed?
- Do they make urine? How much?
- Have they ever had a UTI? With fever? Recurrent?
- Have they ever had urinary stones?
- Are they potty trained? At what age?
- Daytime incontinence history and current status?
- Nighttime incontinence history and current status?
- Any prior urologic surgeries?
- Bowel management and status?
- Any compliance issues?
- Any congenital anomalies or syndromes that are associated with vascular anomalies to alert surgery team to?

Box 2
Indications for pretransplant native nephrectomy

- Significant proteinuria not controlled with medical nephrectomy or angioablation
- Nonfunctioning renal units with symptomatic renal stones that are not able to be cleared easily with minimally invasive techniques or lithotripsy
- Persistent antiglomerular basement membrane antibody levels
- Intractable hypertension
- Recurrent pyelonephritis in nonfunctioning kidneys
- High-grade VUR with recurrent infections in nonfunction kidneys
- Polycystic kidneys that are symptomatic with severe, recurrent symptomatic complications (bleeding, stones, and/or infections) will often need a bilateral nephrectomy
- Polycystic kidneys that are large and need removal for accommodation of a new transplant when the native enlarged kidney extends past the anterior superior iliac spine, do just a unilateral nephrectomy on the intended transplant side
- Malignancy/malignant predisposition (ie, Wilms tumors/Denys-Drash syndrome)

and determine the appropriate timing for these procedures. With experience, it is has been determined that the true indications are less than previously thought, and many of these children can proceed to transplant with their native kidneys in place. Preserving native renal function and clearance of nonconcentrated urine can assist the patient in volume management and limits the need for strict fluid and dietary restrictions. Efforts to preserve urine production may improve the management of hypertension and reduce risk for cardiac complications.[17] Other benefits include production of native erythropoietin to negate the need for exogenous or blood transfusions, improved homeostasis of vitamin D/calcium and cycling of bladder with native urine in the time period before transplantation. Indications and timing must be balanced with risks of observation of native kidneys when left in place. If a living donor is available, bilateral native nephrectomy can be done safely as soon as just 6 weeks before planned renal transplantation to limit time the patient is anuric but to ensure the patient is healed well before the subsequent procedure. Native nephrectomy can be done at the same time as the transplantation procedure, but this may increase perioperative complications and morbidity.[18] In a conservative series with moderate follow-up, only 2% to 5% of renal transplant patients required a posttransplant native nephrectomy.[15] Most of the unilateral or bilateral PTNN can be done laparoscopically or robotically. Because many of these pediatric patients will already be on peritoneal dialysis, the authors prefer a laparoscopic or robotic retroperitoneal approach and have not had an issue resuming peritoneal dialysis on postoperative day 1. This approach, when successful, obviates the need to change to hemodialysis during the recovery period. Not all patients will require a bilateral PTNN. Selective unilateral PTNN, even in cases of refractory proteinuria or hypertension, can be sufficient to manage the underlying indication until transplantation.[15]

Need for Lower Urinary Tract Reconstruction or Diversion

Patients with high-pressure and small-capacity bladders that are refractory to medical and clean intermittent catheterization (CIC) management put a new transplanted kidney at risk for infection and renal dysfunction because of high-pressure storage.[19] Renal transplant patients should have an established reliable urinary drainage system with low-pressure storage and adequate emptying. Urinary diversions with a cutaneous vesicostomy or ureterostomy are at a high risk for stenosis or complications. These diversions should be avoided as the outlet drainage plan, when possible, before renal transplantation, and monitored closely when no other options are feasible. On occasions due to patient size and comorbidities, it is indicated to do the transplantation at a younger age/size than it is for their definitive bladder reconstruction. In these cases, a well-thought-out plan for eventual reconstruction and interim monitoring and management should be in place.

Prolonged percutaneous drainage is prone to repeated infections and development of bacterial resistance. Complications of these infections are commonly a problem, and this should be avoided at all costs.

Patients who have normal bladders but are anuric will usually show small defunctionalized bladders with low capacity on evaluation but can have the reasonable expectation that they will regain normal functional capacity within weeks of transplantation and do not need pretransplantation reconstruction or cycling.[20] However, those with abnormal bladders before transplantation should not have this expectation, and a prior reconstruction or bladder management plan should be in place. Whenever possible, it can be beneficial to start the CIC process before transplantation, even if they have little or no urine output. Identifying issues with the catheterization process before transplantation is important, and working out solutions in a low risk situation is preferred. In general, lower urinary tract reconstruction is better done with adequate urine production to reduce risk for stricture, stones, infections, and loss of compliance but should be balanced with the risks of being done at the same time as the transplantation procedure or in the posttransplantation period.

Patients with severe lower urinary tract dysfunction can have similar outcomes compared with those without bladder dysfunction, after renal transplantation, when properly managed.[19,21] Urinary tract infections (UTI) are more common, but long-term graft outcomes are similar in patients with lower urinary tract reconstruction.[22,23]

The time at which to do the bladder augmentation or reconstruction in the patient with CKD before transplantation is challenging. It is reassuring to see that a bladder augmentation did not accelerate the deterioration of renal function in a single-center review and showed 18% actually had some temporary improvement.[24] Proper management and close monitoring by the urologic and nephrology teams during the perioperative and postoperative period are imperative, and some patients do improve in the short term. This temporary improvement in renal function is likely due to the underestimation of the prior bladder management or diversions ongoing effects on renal function. In multiple reports, there was not a significant difference if the bladder reconstruction was done before or after the renal transplant from a patient safety standpoint.[25]

In select patients with poor renal function and dilated megaureters, the use of these megaureters for ureterocystoplasty can be a useful and a metabolically neutral alternative to the use of bowel segments.[26] Overall, a ureterocystoplasty has less problems with mucus, stones, and infections because no bowel is incorporated but fails to increase capacity and improve compliance at a higher rate compared with traditional enterocystoplasty. Therefore, the use of this is selective and needs to be followed closely in the postoperative period with the understanding that some will fail to achieve the goal of improved storage pressures and bladder compliance.[27] It is, though, still expected that they will require CIC as well.

Drainage of transplanted kidneys into an augmented bladder or urinary conduit is an appropriate management strategy when the native bladder is unsuitable. Patients with kidney transplants drained into augmented bladder or urinary conduit are at increased risk for urine infection. Graft survival is not adversely affected compared with historical controls when a kidney transplant is drained into a urinary conduit or augmented bladder.[28–30]

Patient with Posterior Urethral Valves

In patients with posterior urethral valves (PUV), the associated valve bladder and degree of bladder dysfunction are a dynamic condition. Uncorrected or unmanaged bladder dysfunction can contribute to the transplant graft dysfunction. Polyuria that is commonly seen in PUV with CKD accentuates the bladder dysfunction but can improve after renal transplantation. Overall, the level of evidence to guide the decision as to which patients will ultimately need reconstruction before transplantation is poor. A few principles can be defined by a comprehensive review of the literature.[31] Transplant outcomes in PUV cases with adequate management of bladder dysfunction were comparable to other causes of ESRD, and bladder dysfunction can improve after urinary undiversion in some cases commiserate with understanding that the valve bladder is dynamic in some patients and they need close long-term follow-up. Not all vesicoureteral reflux (VUR) needs to be corrected, nor do all PUV bladders need to be augmented. Those with stable low pressure reflux and emptying with spontaneous voiding or with CIC are likely safe to proceed with renal transplant despite persistent VUR. However, overall, UTIs were more common in transplanted PUV patients.[32] In those patients who were diverted with a vesicostomy, an undiversion can show recovery of bladder function spontaneously. Close follow-up is necessary with the understanding that some will not have this improved function and will require bladder augmentation for persistent high-pressure bladder dysfunction. A review by Jesus and Pippi Salle[31] also showed that bladder augmentation is feasible with similar outcomes, when done before or after renal transplant, and showed outcomes that are consistent with those seen in other causes of lower urinary tract dysfunction that require augmentation as well. Most important to note is that bladder dysfunction with high pressure needs to be corrected before renal transplantation. However, not all VUR requires surgical correction in PUV patients.

Risks After Kidney Transplantation

There is a 40% rate of rehospitalization in the first 6 months after renal transplantation for all causes[12] (**Box 3**). Surgical complications can be seen immediately or in the short term after transplantation. The incidence of vascular thrombosis in pediatric kidney transplantation ranges from 2% to 12% internationally and is about 7% in the United States.[33–35] The development of a lymphocele is common after renal transplantation and occurs in between 1% and 25% of cases. Only approximately 5% are symptomatic and require treatment, especially if there is associated ureteral compression with hydronephrosis or iliac vein compression with thrombosis, which is rare. Typically they are just associated with swelling and pain. First-line therapy is via percutaneous approach for aspiration. If it is very large and causing thrombosis or graft dysfunction, then drain placement is appropriate. Addition of sclerotherapy is typically only necessary when recurrent drainages are needed. Internal drainage laparoscopically for a peritoneal window or open drainage offers the lowest recurrence rate, but these options are not typically indicated as a primary approach.[36]

The incidence of urologic complications seen after renal transplantation is between 3% and 15%, and the most common are urinary obstruction, urinary leak, VUR, hematuria, and urolithiasis. The incidence of urologic complications after transplantation correlates with the presence of pretransplantation obstructing uropathy or bladder dysfunction.[37–41] Surgically treated urologic complications significantly contribute to the posttransplantation morbidity, but they do not seem to affect the long-term graft survival.[42] Of the variety of techniques used for transplant ureter reimplantation, the urologic complications are similar when common extravesical techniques are compared except for potentially higher rates of hematuria with a U-stitch method.[43] The authors use a modified Lich-Gregoir extravesical reimplant traditionally and place a ureteral stent routinely.[43]

Box 3
Risks after kidney transplantation

- Surgical complications
- Rejection
- Infection
- Recurrence of disease
- Noncompliance
- Side effect of immunosuppression

Of the urologic complications, about 80% occur in the first month, but 20% occur late.[44] Urinary fistula or leak typically occurs secondary to necrosis of the distal ureter at the site of the ureteroneocystostomy. Leaks usually occur within the first 2 weeks after surgery and present with a decrease in urine output, decrease in renal function, graft or lower quadrant pain, swelling, and sometimes leakage from the incision. First-line treatment if the ureteral stent is in place would be for replacement of the Foley catheter for prolonged drainage. Those cases that are refractory will require return to the operating room for excision of the devitalized segment and repeat anastomosis to the bladder. Ureteral strictures/obstruction occurs in approximately 1% to 4.5% of renal transplant recipients.[45] Obstruction typically occurs at the ureterovesical anastomosis and can develop several months after the initial transplant. Strictures are typically thought to be related to chronic ischemia but can be infectious and immunologic in nature. Obstructions would typically present with an increase in creatinine and hydronephrosis seen on imaging. First-line attempts at retrograde or antegrade endourologic or interventional radiologic management are appropriate and can be effective. However, in recurrent disease, an open revision of the anastomosis will be required.

Routine placement of a ureteral stent at the time of renal transplantation for the transplant ureter ureteroneocystostomy is shown to decrease the incidence of urologic complications from 8.8% to 3.3% but did increase the incidence of UTIs when compared with a group that was not stented.[46]

Graft rejection that is biopsy proven occurs in about 10% of patients within the first year. Factors that make rejection more likely include some steroid avoidance immunosuppression regimens, medication adherence, and donor-recipient HLA match.

Infections accounted for 33% of all mortality in a French 70-month follow-up after transplantation.[47] Within the first month of transplantation, the organisms causing infection tend to be similar to those associated with major urologic operations (UTIs, wound infections, and respiratory infections).[16] Infections are usually related to complications from surgery and invasive medical devices (urinary catheters and ureteral stents) and most commonly involve the genitourinary tract. Infections can be prevented with normal practices of removing unnecessary drains and catheters in a reasonably timely fashion. For instance, in the authors' practice, the Foley catheter is removed in a typical renal transplant patient on postoperative day 4, and the ureteral stent is removed at 4 weeks after transplant. During this time, trimethoprim-sulfamethoxazole is given as daily prophylaxis for UTIs and more significantly for prevention of pneumocystis pneumonia; this is typically done for 3 to 6 months.

Between 1 to 6 months after surgery, cellular immune system infections are more prevalent. These opportunistic infections include fungilike Candida, Pneumocystis, Aspergillus, and Cryptococcus; bacteria, including Listeria monocytogenes, Nocardia, and Toxoplasmosis; and viruses such as cytomegalovirus, Epstein-Barr virus (EBV), polyomavirus, hepatitis virus, and herpes viruses. The incidence is influenced by a combination of history of pretransplant exposures of the donor and recipient and by the immunosuppression regimen. Many of these are prevented with routine prophylaxis during this time with trimethoprim-sulfamethoxazole, nystatin, and valganciclovir.[48]

After 6 months, infection risk is influenced by graft function and prior infections. UTIs account for more than 15% of hospital readmissions in an adult population within the first 2 years after kidney transplantation.[48] Recurrent UTIs should undergo complete evaluation for anatomic risk factors, such as fistulas, incontinence, urinary retention, VUR, stones, and/or foreign bodies. The authors typically get a baseline transplant renal ultrasound a month after the stent has been removed and annually thereafter. Ultrasound surveillance of the transplanted kidney is especially important in all patients with a urologic history associated with their renal failure. Routine voiding cystourethrogram (VCUG) to assess for reflux into the transplant kidney is not indicated. Among studies that evaluate for VUR after renal transplantation, VUR is common, ranging from 50% to 86%.[45] However, most of this VUR is asymptomatic and did not affect graft outcomes. In those patients with recurrent UTIs after transplantation, there is a need for VCUG to evaluate for VUR into the transplant kidney.[49,50] These patients should also be assessed for voiding dysfunction, and in place of VCUG, video urodynamics are performed for a comprehensive assessment of lower urinary tract function. For those patients with recurrent infections and no bladder dysfunction, some may be candidates for minimally invasive antireflux treatment with injection of dextranomer/hyaluronic acid copolymers, but in the authors' experience, injections into the transplant ureter is extremely challenging. Studies have shown an efficacy of approximately 50% to 57.9% with a single injection and 53.8% to 100% overall after multiple injections.[51–53] In cases with recurrent episodes of pyelonephritis in the transplant kidney and persistent VUR, an ureteroneocystostomy of the transplant ureter or diversion to the native ureter, if it does not have VUR, would be indicated. There is not an expectation that reduction in immunosuppression will improve risk for recurrent UTIs. Focusing on optimal voiding habits and bladder emptying in the pediatric patient is important. In chronic severely immunosuppressed patients, immunoglobulin replacement can help with incidence of recurrent infections, including UTIs, potentially.

Recurrent UTIs are also more common in those patients with lower urinary tract dysfunction, bladder reconstruction, and need for CIC,[22,23] although at least one center using gastric augmentations, antirefluxing reimplantation, and gentamicin irrigations did not have an increase in the incidence of UTIs following renal transplantation in patients with augmented bladders compared with controls.[54]

Viral infections, like adenovirus, which can cause hemorrhagic cystitis, are usually self-limiting and resolve with improved hydration. BK polyoma viral nephropathy is best followed serially with serum polymerase chain reaction and can cause nephropathy and in some cases ureteral strictures. A viral infection is treated with first-line reduction of immunosuppression and monitoring of renal function. BK virus infections occur in 4.6% of children after a kidney transplant secondary to the necessary immunosuppression, and nephropathy associated with BK virus leads to graft loss in up to 11%.[55,56] Asymptomatic BK viruria is seen in 7% of healthy patients and 28% of renal transplant recipients.[56–58]

Recurrence of disease is a significant cause of graft dysfunction in pediatric renal transplant patients. Recurrence of disease is classically considered in renal causes like primary focal segmental glomerulosclerosis or atypical hemolytic uremic syndrome, for instance. However, as pediatric urologists, the authors have seen many patients in whom the primary urologic disease that contributed to their native kidney loss of function is the same problem causing posttransplantation morbidity and graft dysfunction if it was not optimally addressed before transplantation. It is no less important than those renal causes at high risk for recurrence in the graft and by incidence these at-risk urologic cause patients are more common.

Excellent outcomes seen in pediatric patients less than 10 years of age are not necessarily seen in older adolescent patients after transplant. Much of this is thought to be related to teenage issues with adherence and noncompliance, which is an important source of graft loss and mortality after transplantation.[59] Also of concern is that it appears that rejection episodes in this age group are more resistant to therapy for unclear reasons.[60] Graft loss with noncompliance as a contributing factor was found in 0.9% in young children compared with adolescents aged 10 to 14 (2.2%) and older teenagers (2.0%), and this difference was more pronounced in African American recipients compared with other races.[61] Patients who have undergone urinary reconstruction are at an increased risk for infections and urinary complications if noncompliance is an issue as well.[19] These studies illustrates of identifying noncompliant issues before transplantation and being diligent in identifying the red flags for these issues throughout the life of the graft.

Long-term use of high-risk immunosuppressant medications can have side effects for long-term renal dysfunction secondary to calcineurin inhibitor toxicity. No significant long-term side effects have been seen for bladder function to date, however. Secondary to viral infections and immunosuppression, 2% to 4% of pediatric renal recipients experienced a malignancy and more than 50% are posttransplant lymphoproliferative disorders and associated with EBV and immunosuppression. In adult populations, transplant recipients have an about 4% 5-year incidence of cancer, but bladder and urologic malignancies are only slightly increased or similar to the general population.[62,63] There is no known increased risk in the pediatric population.

In conclusion, the pediatric urologist plays an important role in the evaluation process of CKD patients before renal transplantation. A comprehensive urologic evaluation is especially important in the large percentage of pediatric CKD patients with a primary urologic cause for their renal dysfunction. These patients are complex patients that need to be thoroughly evaluated from a multidisciplinary approach and by a pediatric urologist well versed in the transplantation process and potential unique risks seen in these patients in the posttransplantation period.

REFERENCES

1. Murray JE, Merrill JP, Harrison JH. Renal homotransplantations in identical twins. Surg Forum 1955;6: 432–6.
2. Starzl T, Marchioro T, Porter K. The role of the organ transplantation in pediatrics. Pediatr Clin North Am 1966;13:381–422.
3. Starzl TE. The puzzle people: memoirs of a transplant surgeon. Pittsburgh (PA): University of Pittsburgh Press; 1992.
4. Davis ID, Chang PN, Nevis TE. Successful renal transplantation accelerates development in young ureic children. Pediatrics 1990;86:594–600.

5. Suthanthiran M, Strom TB. Renal transplantation. N Engl J Med 1994;331:365–76.

6. Wolfe RA, Ashby VB, Milford EL, et al. Comparison of mortality in all patients on dialysis, patients on dialysis awaiting transplantation and recepients of a first cadaveric transplant. N Engl J Med 1999; 341:1725–30.

7. McDonald SP, Craig JC, Australian and New Zealand Paediatric Nephrology Association. Long-term survival of children with end-stage renal disease. N Engl J Med 2004;350:2654–62.

8. Fennell RS III, Rasbury WC, Fennell EB, et al. Effects of kidney transplantation on cognitive performance in a pediatric population. Pediatrics 1984; 74:273–8.

9. Kasiske BL, Cangro CB, Hariharan S, et al. The evaluation of renal transplantation candidates: a clinical practice guidelines. Am J Transplant 2001; 1(Suppl 2):3–95.

10. Penna FJ, Elder JS. CKD and bladder problems in children. Adv Chronic Kidney Dis 2011;18(5):362–9.

11. Ewalt DH, Allen TD. Urinary tract reconstruction in children undergoing renal transplantation. Adv Ren Replace Ther 1996;3(1):69–76.

12. Matas AJ, Smith JM, Skeans MA, et al. OPTN/SRTR 2012 annual data report: kidney. Am J Transplant 2014;14(S1):11–44.

13. Abecassis M, Adams M, Adams P, et al. Consensus statement on the live organ donor. JAMA 2000;284: 2919–26.

14. Shapiro R. The transplant procedure. In: Shapiro R, Simmons R, Starzl T, editors. Renal transplantation. Stamford (CT): Appleton & Lange; 1998. p. 103–43.

15. Fraser N, Lyon PC, Williams AR, et al. Native nephrectomy in pediatric transplantation – less is more. J Pediatr Urol 2012;9:84–91.

16. Sharma A, Ramanathan R, Posner M, et al. Pediatric kidney transplantation: a review. Transpl Res Risk Manag 2013;5:21–31.

17. Shemin D, Bostom AG, Laliberty P, et al. Residual renal function and mortality risk in hemodialysis patients. Am J Kidney Dis 2001;38(1):85–90.

18. Fuller TF, Brennan TV, Feng S, et al. End stage polycystic kidney disease: indications and timing of native nephrectomy relative to kidney transplantation. J Urol 2005;174(6):2284–8.

19. Bilginer Y, Aki F, Topaloglu R, et al. Renal transplantation in children with lower urinary tract dysfunction of different origin: a single-center experience. Transplant Proc 2008;40(1):85–6.

20. Wu YJ, Veale JL, Gritsch HA. Urological complications of renal transplant in patients with prolonged anuria. Transplantation 2008;86(9):1196–8.

21. Capizzi A, Zanon FG, Zacchello G, et al. Kidney transplantation in children with reconstructed bladder. Transplantation 2004;77(7):1113–6.

22. Aki FT, Aydin AM, Dogan HS, et al. Does lower urinary tract status affect renal transplantation in children? Transplant Proc 2015;47(4):1114–6.

23. Pereria DA, Barroso U Jr, Machado P, et al. Effects of urinary tract infections in patients with bladder augmentation and kidney transplantation. J Urol 2008;180(6):2607–10.

24. Ivancic V, DeFoor W, Jackson E, et al. Progression of renal insufficiency in children and adolescents with neuropathic bladder is not accelerated by lower urinary tract reconstruction. J Urol 2010;184:1768–74.

25. Koo HP, Bunchman TE, Flynn JT, et al. Renal transplantation in children with severe lower urinary tract dysfunction. J Urol 1999;161(1):240–5.

26. Fisang C, Hauser S, Muller SC. Ureterocystoplasty: an ideal method for vesical augmentation in children. Aktuelle Urol 2010;41:S50–2.

27. Husmann DA, Snodgrass WT, Koyle MA, et al. Ureterocystoplasty: indications for a successful augmentation. J Urol 2004;171(1):376–80.

28. Hatch DA, Koyle MA, Baskin LS, et al. Kidney transplantation in children with urinary diversion or bladder augmentation. J Urol 2001;165:2265–8.

29. Rigamonti W, Capizzi A, Zacchello G, et al. Kidney transplantation into bladder augmentation or urinary diversion: long-term results. Transplantation 2005; 80(10):1435–40.

30. Broniszczak D, Ismail H, Nachulewicz P, et al. Kidney transplantation in children with bladder augmentation or ileal conduit diversion. Eur J Pediatr Surg 2010;20(1):5–10.

31. Jesus LE, Pippi Salle JL. Pre-transplant management of valve bladder: a critical literature review. J Pediatr Urol 2015;11(1):5–11.

32. Lopez Pereira P, Ortiz R, Espinosa L, et al. Does bladder augmentation negatively affect renal transplant outcomes in posterior urethral valve patients? J Pediatr Urol 2014;10(5):892–7.

33. Gargah T, Abidi K, Rajhi H, et al. Vascular complications after pediatric kidney transplantation. Tunis Med 2011;89:458–61.

34. Keller AK, Jorgensen TM, Jepersen B. Identification of risk factors for vascular thrombosis may reduce early renal graft loss: a review of recent literature. J Transplant 2012;2012:793461.

35. Afanetti M, Niaudet P, Niel O, et al. Pediatric en bloc kidney transplantation into pediatric recipients: the French experience. Pediatr Transplant 2012;16: 183–6.

36. Lucewicz A, Wong G, Lam VW, et al. Management of primary symptomatic lymphocele after kidney transplanation: a systemic review. Transplantation 2011; 92(6):663–73.

37. Routh JC, Yu RN, Kozinn SI, et al. Urological complications and vesicoureteral reflux following pediatric kidney transplantation. J Urol 2013;189: 1071–6.

38. Nuininga JE, Feitz WF, van Dael KC, et al. Urologic complications in pediatric renal transplantation. Eur Urol 2001;39:598–602.

39. Dalgic A, Boyvat F, Karakayali H, et al. Urologic complications in 1523 renal transplantations: the Baskent University experience. Transplant Proc 2006;38:543–7.

40. Englesbe MJ, Lynch RJ, Heidt DG, et al. Early urologic complications after pediatric renal transplant: a single-center experience. Transplantation 2008; 86:1560–4.

41. Khositseth S, Askiti V, Nevins TE, et al. Increased urologic complications in children after kidney transplants for obstructive and reflux uropathy. Am J Transplant 2007;7:2152–7.

42. Khairoun M, Baranski AG, van der Boog PJM, et al. Urological complications and their impact on survival after kidney transplantation from deceased cardiac death donors. Transpl Int 2009;22:192–7.

43. Kayler L, Kang D, Molmenti E, et al. Kidney transplant ureteroneocystostomy techniques and complications: review of the literature. Transplant Proc 2010;42:1413–20.

44. Neri F, Tsivian M, Coccolini F, et al. Urological complications after kidney transplantation: experience of more than 1,000 transplantations. Transplant Proc 2009;41(4):1224–6.

45. Duty BD, Barry JM. Diagnosis and management of ureteral complications following renal transplantation. Asian J Urol 2015;2:202–7.

46. Harza M, Baston C, Preda A, et al. Impact of ureteral stenting on urological complications after kidney transplantation surgery: a single-center experience. Transplant Proc 2014;8:51.

47. Allain-Launay E, Roussey-Kesler G, Ranchin B, et al. Mortality in pediatric renal transplantation: a study of the French Pediatric Kidney database. Pediatr Transplant 2009;13:725–30.

48. Gritsch HA, Blumberg JM. Renal transplantation. In: Campbell-Walsh urology, vol. 4, 11th edition. Philadelphia: Elsevier; 2016. p. 1069–88.

49. Alam S, Sheldon C. Urological issues in pediatric renal transplantation. Curr Opin Urol 2008;18:413–8.

50. Barrero R, Fijo J, Fernandez-Hurtado M, et al. Vesicoureteral reflux after kidney transplantation in children. Pediatr Transplant 2007;11:498–503.

51. Seifert HH, Mazzola B, Ruszat R, et al. Transurethral injection therapy with dextranomer/hyaluronic acid copolymer (Deflux) for treatment of secondary vesicoureteral reflux after renal transplantation. J Endourol 2007;21:1357–60.

52. Pichler R, Buttazzoni A, Rehder P, et al. Endoscopic application of dextranomer/hyaluronic acid copolymer in the treatment of vesico-ureteric reflux after renal transplantation. BJU Int 2011;107:1967–72.

53. Yucel S, Akin Y, Celik O, et al. Endoscopic vesicoureteral reflux correction in transplanted kidneys: does injection technique matter? J Endourol 2010; 24:1661–4.

54. Traxel E, DeFoor W, Minevich E, et al. Low incidence of urinary tract infections following renal transplantation in children with bladder augmentation. J Urol 2011;186(2):667–71.

55. Smith JM, Dharnidharka VR, Talley L, et al. BK virus nephropathy in pediatric renal transplant recipients: an analysis of the North American Pediatric Renal Trials and Colloborative Studies (NAPRTCS) registry. Clin J Am Soc Nephrol 2007;2:1037–42.

56. Fogeda M, Munoz P, Luque A, et al, BKV Study Group. Cross-sectional study of BK virus infection in pediatric kidney transplant recipients. Pediatr Transplant 2007;11:394–401.

57. Dharnidharka VR, Abdulnour HA, Araya CE. The BK virus in renal transplant recipients – review of pathogenesis, diagnosis and treatment. Pediatr Nephrol 2011;26:1763–74.

58. Egli A, Infanti L, Dumoulin A, et al. Prevalence of polyomavirus BK and JC infection and replication in 400 healthy blood donors. J Infect Dis 2009;199: 837–46.

59. Shaw RJ, Palmer L, Blasey C, et al. A typology of non-adherence in pediatric renal transplant recipients. Pediatr Transplant 2003;7:489–93.

60. Zarkhin V, Kambham N, Li L, et al. Characterization of intra-graft B cells during renal allograft rejection. Kidney Int 2008;74:664–73.

61. Hardy BE, Shah T, Cicciarelli J, et al. Kidney transplantation in children and adolescents: an analysis of united network for organ sharing database. Transplant Proc 2009;41:1533–5.

62. United States Organ Transplantation. OPTN and SRTR annual data report 2011. Available at: http://srtr.transplant.hrsa.gov/annual_reports/2011/pdf/00_intro_12.pdf. Accessed February 1, 2018.

63. Hall EC, Pfeiffer RM, Segev DL, et al. Cumulative incidence of cancer after solid organ transplantation. Cancer 2013;119(12):2300–8.

Neuropathic Bladder and Augmentation Cystoplasty

Joshua D. Roth, MD*, Mark P. Cain, MD

KEYWORDS

- Neuropathic bladder • Neurogenic bladder • Augmentation cystoplasty

KEY POINTS

- A normal lower urinary tract serves 2 functions: low-pressure urine storage and periodic voluntary emptying.
- A neuropathic bladder (NB) is a heterogeneous condition that can result in a variety of conditions that affect the central and/or peripheral nervous systems.
- The management of NB aims to preserve the native bladder to store urine at low pressure and to allow efficient emptying of the bladder.

INTRODUCTION

A normal lower urinary tract serves 2 functions: low-pressure urine storage and periodic voluntary emptying. A neuropathic bladder (NB) is a heterogeneous condition that can result from a variety of conditions affecting the central or peripheral nervous systems. Myelodysplasia, specifically spina bifida, remains the most common cause of NB in the pediatric population. Spina bifida has an incidence of 3.7 per 10,000 live births in the United States.[1] Other conditions that can result in NB include tethered cord, sacral agenesis, spinal cord injury, cerebral palsy, bladder exstrophy, cloacal anomalies, and anorectal malformations.[2]

The management of NB aims to preserve the native bladder to store urine at low pressure and to allow efficient emptying of the bladder. Early management is usually focused on preventing irreversible injury to either the upper or lower urinary tract. As children age, it is also important to consider the quality of life of the child and caregiver with regard to urinary continence and independence in bladder management. Because each patient and family is unique, it is important for urologists to understand the numerous medical and surgical options available to manage NB and

also to appreciate that the life expectancy for these patients requires careful decision making at each stage in their lives.

EVALUATION OF NEUROPATHIC BLADDER

NB dysfunction may lead to recurrent urinary tract infections, vesicoureteral reflux, loss of renal parenchyma, renal scar formation, and chronic renal failure.[3] Thus, NB and especially the upper urinary tracts must be closely monitored. The NB and upper tracts can be evaluated radiographically by ultrasonography, fluoroscopy, or nuclear medicine imaging and functionally by urodynamics. The goal of evaluation is to prevent long-term renal failure by assessing for renal/bladder changes so that intervention can occur before irreversible renal scars develop.

In evaluating the NB, the goal is to detect early upper tract (or ideally lower tract) changes that may precede deterioration, which is key to long-term prevention of renal failure. Upper tracts are routinely monitored with renal bladder ultrasonography (RBUS), which often fails to detect renal scarring. One study of adults with spinal dysraphism observed renal scars on ultrasonography in 10% of cases but also observed scarring on

Disclosure: The authors have no disclosures.
Department of Pediatric Urology, 705 Riley Hospital Drive, Suite 4230, Indianapolis, IN 46202, USA
* Corresponding author. Riley Hospital for Children at Indiana University Health, 535 North Barnhill Drive Suite 150, Indianapolis, IN 46202.
E-mail address: joshroth@iupui.edu

dimercaptosuccinic acid (DMSA) scans in 46% of cases.[4] However, other series cite rates of renal scarring as 10% to 25% of children and young adults with myelodysplasia via DMSA scans.[5–7] These studies report that, of the patients with renal scarring, 75% to 100% had associated vesicoureteral reflux. The overall rate of reflux in patients with lower urinary tract dysfunction and myelodysplasia is 40% to 48%.[5–7] Because of an evaluation strategy that is reliant on RBUS changes, providers may fail to recognize early scarring, especially in high-risk populations like patients with NB and vesicoureteral reflux.

Urodynamics allow precise measurements of intravesical pressures, abdominal pressures, detrusor pressures, electromyography, and fluoroscopic voiding cystourethrography. A detrusor leak point pressure (DLPP)/end fill pressure (EFP) of 40 cm H_2O has generally been recognized as a threshold that, once passed, can transmit increased pressures to the upper tracts and portend renal injury. This threshold is based on a study of 42 patients with myelodysplasia that showed high rates of both vesicoureteral reflux (68%) and ureteral dilatation (81%) in 22 children with DLPP/EFP greater than 40 cm H_2O. No patient with pressures less than 40 cm H_2O had vesicoureteral reflux and only 10% had ureteral dilatation.[8] Recent studies that attempted to corroborate these claims have shown that more than half of the almost 200 children with myelodysplasia had normal upper tract function at age 3 years, even with a DLPP/EFP greater than 40 cm H_2O. However, a DLPP/EFP of 20 cm H_2O showed a higher sensitivity to predict upper tract damage.[9] Although there is an association between increased detrusor pressures and upper tract deterioration, more research is needed to determine a cutoff point at which the upper tracts are reliably protected from damage. It is clear that the storage time at increased pressure, especially with the presence of vesicoureteral reflux, is more important than single measurements.

Because of the difficulties in early assessment of upper tract scarring, there have been attempts at identifying early alterations in the bladder wall on imaging. Several studies have attempted to evaluate bladder wall thickness to determine whether identifying a thick-walled bladder on ultrasonography could reliably predict renal outcomes or urodynamic parameters. Bladder wall hypertrophy may decrease compliance through effects on smooth muscle, connective tissue, innervation, and tissue hypoxia. Studies have concluded that bladder wall thickness is a sensitive screening tool for increased DLPP/EFP on urodynamics that can pose a risk for deterioration in the upper urinary tract in children with spina bifida.[3,10] One study also found that urinary levels of transforming growth factor β1, nerve growth factor, and tissue inhibitor of metalloproteinase-2 were also significantly increased in patients with DLPPs greater than 40 cm H_2O and those with renal scarring on DMSA.[3] However, another study of the same pediatric population failed to find an association between bladder wall thickness and any urodynamic parameter other than bladder trabeculation.[11] This finding is corroborated by the largest study to date evaluating the utility of bladder wall thickness in adults measured by ultrasonography. No threshold wall thickness was predictive of urodynamic findings, and thus it could not replace urodynamic testing to evaluate for increased DLPP/EFP. Bladder wall thickness was significantly increased in individuals with low bladder compliance and neurogenic detrusor overactivity associated with detrusor sphincter dyssynergia.[12] There is yet to be a reliable, noninvasive way to evaluate when the upper tracts of children with NB are at risk for deterioration.

INITIAL MANAGEMENT OF NEUROPATHIC BLADDER

In 1971, Lapides and colleagues[110] described performing clean intermittent catheterization (CIC) on 14 patients with neuropathic and atonic bladders. Before the widespread use of CIC, renal failure was the most common cause of death at all ages in those with NB caused by spina bifida.[13] In sharp contrast, 74% of patients with NB caused by spina bifida at centers participating in the National Spina Bifida Registry use CIC.[14] The combination of CIC, medical management, and surgical management has greatly reduced mortality related to renal failure.[15–18] The optimal timing of initiation of CIC, medication, and when to offer surgical intervention is often based on the clinical discretion of the provider after consideration of urodynamic parameters, imaging studies, family compliance, and social situations.

MEDICAL MANAGEMENT OF NEUROPATHIC BLADDER

In addition to CIC, anticholinergic medications, such as oxybutynin, are used to ensure low intravesical pressures by maintaining a sizable, continent, and compliant urinary reservoir.[16] Oral anticholinergic medication has been shown to significantly improve maximal cystometric capacity and EFP with minimal side effects of constipation and facial flushing reported. In one study, 63% of children with pretreatment EFP greater than 40 cm H_2O had EFP that decreased to and remained less than 40 cm H_2O throughout treatment.[19] In children unable to tolerate oral anticholinergic medication, intravesical instillation of oxybutynin has also been shown to improve cystometric capacity and reduce EFP with no reported side effects.[20] Recently, β3-adrenoreceptor agonists, like mirabegron, have been approved for monotherapy for idiopathic overactive bladder. Initial studies in pediatric patients with overactive bladder show increases in bladder capacity with side effects of transient abdominal colic, constipation, and blurred vision reported in less than 10% of patients.[21] Although oral anticholinergic therapy is currently the mainstay of medical management for pediatric NB, more research into manipulation of the adrenergic pathway and intravesical administration of known pharmacologic therapies may provide additional medical options for children with NBs.

INTRADETRUSOR onabotulinumtoxinA

In 2011, onabotulinumtoxinA was approved by the US Food and Drug Administration (FDA) in adults for intravesical injection for the treatment of urinary incontinence secondary to neurogenic detrusor overactivity. Several studies have shown similar benefits in children with regard to improved continence, bladder capacity, and compliance following injection.[22–24] Of those who failed medical management, patients with anticholinergic intolerance who were treated with onabotulinumtoxinA had higher continence rates than those refractory to anticholinergic treatment.[24]

Consensus opinion is that 10 to 12 units/kg onabotulinumtoxinA (up to 300 units maximum) can be safely administered in children.[24] OnabotulinumtoxinA can be used to treat a variety of conditions, such as chronic migraine, upper limb spasticity, cervical dystonia, primary axillary hyperhidrosis, blepharospasms, and strabismus. Urologists must be aware if this agent is being injected into other sites for these indications because the highest dose of onabotulinumtoxinA studied in an FDA trial is 360 cumulative units within a 3-month interval.[24,25] With injection of onabotulinumtoxinA, there is a risk of spread of toxin, which can result in symptoms of asthenia, generalized muscle weakness, diplopia, ptosis, dysphagia, dysarthria, breathing difficulties, and dysphagia and can result in aspiration pneumonia and paralysis of respiratory muscles, which can require intubation.[26–28]

OnabotulinumtoxinA presents a promising minimally invasive option to manage children who have failed medical management of NB. However, no

improvement in incontinence is observed in up to 50% of children.[24] In those in whom a response was observed, mean duration of efficacy ranged from 4.6 to 7 months.[24,25] The poorest response for intravesical onabotulinumtoxinA injections in children with NB has been observed in children with severely impaired bladder compliance, particularly those without detrusor overactivity (**Fig. 1**).[26–28] This finding may represent a timing problem, because this therapy is often reserved for treatment after failure of medical management, and the bladder may already have increased collagen deposition in addition to muscular hypertrophy. In reviewing the Pediatric Health Information System (PHIS) data through 2015, the use of intradetrusor onabotulinumtoxinA has increased dramatically, but the incidence of bladder augmentation has not changed during the same time period (**Figs. 2** and **3**). Whether this represents the inevitable need for augmentation in a small subset of patients or late introduction of onabotulinumtoxinA therapy, before the terminal changes of poor compliance, is yet to be determined.

There are concerns about onabotulinumtoxinA as a chronic management strategy because it requires regular injections that require repeated anesthesia in young patients. The costs and risks of repeated anesthesia exposure are not minimal. Further, there may be a loss of efficacy over time.[29] Although it is not currently FDA approved for treatment in children, onabotulinumtoxinA is an accepted minimally invasive alternative to more invasive procedures. However, more research is needed to understand the optimal candidates, timing, and benefits of treatment with onabotulinumtoxinA in children with NB. The repeated costs of procedures and anesthetics, along with the decreased efficacy over time, may just be delaying the time until definitive treatment in the form of augmentation cystoplasty is offered to families. This delay may ultimately prove to be beneficial because it will give children more time to mature and families more time to understand the risks associated with, and care needed to maintain, a bladder augmentation. Despite the controversy, onabotulinumtoxinA does seem to be a very good alternative for initial intervention in children, especially in patients with marked detrusor overactivity.

SURGICAL RECONSTRUCTION FOR NEUROPATHIC BLADDER

In individuals who have failed medical and intravesical treatment options, more definitive procedures may be performed to create a reservoir that

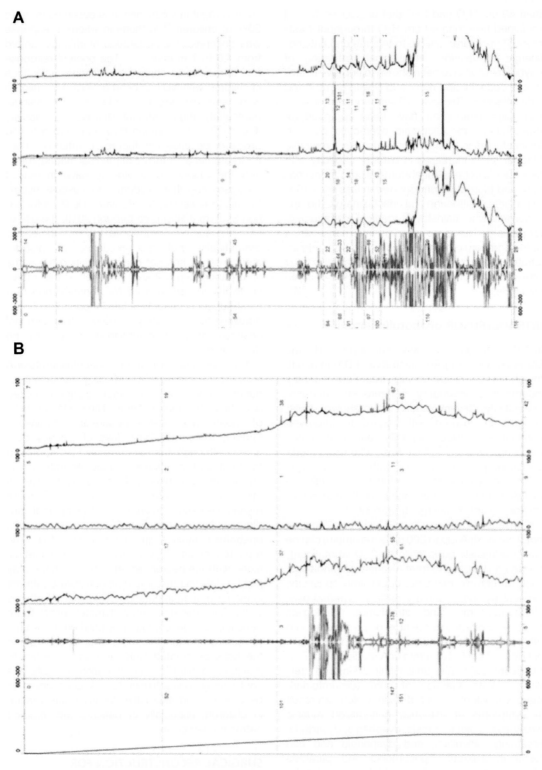

Fig. 1. (*A*) Urodynamics showing detrusor overactivity that would be a good candidate for intradetrusor onabotulinumtoxinA. (*B*) Urodynamics showing poor terminal compliance suggesting the patient may have a poor response to intradetrusor onabotulinumtoxinA.

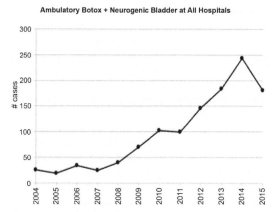

Ambulatory Botox + Neurogenic Bladder at All Hospitals

Fig. 2. Annual rates of ambulatory onabotulinumtoxinA from PHIS hospitals.

will store urine at low pressure and help achieve continence, while protecting the upper tracts. For patients with bladder failure but intact sphincter and ability to independently catheterize per urethra, bladder augmentation with correction of associated high-grade vesicoureteral reflux is the next option. In the scenario in which the bladder is a poor reservoir and continence is desired, and the patient and family are willing to accept the required lifelong maintenance, continence can be achieved by a combination of augmentation cystoplasty; bladder outlet procedures such as bladder neck slings, artificial urinary sphincters, bladder neck reconstruction, or bladder neck closure; and creation of a catheterizable channel. In patients who are risk averse or who are unable to perform the necessary upkeep with some of the procedures mentioned earlier, incontinent diversion options including vesicostomy, ileal chimney, and ileal conduit can be considered.

Surgical indications for individuals with NB include unsafe urinary storage pressures, progressive upper tract deterioration, or continued urinary incontinence that is recalcitrant to oral pharmacologic therapy and intermittent catheterization. In a few select patients with favorable urodynamics and low outlet resistance, a bladder neck procedure can be performed without bladder augmentation to achieve continence. However, it is difficult to consistently identify which patients have favorable urodynamics on preoperative studies, and all patients with bladder neck procedures without augmentation require close observation because many have deterioration of the bladder and sometimes rapid onset of upper tract problems (hydronephrosis and vesicoureteral reflux) caused by the increased outlet resistance.[30–32] Following isolated bladder neck procedures, some patients develop rapid bladder thickening, likely caused by collagen deposition, and require bladder augmentation (**Fig. 4**).

AUGMENTATION CYSTOPLASTY

Initially, many children with neurogenic bladder were managed with an ileal conduit. However, in the mid-1970s, many of these patients underwent so-called undiversion to an augmented bladder with bowel.[33] Initially described at the end of the nineteenth century,[34] ileocystoplasty was refined by Goodwin in the 1950s,[35–37] and continued to be refined into the 1980s, when the detubularized and reconfigured clam enterocystoplasty, now commonly used, was described.[18] Bladder augmentation is currently the gold standard surgical procedure used to increase bladder capacity and reduce storage pressures. Small bowel, colonic, and gastric segments have all been used to augment the bladder.[38–42] However, the use of

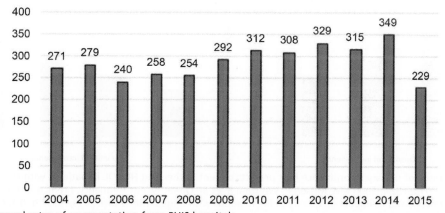

Fig. 3. Annual rates of augmentation from PHIS hospitals.

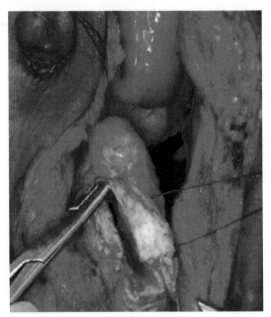

Fig. 4. Thick-walled bladder observed less than 1 year after an isolated bladder neck procedure in a bladder with prior normal wall thickness.

gastric segments has been almost entirely abandoned because of the development of hematuria-dysuria syndrome in approximately 25%, refractory metabolic alkalosis in 7%, and increased risk of aggressive neoplasia compared with other forms of augmentation, requiring takedown of the gastric segment in greater than 20%.[43] The concern of increased relative risk of gastrocystoplasty and bladder cancer has led many institutions to avoid using stomach for augmentation.

Augmentation cystoplasty increases bladder capacity, which allows urine to be stored at low pressures with excellent long-term results. Renal failure, secondary to the abnormal neurogenic

bladder, was the leading cause of mortality in the spina bifida population in the era immediately after the ventriculoperitoneal shunt (VPS) was developed. However, recent studies have shown the that renal failure was the cause of mortality in only 0.5% of patients with spina bifida who underwent augmentation cystoplasty at a mean follow-up of 10 years.[30–32]

Bladder reconstruction has shown positive effects on health-related quality of life (HRQOL), including improved self-image and self-esteem.[44] The positive effects on HRQOL are driven by urinary continence. Specifically in the spina bifida population, HRQOL was improved with decreased amounts of urinary incontinence.[45] The quantity of urinary incontinence has been shown to be the best predictor of patient bother and HRQOL in patients with NB caused by spina bifida (**Fig. 5**).[46]

The benefits of improved quality of life and decreased risk of renal failure are weighed against the significant long-term risks associated with bladder augmentation, including calculi, acid/base disturbances caused by absorption of urine by bowel, bladder perforation, B_{12} deficiency, bowel obstruction, and increased risk of malignancy. Bladder reconstruction should be considered a permanent alteration to the lower urinary tract requiring close and lifelong observations. In the largest published series, complications were observed in 169 of 500 bladder augmentations (34%), resulting in an additional 254 surgeries, for a cumulative risk of further bladder-level surgery of 0.04 operations per patient per year following bladder reconstruction. However, two-thirds of patients with bladder augmentations did not require additional procedures.[47] Our impression is that the true reoperation rate currently is lower, because this large series included patients who would currently be considered of historical value only, because some patients had

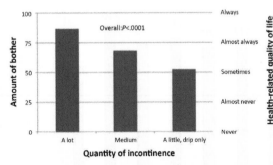
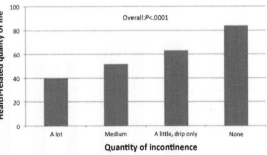

Fig. 5. Quantity of urinary incontinence best predicts patient bother and HRQOL in patients with NB caused by spina bifida. (*From* Szymanski KM, Misseri R, Whittam B, et al. Quantity, not frequency, predicts bother with urinary incontinence and its impact on quality of life in adults with spina bifida. J Urol 2016;195(4 Pt 2):1263–9; with permission.)

nonreconfigured/nondetubularized bowel segments early in the series.

Other methods have been described to augment the bladder without the use of bowel. Ureterocystoplasty, similar to enterocystoplasty, provides durable functional improvement in urodynamic parameters without the risks of long-term metabolic complications.[48,49] Ureterocystoplasty can be used in patients with any single or double collecting system, without reflux, and with a ureteral width of 1.5 cm or more, and in patients with vesicoureteral reflux and mild noncompliance (greater than 20 mL/cm H_2O) on urodynamics.[50] Autoaugmentation, which is performed by vesicomyotomy or detrusorotomy, has been advocated by some clinicians to avoid the long-term complications of enterocystoplasty. However, although short-term results have been promising, there has been debate over the durability of the repair.[51] Compared with enterocystoplasty, patients undergoing autoaugmentation had significantly less improvement in bladder capacity following the procedure, without any difference in continence, antimuscarinic use, or condition of the upper tract. If bladder volume is adequate, autoaugmentation can be considered to help decrease compliance.[52]

BLADDER CALCULI

Bladder calculi are the most commonly observed complication observed in 11% to 52% patients following bladder augmentation,[47,53–56] and represent the highest risk for additional procedures following augmentation. Calculi typically form in bladders augmented with ileum and/or colon, when absorbable staples are used, in the setting of incomplete bladder emptying, and in patients with a metabolic predisposition for stone formation (eg, hypocitraturia). Because of the acidic urine, bladder calculi are rare in gastric augments.[36,57–59] Recurrent urinary tract infections, NB caused by exstrophy, noncompliance with catheterizations or irrigations, and poor adherence to follow-up have also been shown to increase the risk of bladder calculi in patients with bladder augmentations.[60–62] Although most of the bladder calculi have an infectious cause, 31% of bladder stones following bladder augmentation have been found to be noninfectious. Several factors may contribute to stone formation, including chronic metabolic acidosis, resultant chronic kidney disease, and hypercalciuria related to wheelchair-dependence-related osteodystrophy.[63] Bladder stones are less likely when an individual catheterizes per urethra compared with an abdominal stoma.[47] High-volume (>240 mL) irrigations have been shown to prevent bladder stones; however, individuals who still developed bladder calculi recalcitrant to high-volume irrigations did not benefit from correction of underlying metabolic abnormalities or mucolytic agents.[64]

Bladder stones form on average 37.5 months (range, 11–120 months) after augmentation.[62] They have a high recurrence rate, with 15% to 29% recurring in less than 2 years after treatment and almost half of patients having recurrence following initial stone surgery independent of treatment modality or patient characteristics.[54,65] Depending on stone size and burden, multiple treatment modalities exist, ranging from endoscopic management to open cystolithotomy. Endoscopy for appropriately sized stones has shown high rates of stone clearance with a low rate of complications while preventing the morbidity of open surgery.[62,66,67] Endoscopy via channel or urethra may result in injury to the channel or to a reconstructed bladder neck. Percutaneous cystolithotomy offers another alternative form of endoscopy that eliminates potential injury to the channel and urethra while also saving patients the increased convalescence of an open procedure.[67] After stone removal, patients should undergo a 24-h urine collection and evaluation in a multidisciplinary stone clinic to facilitate coordinated management with urology and nephrology.[65]

METABOLIC DERANGEMENTS

Metabolic derangements can occur following inclusion of bowel segments into the urinary tract because of the absorptive nature of the bowel segments. Symptomatic metabolic acidosis is rare in patients with normal renal function who have undergone a bladder augmentation with a small bowel segment but may require treatment in patients with preexisting renal insufficiency.[41,68] The metabolic derangements that can occur are very predictable based on the bowel segment used. After incorporating ileal and/or colonic segments into the urinary tract, hyperchloremic metabolic acidosis can occur secondary to the loss of bicarbonate and potassium. This process results from the reabsorption of ionized ammonium and chloride; ammonium is exchanged for a hydrogen proton, and bicarbonate is exchanged for a chloride ion. Ionized ammonium can then be absorbed into the blood through potassium channels.[69,70] Hypochloremic hypokalemic metabolic alkalosis can occur with the use of gastric segments and hyponatremic hypochloremic hyperkalemic metabolic acidosis develops with the use of jejunum, both of which are more difficult to manage clinically.[36,70]

Chronic metabolic acidosis can lead to decreased bone mineral density and has raised concern for impaired linear growth following bladder augmentation in children; however, no studies have validated this theoretic complication.[71] Prolonged acidosis may lead to osteomalacia or osteoporosis in adulthood.[72] Metabolic acidosis should be corrected when diagnosed and patients should be provided calcium and vitamin D supplements. In some cases, bisphosphonates become necessary to prevent loss of bone mass.[71,73–75] Although there are no current guidelines for monitoring the increased risk of bone demineralization following augmentation, clinicians should discuss this with patients, especially adult women.

PERFORATION

Although not common, bladder perforation represents the most morbid and catastrophic complication following bladder augmentation. Perforation may culminate in peritonitis, sepsis, and even death. Reported rates of bladder perforation following augmentation range between 6% and 13%.[76–81] Perforation occurs because of increased intravesical pressure, which may result from chronic bladder overdistention, chronic infection, traumatic catheterization, and ischemic necrosis of the intestinal segment used for the augmentation.[82–87] Bladder perforation usually demands exploratory laparotomy with externalization of VPS, if present, to reduce the risk of a central nervous system infection.[88]

In the largest published series to date, 43 out of the 500 patients (8.6%) who underwent bladder augmentation experienced a perforation. Increased risk of perforation was associated with the use of nondetubularized sigmoid colon, presence of a bladder neck procedure, and history of prior bladder perforation, whereas presence of a continent catheterizable channel was protective for perforation, likely because of the easier access to the bladder. Bladder perforation remains a lifelong risk following bladder augmentation, with one-third occurring within 2 years, another third between 2 and 6 years, and the final third occurring after 6 years following initial surgery.[76] This risk continues throughout the patient's life and may increase in adulthood because of the recognized risk of poor patient compliance associated with increased risk of substance abuse and noncompliance with intermittent catheterization in this patient population.[64,89]

Physicians must possess a high clinical suspicion for a perforated bladder augmentation because of impaired sensation in patients with spina bifida. A detailed history, physical examination to assess for peritonitis, and laboratory analysis including white blood count and serum creatinine are useful when diagnosing bladder perforation. Patients with history of bladder augmentation who present with acute abdominal pain, poor urine output, increased serum creatinine level, and increased white blood count should be urgently evaluated for possible bladder perforation. A low-pressure computed tomography cystogram, including postdrainage film, remains the gold standard for diagnosing bladder perforation by evaluating for contrast extravasation.[76,87] Recently, a large series showed that increased intraperitoneal fluid and unexplained pneumoperitoneum were the most sensitive findings in symptomatic patients, detecting bladder perforation in individuals without contrast extravasation. Thus, bladder perforation should be suspected in any patient following bladder augmentation with a moderate or large amount of pelvic fluid or unexplained pneumoperitoneum.[90]

VITAMIN B_{12} DEFICIENCY

Hypocobalaminemia, or vitamin B_{12} deficiency, occurs when serum B_{12} concentration decreases to less than 200 pg/mL. This condition can occur after bladder augmentation with symptoms ranging from subtle to dramatic. Patients with B_{12} deficiency may present with pernicious anemia, characterized by megaloblastic anemia, gastrointestinal symptoms, and potentially irreversible neurologic symptoms, including peripheral neuropathy, loss of positional and vibrational sense, ataxia, seizures, and dementia.[91,92] The risk of hypocobalaminemia increases approximately 5 years after augmentation and continues to escalate over time, as the body's stores of B_{12} are depleted.[93,94]

Vitamin B_{12} can be replaced orally or parenterally. Oral replacement is generally well tolerated and effective in increasing serum B_{12} levels for the short term. However, long-term oral replacement success is poor, possibly because of reduced patient compliance.[42,95] Although hypocobalaminemia is often asymptomatic, the potentially devastating, irreversible neurologic complications make the diagnosis and treatment essential. A review of 23 patients with augmented bladders with serum B_{12} levels less than 300 pg/mL revealed no evidence of pernicious anemia at a mean of 49 months following initial abnormal B_{12} level.[95] Vitamin B_{12} levels should be checked annually starting 5 years after bladder augmentation and, if hypocobalaminemia persists on oral medication, there should be a low threshold to transition the patient to a parenteral regimen.

MALIGNANCY

Although rare, bladder cancer has been reported in augmented bladders at an incidence of 1.1% to 4.5%.[40,96–104] Bladder cancer has been found to be deadly and rapidly progressive in patients with congenital bladder anomalies.[104] Higher rates of bladder cancer were associated with well-known carcinogenic stimuli; for example, prolonged tobacco exposure, chronic immunosuppression, and bladder exstrophy.[105] Patients with gastric augmentation seem to develop tumors more frequently and earlier after surgery compared with patients with ileal augmentation. Whether this association is just caused by the interposition of a gastric segment, or because gastrocystoplasty was preferred in a high-risk population (ie, patients with renal failure and/or renal transplant) remains unclear.[101] Patients with neurogenic bladder managed solely with CIC have also shown an increased risk of bladder cancer, and ileal/colonic bladder augmentation does not seem to increase the risk of bladder malignancy beyond the inherent cancer risk associated with the underlying congenital abnormality.[39,104]

Although yearly endoscopy was previously used for cancer surveillance, it has since fallen out of favor, because it is not cost-effective and the potential morbidity makes it an ineffective screening procedure.[106–108] Current recommendations are to perform cystoscopy in patients with 4 or more symptomatic urinary tract infections per year, gross hematuria, microscopic hematuria with 50 or more red blood cells per high-power field, abnormal radiographic screening studies, chronic perineal, pelvic or bladder pain, and colonic augments aged 50 years or older (consistent with colonoscopy recommendations).[107,109] Any significant change in a patient's baseline function may merit investigation with anatomic or functional studies for this vulnerable population at the clinical discretion of the urologist.

CATHETERIZABLE CHANNEL

CIC, popularized by Lapides and colleagues,[110] allowed the development of bladder augmentations and continent urinary reservoirs by creating an effective means to drain urine[111] separate from the reconstructed urethra/bladder neck. Catheterizable channels or Mitrofanoff procedures are often created to facilitate ease of intermittent catheterization, which is especially important in wheelchair-confined patients with spina bifida who undergo bladder augmentation. Catheterizable channels allow patients to independently and more discretely empty their bladders, but these channels carry their own long-term risks that require monitoring. Channels may be created from appendix (appendicovesicostomy) or a segment of retubularized ileum (Yang-Monti ileovesicostomy or Casale procedure/spiral Monti).[112–115] All catheterizable channels have a low rate of stomal stenosis, at less than 10%, and a high rate of continence, at greater than 95%. Other complications observed with catheterizable channels include inability to catheterize, channel perforation, and diverticulum formation. Although stomal stenosis, stomal revision procedures, and channel continence were similar between the various channels, patients with Yang-Monti catheterizable channels, especially those placed in the umbilicus, are twice as likely to require subfascial revision at 10-year follow-up. The longer spiral Monti channels to the umbilicus carried the greatest risk for subfascial revision.[116,117] Complications can continue to occur at any point following channel creation, but most occur in the first 5 years.[116]

URETERAL REIMPLANTATION

In patients with concurrent vesicoureteral reflux and neurogenic bladder, approximately half resolve their reflux by decreasing detrusor pressures with appropriate medical interventions and the simultaneous institution of intermittent catheterization.[118] In the remainder, the persistence of vesicoureteral reflux increases the risk of pyelonephritis and renal scarring. It can occur through either a defective ureterovesical junction (primary reflux) or through a normal vesicoureteral junction that has been overwhelmed, as in the case of a high-pressure neurogenic bladder (secondary reflux). Surgical intervention is indicated if reflux persists following the institution of medical therapy and intermittent catheterization and the upper tracts are at risk because of repeat urinary tract infections. Persistent vesicoureteral reflux may be approached by endoscopic methods, with reported success rates of 53% to 86% in children with neurogenic bladder, with success inversely proportional to the grade of reflux.[119,120] In comparison, open ureteral reimplantation has reported success rates approaching 100% for primary reflux and 85% to 96% for secondary reflux.[120–122] Subureteral injection has been popularized because of relative ease of use; however, parents should be counseled about the risk of recurrence.

Surgery should also be considered to address vesicoureteral reflux as part of larger operations that increase bladder capacity and manage outlet resistance to limit repeat operations, which may be important in patients following bladder augmentation, because the reflux of mucus/bacteria may increase the risk of upper tract infections and stones. In these cases, creating a longer submucosal ureteral tunnel intravesically via the Leadbetter-Politano or Cohen techniques is indicated. The role for other techniques, such as the Glenn-Anderson technique or the extravesical Lich-Gregoire, has been poorly described in neurogenic bladders.[120]

VESICOSTOMY

Vesicostomy has long been described as a viable treatment option in neurogenic bladder.[123] It is created by bringing the dome of the bladder to the skin to allow continuous bladder drainage. Although medical and surgical advances have decreased its use recently, some families are unwilling or unable to accept the consequences of bladder augmentations, bladder neck reconstructions, and catheterizable channels. In these instances, a vesicostomy helps preserve renal function by creating a pop-off valve, which helps to maintain bladder pressures in an acceptable range. Alternatively, vesicostomy is an attractive alternative for infants with a hostile bladder with upper tract changes, especially with a noncompliant family.

In patients who have physical or cognitive barriers to compliance with CIC, vesicostomy is a workable alternative because it is not dependent on a catheterization schedule or caregiver. However, it can be associated with ostomy prolapse, bladder lithiasis, urinary stasis and infections, and stomal stenosis. Further, because of size and location, it is often difficult to adequately collect urine drainage in a pouch with a flush vesicostomy. As such, most children with a vesicostomy wear diapers to collect urinary drainage.

Ileovesicostomy, initially described in the 1950s, uses a piece of bowel that is anastomosed to the bladder on one end and to the skin on the other in peristaltic fashion to allow drainage of the bladder into a bag. This approach enables the use of a stomal appliance as opposed to diapers, which could improve quality of life by removing the nidus for a strong unpleasant odor associated with continuous leakage into a diaper. From a surgical perspective, the morbidity of a cystectomy is avoided, and an ileovesicostomy is a technically easier operation to perform. Further, the native trigone remains in situ, along with the native ureter's antirefluxing mechanism. Because the bladder remains in place, the procedure is reversible. However, ileovesicostomies can be associated with stomal stenosis, parastomal hernia, poor drainage, urinary tract infections, urolithiasis, ileal limb kinking/structuring, and mucous plugging, especially with long-term use.[124]

INCONTINENT URINARY DIVERSION

Bladder management by urinary diversion is considerably simpler compared with bladder augmentation. It is an attractive alternative in individuals with a hostile bladder with upper tract changes, especially with a noncompliant family. With urinary diversion, patients and caregivers are not required to catheterize the bladder to drain it and do not need to irrigate the bladder. Instead, the urine flows through the bowel conduit to an incontinent stoma. The patient or caregiver only needs to periodically change the external appliance. Cystectomy can be performed at the same time as urinary diversion to eliminate the risk of pyocystis, or the bladder can be left in situ. However, bowel conduit urinary diversions have been associated with an altered body image, recurrent pyelonephritis, metabolic derangements, nephrolithiasis, vitamin B_{12} deficiency if the ileum is used, and delayed anastomotic ureteroenteric stricture. Of note, older patients and women are more likely to undergo urinary diversion. It is thought that this is caused by a lack of social support and more difficulties with catheterization, respectively.[125] However, this procedure was almost universally abandoned for use in children in the 1970s because of the risk of renal deterioration caused by the combination of stomal, midloop, and ureteroenteric strictures, which was observed in 42% to 61% of patients.[126–130] In addition to renal deterioration, many centers also reported other long-term complications, such as chronic bacilluria, stones, and pyocystis in cases in which cystectomy was not performed.[131–137] The ileal conduit was replaced by use of a colon segment because conduit stenosis is much less common with a colon conduit.[111] Absence of reflux by creating nonrefluxing tunneled ureteral anastomoses and avoidance of stomal obstruction were the keys to the long-term success of colon conduits.[138–140]

SUMMARY

Although bladder augmentation carries significant long-term morbidity, it has drastically reduced mortality caused by renal failure in the NB population, while preserving the native bladder. Counseling the patient and family and delaying surgery, if possible, until the patient is mature enough to understand the associated risks are of the utmost importance when considering bladder augmentation.

REFERENCES

1. Parker SE, Mai CT, Canfield MA, et al. Updated national birth prevalence estimates for selected birth defects in the United States, 2004-2006. Birth Defects Res A Clin Mol Teratol 2010;88(12):1008–16.

2. Bauer SB. Neurogenic bladder: etiology and assessment. Pediatr Nephrol 2008;23(4):541–51.

3. Şekerci ÇA, İşbilen B, İşman F, et al. Urinary NGF, TGF-β1, TIMP-2 and bladder wall thickness predict neurourological findings in children with myelodysplasia. J Urol 2014;191(1):199–205.

4. Veenboer PW, Hobbelink MGG, Ruud Bosch JLH, et al. Diagnostic accuracy of Tc-99m DMSA scintigraphy and renal ultrasonography for detecting renal scarring and relative function in patients with spinal dysraphism. Neurourol Urodyn 2015; 34(6):513–8.

5. Cohen RA, Rushton HG, Belman AB, et al. Renal scarring and vesicoureteral reflux in children with myelodysplasia. J Urol 1990;144(2 Pt 2):541–4 [discussion: 545].

6. DeLair SM, Eandi J, White MJ, et al. Renal cortical deterioration in children with spinal dysraphism: analysis of risk factors. J Spinal Cord Med 2007; 30(Suppl 1):S30–4.

7. Shiroyanagi Y, Suzuki M, Matsuno D, et al. The significance of 99mtechnetium dimercapto-succinic acid renal scan in children with spina bifida during long-term followup. J Urol 2009;181(5):2262–6 [discussion: 2266].

8. McGuire EJ, Woodside JR, Borden TA, et al. Prognostic value of urodynamic testing in myelodysplastic patients. J Urol 1981;126(2):205–9.

9. Tarcan T, Şekerci ÇA, Akbal C, et al. Is 40 cm H2O detrusor leak point pressure cut-off reliable for upper urinary tract protection in children with myelodysplasia? Neurourol Urodyn 2017;36(3):759–63.

10. Tanaka ST, Grantham JA, Thomas JC, et al. A comparison of open vs laparoscopic pediatric pyeloplasty using the pediatric health information system database—do benefits of laparoscopic approach recede at younger ages? J Urol 2008; 180(4):1479–85.

11. Kim WJ, Shiroyanagi Y, Yamazaki Y. Can bladder wall thickness predict videourodynamic findings in children with spina bifida? J Urol 2015;194(1): 180–3.

12. Silva JAF, Gonsalves M, de CD, et al. Association between the bladder wall thickness and urodynamic findings in patients with spinal cord injury. World J Urol 2015;33(1):131–5.

13. Woodhouse CRJ. Myelomeningocele in young adults. BJU Int 2005;95(2):223–30.

14. Sawin KJ, Liu T, Ward E, et al. The national spina bifida patient registry: profile of a large cohort of participants from the first 10 clinics. J Pediatr 2015;166(2):444–50.e1.

15. Diokno AC, Sonda LP, Hollander JB, et al. Fate of patients started on clean intermittent self-catheterization therapy 10 years ago. J Urol 1983; 129(6):1120–2.

16. Dik P, Klijn AJ, van Gool JD, et al. Early start to therapy preserves kidney function in spina bifida patients. Eur Urol 2006;49(5):908–13.

17. de Jong TPVM, Chrzan R, Klijn AJ, et al. Treatment of the neurogenic bladder in spina bifida. Pediatr Nephrol 2008;23(6):889–96.

18. Szymanski KM, Misseri R, Whittam B, et al. Mortality after bladder augmentation in children with spina bifida. J Urol 2015;193(2):643–8.

19. Lee JH, Kim KR, Lee YS, et al. Efficacy, tolerability, and safety of oxybutynin chloride in pediatric neurogenic bladder with spinal dysraphism: a retrospective, multicenter, observational study. Korean J Urol 2014;55(12):828–33.

20. Humblet M, Verpoorten C, Christiaens M-H, et al. Long-term outcome of intravesical oxybutynin in children with detrusor-sphincter dyssynergia: with special reference to age-dependent parameters. Neurourol Urodyn 2015;34(4):336–42.

21. Blais A-S, Nadeau G, Moore K, et al. Prospective pilot study of mirabegron in pediatric patients with overactive bladder. Eur Urol 2016;70(1):9–13.

22. Riccabona M, Koen M, Schindler M, et al. Botulinum-A toxin injection into the detrusor: a safe alternative in the treatment of children with myelomeningocele with detrusor hyperreflexia. J Urol 2004;171(2 Pt 1):845–8 [discussion: 848].

23. Figueroa V, Romao R, Pippi Salle JL, et al. Single-center experience with botulinum toxin endoscopic detrusor injection for the treatment of congenital neuropathic bladder in children: effect of dose adjustment, multiple injections, and avoidance of reconstructive procedures. J Pediatr Urol 2014; 10(2):368–73.

24. Khan MK, VanderBrink BA, DeFoor WR, et al. Botulinum toxin injection in the pediatric population with medically refractory neuropathic bladder. J Pediatr Urol 2016;12(2):104. e1–e6.

25. Greer T, Abbott J, Breytenbach W, et al. Ten years of experience with intravesical and intrasphincteric onabotulinumtoxinA in children. J Pediatr Urol 2016;12(2):94. e1–e6.

26. Tiryaki S, Yagmur I, Parlar Y, et al. Botulinum injection is useless on fibrotic neuropathic bladders. J Pediatr Urol 2015;11(1):27. e1–e4.

27. Kim SW, Choi JH, Lee YS, et al. Preoperative urodynamic factors predicting outcome of botulinum

toxin-A intradetrusor injection in children with neurogenic detrusor overactivity. Urology 2014; 84(6):1480–4.

28. Kask M, Rintala R, Taskinen S. Effect of onabotuli-numtoxinA treatment on symptoms and urodynamic findings in pediatric neurogenic bladder. J Pediatr Urol 2014;10(2):280–3.

29. Chohan N, Hilton P, Brown K, et al. Efficacy and duration of response to botulinum neurotoxin A (onabotulinumA) as a treatment for detrusor overactivity in women. Int Urogynecol J 2015;26(11): 1605–12.

30. Grimsby GM, Menon V, Schlomer BJ, et al. Long-term outcomes of bladder neck reconstruction without augmentation cystoplasty in children. J Urol 2016;195(1):155–61.

31. Dave S, Pippi Salle JL, Lorenzo AJ, et al. Is long-term bladder deterioration inevitable following successful isolated bladder outlet procedures in children with neuropathic bladder dysfunction? J Urol 2008;179(5):1991–6 [discussion: 1996].

32. Whittam B, Szymanski K, Misseri R, et al. Long-term fate of the bladder after isolated bladder neck procedure. J Pediatr Urol 2014;10(5):886–91.

33. Mundy AR, Stephenson TP. "Clam" ileocystoplasty for the treatment of refractory urge incontinence. Br J Urol 1985;57(6):641–6.

34. Adams MC, Mitchell ME, Rink RC. Gastrocysto-plasty: an alternative solution to the problem of urological reconstruction in the severely compromised patient. J Urol 1988;140(5 Pt 2):1152–6.

35. Kurzrock EA, Baskin LS, Kogan BA. Gastrocysto-plasty: is there a consensus? World J Urol 1998; 16(4):242–50.

36. Hubert KC, Large T, Leiser J, et al. Long-term renal functional outcomes after primary gastrocysto-plasty. J Urol 2015;193(6):2079–84.

37. Castellan M, Gosalbez R, Bar-Yosef Y, et al. Complications after use of gastric segments for lower urinary tract reconstruction. J Urol 2012;187(5): 1823–7.

38. Schlomer BJ, Copp HL. Cumulative incidence of outcomes and urologic procedures after augmentation cystoplasty. J Pediatr Urol 2014;10(6): 1043–50.

39. Higuchi TT, Granberg CF, Fox JA, et al. Augmentation cystoplasty and risk of neoplasia: fact, fiction and controversy. J Urol 2010;184(6):2492–6.

40. Soergel TM, Cain MP, Misseri R, et al. Transitional cell carcinoma of the bladder following augmentation cystoplasty for the neuropathic bladder. J Urol 2004;172(4 Pt 2):1649–51 [discussion: 1651–2].

41. Hafez AT, McLorie G, Gilday D, et al. Long-term evaluation of metabolic profile and bone mineral density after ileocystoplasty in children. J Urol 2003;170(4 Pt 2):1639–41 [discussion: 1641–2].

42. Vanderbrink BA, Cain MP, King S, et al. Is oral vitamin B(12) therapy effective for vitamin B(12) deficiency in patients with prior ileocystoplasty? J Urol 2010;184(4 Suppl):1781–5.

43. Szymanski KM, Rink RC, Whittam B, et al. Long-term outcomes of the Kropp and Salle urethral lengthening bladder neck reconstruction procedures. J Pediatr Urol 2016;12(6):403.e1–7.

44. Watanabe T, Rivas DA, Smith R, et al. The effect of urinary tract reconstruction on neurologically impaired women previously treated with an indwelling urethral catheter. J Urol 1996;156(6): 1926–8.

45. Szymanski KM, Cain MP, Whittam B, et al. All incontinence is not created equal: impact of urinary and fecal incontinence on quality of life in adults with spina bifida. J Urol 2017;197(Part 2):885–91.

46. Szymanski KM, Misseri R, Whittam B, et al. Quantity, not frequency, predicts bother with urinary incontinence and its impact on quality of life in adults with spina bifida. J Urol 2016;195(4 Pt 2): 1263–9.

47. Metcalfe PD, Cain MP, Kaefer M, et al. What is the need for additional bladder surgery after bladder augmentation in childhood? J Urol 2006; 176(4 Pt 2):1801–5 [discussion: 1805].

48. Hitchcock RJ, Duffy PG, Malone PS. Ureterocysto-plasty: the "bladder" augmentation of choice. Br J Urol 1994;73(5):575–9.

49. Johal NS, Hamid R, Aslam Z, et al. Ureterocysto-plasty: long-term functional results. J Urol 2008; 179(6):2373–5 [discussion: 2376].

50. Husmann DA, Snodgrass WT, Koyle MA, et al. Ureterocystoplasty: indications for a successful augmentation. J Urol 2004;171(1):376–80.

51. MacNeily AE, Afshar K, Coleman GU, et al. Autoaugmentation by detrusor myotomy: its lack of effectiveness in the management of congenital neuropathic bladder. J Urol 2003;170(4 Pt 2): 1643–6 [discussion: 1646].

52. Veenboer PW, Nadorp S, de Jong TPVM, et al. Enterocystoplasty vs detrusorectomy: outcome in the adult with spina bifida. J Urol 2013;189(3): 1066–70.

53. Blyth B, Ewalt DH, Duckett JW, et al. Lithogenic properties of enterocystoplasty. J Urol 1992;148(2 Pt 2):575–7 [discussion: 578–9].

54. Palmer LS, Franco I, Reda EF, et al. Endoscopic management of bladder calculi following augmentation cystoplasty. Urology 1994;44(6):902–4.

55. Mathoera RB, Kok DJ, Nijman RJ. Bladder calculi in augmentation cystoplasty in children. Urology 2000;56(3):482–7.

56. DeFoor W, Minevich E, Reddy P, et al. Bladder calculi after augmentation cystoplasty: risk factors and prevention strategies. J Urol 2004; 172(5 Pt 1):1964–6.

57. Kaefer M, Hendren WH, Bauer SB, et al. Reservoir calculi: a comparison of reservoirs constructed from stomach and other enteric segments. J Urol 1998;160(6 Pt 1):2187–90.

58. Kronner KM, Casale AJ, Cain MP, et al. Bladder calculi in the pediatric augmented bladder. J Urol 1998;160(3 Pt 2):1096–8 [discussion: 1103].

59. Palmer LS, Franco I, Kogan SJ, et al. Urolithiasis in children following augmentation cystoplasty. J Urol 1993;150(2 Pt 2):726–9.

60. Khoury AE, Salomon M, Doche R, et al. Stone formation after augmentation cystoplasty: the role of intestinal mucus. J Urol 1997;158(3 Pt 2):1133–7.

61. Clark T, Pope JC, Adams MC, et al. Factors that influence outcomes of the Mitrofanoff and Malone antegrade continence enema reconstructive procedures in children. J Urol 2002;168(4 Pt 1):1537–40 [discussion: 1540].

62. Kisku S, Sen S, Karl S, et al. Bladder calculi in the augmented bladder: a follow-up study of 160 children and adolescents. J Pediatr Urol 2015;11(2):66. e1–e6.

63. Szymanski KM, Misseri R, Whittam B, et al. Bladder stones after bladder augmentation are not what they seem. J Pediatr Urol 2016;12(2):98. e1–e6.

64. Husmann DA. Long-term complications following bladder augmentations in patients with spina bifida: bladder calculi, perforation of the augmented bladder and upper tract deterioration. Transl Androl Urol 2016;5(1):3–11.

65. Szymanski KM, Misseri R, Whittam B, et al. Cutting for stone in augmented bladders–what is the risk of recurrence and is it impacted by treatment modality? J Urol 2014;191(5):1375–80.

66. Salah MA, Holman E, Khan AM, et al. Percutaneous cystolithotomy for pediatric endemic bladder stone: experience with 155 cases from 2 developing countries. J Pediatr Surg 2005;40(10):1628–31.

67. Rhee AC, Cain MP. Percutaneous cystolithotomy in the pediatric neuropathic bladder with laparoscopic trocar access: a modified approach useful for the augmented and native bladder, and continent urinary reservoir. J Pediatr Urol 2013;9(3):289–92.

68. Mingin GC, Nguyen HT, Mathias RS, et al. Growth and metabolic consequences of bladder augmentation in children with myelomeningocele and bladder exstrophy. Pediatrics 2002;110(6):1193–8.

69. Koch MO, McDougal WS, Thompson CO. Mechanisms of solute transport following urinary diversion through intestinal segments: an experimental study with rats. J Urol 1991;146(5):1390–4.

70. Roth JD, Koch MO. Metabolic and nutritional consequences of urinary diversion using intestinal segments to reconstruct the urinary tract. Urol Clin North Am 2018;45(1):19–24.

71. Mingin G, Maroni P, Gerharz EW, et al. Linear growth after enterocystoplasty in children and adolescents: a review. World J Urol 2004;22(3):196–9.

72. Stein R, Schröder A, Thüroff JW. Bladder augmentation and urinary diversion in patients with neurogenic bladder: non-surgical considerations. J Pediatr Urol 2012;8(2):145–52.

73. Richards P, Chamberlain MJ, Wrong OM. Treatment of osteomalacia of renal tubular acidosis by sodium bicarbonate alone. Lancet 1972;2(7785):994–7.

74. Siklos P, Davie M, Jung RT, et al. Osteomalacia in ureterosigmoidostomy: healing by correction of the acidosis. Br J Urol 1980;52(1):61–2.

75. Perry W, Allen LN, Stamp TC, et al. Vitamin D resistance in osteomalacia after ureterosigmoidostomy. N Engl J Med 1977;297(20):1110–2.

76. Metcalfe PD, Casale AJ, Kaefer MA, et al. Spontaneous bladder perforations: a report of 500 augmentations in children and analysis of risk. J Urol 2006;175(4):1466–70 [discussion: 1470–1].

77. Krishna A, Gough DC, Fishwick J, et al. Ileocystoplasty in children: assessing safety and success. Eur Urol 1995;27(1):62–6.

78. Flood HD, Malhotra SJ, O'Connell HE, et al. Long-term results and complications using augmentation cystoplasty in reconstructive urology. Neurourol Urodyn 1995;14(4):297–309.

79. Bertschy C, Bawab F, Liard A, et al. Enterocystoplasty complications in children. A study of 30 cases. Eur J Pediatr Surg 2000;10(1):30–4.

80. Shekarriz B, Upadhyay J, Demirbilek S, et al. Surgical complications of bladder augmentation: comparison between various enterocystoplasties in 133 patients. Urology 2000;55(1):123–8.

81. DeFoor W, Tackett L, Minevich E, et al. Risk factors for spontaneous bladder perforation after augmentation cystoplasty. Urology 2003;62(4):737–41.

82. Elder JS, Snyder HM, Hulbert WC, et al. Perforation of the augmented bladder in patients undergoing clean intermittent catheterization. J Urol 1988;140(5 Pt 2):1159–62.

83. Rushton HG, Woodard JR, Parrott TS, et al. Delayed bladder rupture after augmentation enterocystoplasty. J Urol 1988;140(2):344–6.

84. Anderson PA, Rickwood AM. Detrusor hyperreflexia as a factor in spontaneous perforation of augmentation cystoplasty for neuropathic bladder. Br J Urol 1991;67(2):210–2.

85. Crane JM, Scherz HS, Billman GF, et al. Ischemic necrosis: a hypothesis to explain the pathogenesis of spontaneously ruptured enterocystoplasty. J Urol 1991;146(1):141–4.

86. Rosen MA, Light JK. Spontaneous bladder rupture following augmentation enterocystoplasty. J Urol 1991;146(5):1232–4.

87. Bauer SB, Hendren WH, Kozakewich H, et al. Perforation of the augmented bladder. J Urol 1992;148(2 Pt 2):699–703.

88. Yerkes EB, Rink RC, Cain MP, et al. Shunt infection and malfunction after augmentation cystoplasty. J Urol 2001;165(6 Pt 2):2262–4.

89. Fox JA, Husmann DA. Continent urinary diversion in childhood: complications of alcohol abuse developing in adulthood. J Urol 2010;183(6): 2342–6.

90. Karmazyn B, Gurram S, Marine MB, et al. Is CT cystography an accurate study in the evaluation of spontaneous perforation of augmented bladder in children and adolescents? J Pediatr Urol 2015; 11(5):267. e1–e6.

91. Lindenbaum J, Healton EB, Savage DG, et al. Neuropsychiatric disorders caused by cobalamin deficiency in the absence of anemia or macrocytosis. N Engl J Med 1988;318(26):1720–8.

92. Healton EB, Savage DG, Brust JC, et al. Neurologic aspects of cobalamin deficiency. Medicine (Baltimore) 1991;70(4):229–45.

93. Rosenbaum DH, Cain MP, Kaefer M, et al. Ileal enterocystoplasty and B12 deficiency in pediatric patients. J Urol 2008;179(4):1544–7 [discussion: 1547–8].

94. Blackburn SC, Parkar S, Prime M, et al. Ileal bladder augmentation and vitamin B12: levels decrease with time after surgery. J Pediatr Urol 2012;8(1):47–50.

95. Keenan A, Whittam B, Rink R, et al. Vitamin B12 deficiency in patients after enterocystoplasty. J Pediatr Urol 2015;11(5):273. e1–e5.

96. Golomb J, Klutke CG, Lewin KJ, et al. Bladder neoplasms associated with augmentation cystoplasty: report of 2 cases and literature review. J Urol 1989;142(2 Pt 1):377–80.

97. Nurse DE, Mundy AR. Assessment of the malignant potential of cystoplasty. Br J Urol 1989;64(5): 489–92.

98. Filmer RB, Spencer JR. Malignancies in bladder augmentations and intestinal conduits. J Urol 1990;143(4):671–8.

99. Barrington JW, Fulford S, Griffiths D, et al. Tumors in bladder remnant after augmentation enterocystoplasty. J Urol 1997;157(2):482–5 [discussion: 485–6].

100. Lane T, Shah J. Carcinoma following augmentation ileocystoplasty. Urol Int 2000;64(1):31–2.

101. Castellan M, Gosalbez R, Perez-Brayfield M, et al. Tumor in bladder reservoir after gastrocystoplasty. J Urol 2007;178(4 Pt 2):1771–4 [discussion: 1774].

102. Balachandra B, Swanson PE, Upton MP, et al. Adenocarcinoma arising in a gastrocystoplasty. J Clin Pathol 2007;60(1):85–7.

103. Vemulakonda VM, Lendvay TS, Shnorhavorian M, et al. Metastatic adenocarcinoma after augmentation gastrocystoplasty. J Urol 2008;179(3):1094–6 [discussion: 1097].

104. Rove KO, Husmann DA, Wilcox DT, et al. Systematic review of bladder cancer outcomes in patients with spina bifida. J Pediatr Urol 2017; 13(5):456.e1–9.

105. Husmann DA, Rathbun SR. Long-term follow up of enteric bladder augmentations: the risk for malignancy. J Pediatr Urol 2008;4(5):381–5 [discussion: 386].

106. Gerharz EW, Turner WH, Kälble T, et al. Metabolic and functional consequences of urinary reconstruction with bowel. BJU Int 2003;91(2):143–9.

107. Higuchi TT, Fox JA, Husmann DA. Annual endoscopy and urine cytology for the surveillance of bladder tumors after enterocystoplasty for congenital bladder anomalies. J Urol 2011;186(5):1791–5.

108. Kokorowski PJ, Routh JC, Borer JG, et al. Screening for malignancy after augmentation cystoplasty in children with spina bifida: a decision analysis. J Urol 2011;186(4):1437–43.

109. Austin JC, Elliott S, Cooper CS. Patients with spina bifida and bladder cancer: atypical presentation, advanced stage and poor survival. J Urol 2007; 178(3 Pt 1):798–801.

110. Lapides J, Diokno AC, Silber SJ, et al. Clean, intermittent self-catheterization in the treatment of urinary tract disease. Trans Am Assoc Genitourin Surg 1971;63:92–6.

111. Hendren WH. Historical perspective of the use of bowel in urology. Urol Clin North Am 1997;24(4): 703–13.

112. Mitrofanoff P. Trans-appendicular continent cystostomy in the management of the neurogenic bladder. Chir Pediatr 1980;21(4):297–305 [in French].

113. Yang WH. Yang needle tunneling technique in creating antireflux and continent mechanisms. J Urol 1993;150(3):830–4.

114. Monti PR, Lara RC, Dutra MA, et al. New techniques for construction of efferent conduits based on the Mitrofanoff principle. Urology 1997;49(1): 112–5.

115. Casale AJ. A long continent ileovesicostomy using a single piece of bowel. J Urol 1999;162(5):1743–5.

116. Szymanski KM, Whittam B, Misseri R, et al. Long-term outcomes of catheterizable continent urinary channels: what do you use, where you put it, and does it matter? J Pediatr Urol 2015;11(4):210. e1–e7.

117. Whittam BM, Szymanski KM, Flack C, et al. A comparison of the Monti and spiral Monti procedures: a long-term analysis. J Pediatr Urol 2015; 11(3):134. e1–e6.

118. Merlini E, Beseghi U, De Castro R, et al. Treatment of vesicoureteric reflux in the neurogenic bladder. Br J Urol 1993;72(6):969–71.

119. Engel JD, Palmer LS, Cheng EY, et al. Surgical versus endoscopic correction of vesicoureteral reflux in children with neurogenic bladder dysfunction. J Urol 1997;157(6):2291–4.

120. Wu CQ, Franco I. Management of vesicoureteral reflux in neurogenic bladder. Investig Clin Urol 2017;58(Suppl 1):S54–8.

121. Kondo A, Otani T. Correction of reflux with the ureteric crossover method. Clinical experience in 50 patients. Br J Urol 1987;60(1):36–8.

122. Granata C, Buffa P, Di Rovasenda E, et al. Treatment of vesico-ureteric reflux in children with neuropathic bladder: a comparison of surgical and endoscopic correction. J Pediatr Surg 1999;34(12):1836–8.

123. Karafin L, Kendall AR. Vesicostomy in the management of neurogenic bladder disease secondary to meningomyelocele in children. J Urol 1966;96(5):723–8.

124. Zimmerman WB, Santucci RA. Ileovesicostomy update: changes for the 21st century. Adv Urol 2009;801038. https://doi.org/10.1155/2009/801038.

125. Wiener JS, Antonelli J, Shea AM, et al. Bladder augmentation versus urinary diversion in patients with spina bifida in the United States. J Urol 2011;186(1):161–5.

126. Smith ED. Follow-up studies on 150 ileal conduits in children. J Pediatr Surg 1972;7(1):1–10.

127. Dunn M, Roberts JB, Smith PJ, et al. The long-term results of ileal conduit urinary diversion in children. Br J Urol 1979;51(6):458–61.

128. Orr JD, Shand JE, Watters DA, et al. Ileal conduit urinary diversion in children. An assessment of the long-term results. Br J Urol 1981;53(5):424–7.

129. Middleton AW, Hendren WH. Ileal conduits in children at the Massachusetts General Hospital from 1955 to 1970. J Urol 1976;115(5):591–5.

130. Abdelhalim A, Elshal AM, Elsawy AA, et al. Bricker conduit for pediatric urinary diversion–should we still offer it? J Urol 2015;194(5):1414–9.

131. Arnarson O, Straffon RA. Clinical experience with the ileal conduit in children. J Urol 1969;102(6):768–71.

132. Delgado GE, Muecke EC. Evaluation of 80 cases of ileal conduits in children: indication, complication and results. J Urol 1973;109(2):311–4.

133. Pitts WR, Muecke EC. A 20-year experience with ileal conduits: the fate of the kidneys. J Urol 1979;122(2):154–7.

134. Retik AB, Perlmutter AD, Gross RE. Cutaneous ureteroileostomy in children. N Engl J Med 1967;277(5):217–22.

135. Shapiro SR, Lebowitz R, Colodny AH. Fate of 90 children with ileal conduit urinary diversion a decade later: analysis of complications, pyelography, renal function and bacteriology. J Urol 1975;114(2):289–95.

136. Schwarz GR, Jeffs RD. Ileal conduit urinary diversion in children: computer analysis of followup from 2 to 16 years. J Urol 1975;114(2):285–8.

137. Straffon RA, Turnbull RB, Mercer RD. The ileal conduit in the management of children with neurogenic lesions of the bladder. J Urol 1963;89:198–206.

138. Althausen AF, Hagen-Cook K, Hendren WH. Nonrefluxing colon conduit: experience with 70 cases. J Urol 1978;120(1):35–9.

139. Altwein JE, Hohenfellner R. Use of the colon as a conduit for urinary diversion. Surg Gynecol Obstet 1975;140(1):33–8.

140. Mogg RA. The treatment of urinary incontinence using the colonic conduit. J Urol 1967;97(4):684–92.

Fertility Issues in Pediatric Urology

Kathleen Kieran, MD, MS, MME*, Margarett Shnorhavorian, MD, MPH

KEYWORDS

- Fertility • Oncology • Differences in sexual differentiation • Pediatric

KEY POINTS

- Improved understanding of the pathophysiology of many medical and surgical conditions and the mechanisms of action and side effects of pharmaceutical agents have identified opportunities to recognize and mitigate.
- Although pediatric urologists should be aware of the many causes of and treatment for fertility concerns, a multidisciplinary, patient-centered approach is crucial to helping providers, patients, and families identify and achieve fertility goals.
- Threats to potential fertility can arise at any point along the hypothalamic-pituitary-gonadal axis, or may be the result of direct end-organ damage.

Although infertility was once considered a disease of adults, improved understanding of the pathophysiology of many medical and surgical conditions and the mechanisms of action and side effects of pharmaceutical agents have identified opportunities to recognize and mitigate potential barriers to fertility at an earlier age, in some cases even before puberty. Despite the fact that many factors influencing fertility arise in children, many pediatric and early-career specialists are not comfortable discussing fertility concerns with patients.[1] This may lead to absent or incorrect information provided to patients and families, and missed opportunities to preserve fertility in time-sensitive settings. Although pediatric urologists should be aware of the many causes of and treatment for fertility concerns, a multidisciplinary, patient-centered approach is crucial to helping providers, patients, and families identify and achieve fertility goals.

In adults, "infertility" is defined as the inability to conceive a child after 1 year of unprotected intercourse, or 6 months if the female partner is older than 35.[2] In the pediatric population, many of whom have not reached sexual maturity and/or are less likely to have attempted conception, fertility concerns are better characterized as changes in fertility potential. These threats to potential fertility can arise at any point along the hypothalamic-pituitary-gonadal axis, or may be the result of direct end-organ damage. Although altered fertility potential can arise from multiple causes, those most relevant to pediatric urologists are described in this article.

Although an evolving understanding of the underlying mechanisms of and optimal treatments for potentially altered fertility mandates that this list should not be considered exhaustive, it provides a reference point for pediatric urology providers caring for these children.

FERTILITY CONSIDERATIONS IN PEDIATRIC ONCOLOGY PATIENTS

Fertility preservation is an increasingly important topic in the treatment of pediatric cancers as

---

Disclosure: None.

Division of Urology, Seattle Children's Hospital, 4800 Sand Point Way Northeast, OA.9.220, Seattle, WA 98105, USA

* Corresponding author. Division of Urology, Seattle Children's Hospital, 4800 Sand Point Way Northeast, OA. 9.220, Seattle, WA 98105.

E-mail address: kathleen.kieran@seattlechildrens.org

Urol Clin N Am 45 (2018) 587–599
https://doi.org/10.1016/j.ucl.2018.06.006

survival rates have improved and quality of life, particularly related to late effects, has become a focal point for survivors and their families.[3–5] Surgical intervention (eg, prostatectomy or orchiectomy), chemotherapy (particularly alkylating agents), and radiotherapy (especially cranial or testicular) have all been implicated in altered fertility in patients with childhood cancer. Replacement of gonads by tumor (as in **Fig. 1**) may also negatively impact fertility potential. Fertility compromise in the oncologic setting can arise from alterations at the hormonal (steroidogenic) or end-organ levels.[6–8] Hormonal derangements can arise at the hypothalamic, pituitary, or gonadal levels; in one series, one-quarter of childhood cancer survivors had hypogonadism (defined as elevations in serum follicle-stimulating hormone [FSH] and luteinizing hormone [LH]), as did more than one-third of survivors of testicular cancer.[9] Patients undergoing bone-marrow transplantation, particularly myeloablative regimens incorporating whole-body radiotherapy, are also at high risk of fertility loss; myeloablative regimens are associated with high rates of ovarian failure, whereas one-third of women receiving nonmyeloablative regimens in one study had successful pregnancies following treatment.[10,11]

Within the testis, spermatogenesis is more likely to be disrupted than steroidogenesis owing to the differential sensitivity of the germinal epithelium (which fosters sperm maturation) to cytotoxic agents compared with the Leydig cells, which secrete testosterone.[12] The direct and dose-dependent gonadal toxicity of chemotherapeutic agents is best understood for alkylating and alkylatinglike agents (eg, cyclophosphamide, chlorambucil, busulfan).[7,8,13–16] Much less robust data are available regarding the impact of contemporary chemotherapy regimens on spermatogenesis and steroidogenesis. In particular, limited fertility data are available for cisplatin, which comprises the backbone of modern chemotherapeutic

regiments for common childhood cancers, including germ cell tumors, osteosarcoma, Ewing sarcoma, and central nervous system malignancies; however, exposure to these agents is associated with lower pregnancy rates for male but not female cancer survivors compared with sibling controls.[17] Although exposure to platinum-based chemotherapy, particularly over multiple cycles, is associated with a 17-fold increased risk of hypogonadism in testicular cancer survivors,[9] much less is known about the spermatogenic and steroidogenic effects of platinum-based chemotherapy in non–germ cell patients. Similar studies of patients receiving ifosfamide alone or in combination with cisplatin are also plagued by small numbers, variability in treatment regimens, inconsistent semen analysis collection, and lack of healthy controls for comparison.[18–20] Bleomycin has been correlated with impaired fertility in some studies.[21]

One promising avenue to understand how exposure to chemotherapy may lead to alterations in fertility is differential methylation of spermatozoal DNA. In normal spermatogenesis, DNA methylation of specific loci is known to play a role in germ cell development[22,23]; variations in DNA methylation patterns have been associated with decreased sperm counts and clinically decreased fertility.[24,25] Altered (both hyper- and hypo-) methylation patterns have been observed in animal models exposed to multiple antineoplastic agents, including cyclophosphamide; these changes persist in future generations, supporting the ability of chemotherapeutic agents to induce an epigenetic shift through differential spermatozoal DNA methylation patterns.[26,27] Differential DNA methylation patterns in chemotherapy-exposed cancer survivors suggest that oncologic treatment may have the potential to influence epigenetic inheritance.[28]

Female patients with cancer may also have fertility challenges arising after chemotherapy,

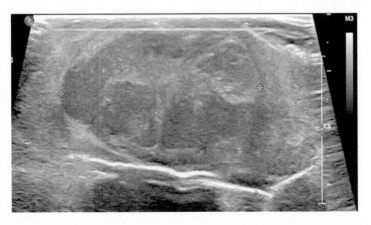

Fig. 1. Testis replaced by leukemia in post-chemotherapy relapse.

radiation therapy, or pelvic surgery. Premature ovarian failure is described as the loss of ovarian function before the age of 40.[29] Unlike testes, which constantly generate new spermatozoa, ovaries have a maximal number of follicles at birth and thus the supply of oocytes cannot be replenished.[30] Like the testis, the ovarian follicles are exquisitely sensitive to the effects of alkylating agents; compared with alternative chemotherapy regimens, those involving alkylating agents are 4 times as likely to be associated with gonadal injury, although platinum-based and other nonalkylating regimens should not be considered to be completely free from potential gonadal toxicity.[31]

Both oocyte cryopreservation and ovarian tissue cryopreservation are options for preservation of fertility in female patients being treated for cancer.[32–35] Oocyte cryopreservation is beneficial in that only oocytes (and not gonadal tissue) are harvested, but to do so requires ovarian stimulation, a process that can take several weeks and may delay the initiation of oncology treatment. Ovarian tissue cryopreservation can be offered to all patients and does not require a delay or hyperstimulation, but carries the risk of potentially preserving neoplastic cells (if any are present within the ovary), as well as failure of the immature follicles contained in ovarian tissue to mature properly. Even when fertilization can be successfully achieved, female patients may not have a uterus capable of carrying a child to term: pelvic radiation or surgery may damage the uterine lining, compliance, and vasculature.[31,36]

As the mechanisms of fertility changes in childhood cancers are further elucidated, fertility preservation through the acquisition and storage of testicular tissue and/or semen samples remains an option for patients and their families. For fertility preservation programs to be successful, however, tissue must be collected before the start of treatment; this requires a motivated and educated provider who recognizes the need to discuss fertility preservation at an often emotionally charged time, as well as a family (and patient) with the interest in and financial resources to preserve genetic material. One particular challenge is the potentially prolonged period between cancer treatment and desired fertility; for example, one study[37] found that although 80% of newly diagnosed adolescents and young adult oncology patients were interested in biologic parenthood, fewer than one-third ranked having a child as a significant life goal, and fewer than half had discussed fertility with their physician. Another study found that patients without insurance, female patients, those receiving treatment regimens classified as "low risk" to fertility, and those raising children younger

than 18 years were less likely to discuss fertility preservation with providers and to make arrangements for fertility preservation.[38] In one study, only approximately 1 in 4 pediatric oncologists routinely referred pubertal female patients for consideration of fertility preservation.[39]

Because children with cancer are younger than the age of consent, parental values and desires may influence treatment choices, including fertility preservation. Although parents are charged with acting in their child's best interest, the priorities of parents and children may not be identical,[40] although discerning whether this is a true difference in values can be challenging. However, one study[41] of cancer survivors found uniform value placed on fertility preservation by both patients and parents. These findings underscore the need for fertility preservation to be uniformly offered to all newly diagnosed patients regardless of cost, for provider education on fertility preservation at a patient-appropriate level, and to use a multidisciplinary approach wherein the responsibility for discussing fertility considerations does not fall on a single provider. Many of the pitfalls and challenges of fertility preservation can be avoided with a standardized process of care[42] even soon after diagnosis, many families will choose to pursue sperm or tissue banking and are satisfied with the process.[43] The American Society for Clinical Oncology published guidelines for fertility preservation in patients with cancer in 2006 and updated these guidelines in 2013; the most current version of the guidelines encourages active assessment of patient/family interest in fertility preservation, referral of interested and ambivalent patients to fertility specialists, and collection and banking of appropriate tissue at the earliest available opportunity (ideally before the initiation of treatment).[44] There are no guidelines on how long banked tissue should be preserved, particularly if the donor patient has died[45]; although this debate is beyond the scope of this article, providers should be aware that simply collecting and banking tissue is not an endpoint for patients and families.

FERTILITY PRESERVATION IN PEDIATRIC PATIENTS WITH DIFFERENCES IN SEX DEVELOPMENT

Addressing fertility concerns of individuals and families with differences in sex development (DSD), given the heterogeneity of this group of patients, ideally is based on genetic and molecular as well as anatomic understanding of each individual with a DSD. DSD is the current nomenclature for patients in whom the chromosomal sex (eg, XX or XY) differs from the gonadal and/or phenotypic sex. DSDs are generally stratified chromosomally: 46,XX; 46,XY; and other abnormalities of sex chromosomes, such as Klinefelter syndrome (47,XXY) and Turner syndrome (45,XO). Abnormal tissue receptivity (complete and partial androgen insensitivity syndrome) are also considered forms of DSD.

The most common cause of DSD is congenital adrenal hyperplasia (CAH) caused by 21-hydroxylase deficiency (salt-wasting and non–salt-wasting), an autosomal recessive condition; 11-beta-hydroxylase deficiency is the second most common subtype of CAH. In this condition, the increased androgen production as a result of insufficient enzyme levels results in masculinization of 46,XX female individuals (**Fig. 2**); in 46,XY male individuals, the phenotype may be less apparent. Impaired fertility is more common in the salt-wasting variant of 21-hydroxylase deficiency and in 11-beta-hydroxylase deficiency, but improved fertility rates can be achieved with suppression of adrenal hormones through exogenous mineralocorticoid administration, thereby relieving the suppression of the hypothalamic-pituitary-gonadal axis and promoting ovulation.[46–49] Male individuals with CAH may also develop adrenal rests that can enlarge and sterically block the reproductive tract.[46,47] Patients with less common, more severe abnormalities of steroid synthesis, such as 3-beta-hydroxysteroid dehydrogenase deficiency, StAR (steroidogenic acute regulatory) protein deficiency, and abnormalities of cytochrome P450 enzymatic pathways, are generally considered infertile.[50–52]

Undervirilization of 46,XY male individuals (**Fig. 3**) may also be secondary to defects in testosterone biosynthesis, in Leydig cell hypoplasia or failure, or in reduced or absent androgen receptivity of target tissue. Patients with inability to endogenously synthesize testosterone are typically infertile, although paternity has been reported in one patient with Leydig cell hypoplasia in whom sperm harvesting was performed after human chorionic gonadotropin (hCG) stimulation.[53–55] Complete androgen insensitivity syndrome typically presents as a phenotypic female without Mullerian structures and with a blind-ending vagina. Histopathology of testes in these patients shows Leydig cell hyperplasia (consistent with increased testosterone secretion in the absence of an intact feedback loop), local fibrosis, and a decreased number of Type Ad spermatogonia.[56] Removal of these gonads following puberty is discussed owing to the increased risk of neoplasia; thus, making fertility potential an important topic of discussion before surgery. Partial androgen insensitivity and 5-alpha reductase insensitivity syndromes have a broader range of phenotypes commensurate with variations in local tissue sensitivity, but abnormal development of Wolffian structures and poor spermatogenesis secondary to

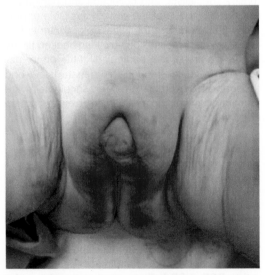

Fig. 2. Masculinized female individual with classic CAH (21-hydroxylase deficiency). Note enlarged clitorophallic structure.

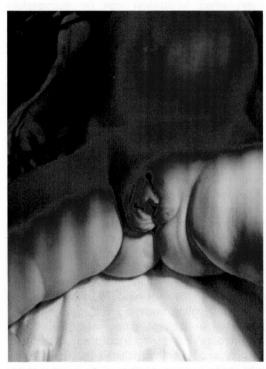

Fig. 3. Patient with partial androgen insensitivity syndrome. Note penoscrotal transposition, poorly rugated and underdeveloped scrotum. This patient also has penoscrotal hypospadias (not pictured).

limited androgen activity may compromise fertility.[57–59] Testes in these patients have a much higher risk of malignant transformation and thus gonadectomy at the time of diagnosis in patients reared female or shortly after puberty in those reared male is recommended.[60]

Ovotesticular DSD is associated with the presence of both ovarian and testicular tissue. In some cases, one of each gonad is present, and in other cases, and ovotestis (both ovarian and testicular tissue in the same gonad). Fertility potential largely reflects the integrity of the internal genitalia; ovarian tissue is often adequate for ovulation, although most children with this condition are raised male.[61,62] However, the risk of gonadoblastoma in ovotestes often prompts consideration for early gonadectomy, which may negatively impact future fertility.[60]

Individuals with DSDs are at risk for hypogonadism that increase their risk of infertility. Male individuals with a 46,XX genotype usually have testes, but these testes have no Leydig cells and no spermatogenesis, and these men are considered infertile.[53,63] Male individuals with Klinefelter syndrome (genotype 47,XXY) typically present with a tall, thin body habitus as well as smaller, firmer testicles at puberty, although many patients will have subtle presentations and may remain undiagnosed. Men with Klinefelter syndrome have low serum testosterone levels but elevated levels of pituitary hormones (LH and FSH), and typically have small, firm testes developing as germ cells are lost beginning in early childhood and replaced with firmer fibrotic tissue[64,65]; as a result, most men with this syndrome have abnormally low or absent sperm counts on semen analysis. Although sperm can be found, microscopically extracted, and preserved (or used for intracytoplasmic injection) in approximately half of patients with Klinefelter syndrome, there is continued debate about whether this procedure should be routinely offered to young men with this condition.[66,67] As with other conditions in which sperm banking should be considered, the interest in and knowledge of future fertility by the adolescent patient and his family, as well as cost, are important considerations for providers and families.

Streak gonads, associated with gonadal failure, have been reported in Turner syndrome (genotype 45,XO) and in mixed gonadal dysgenesis (variable genotype). In Turner syndrome, patients are phenotypically female but have few ovarian follicles at birth. The ovarian failure also necessitates exogenous estrogen replacement in most patients. Women with this condition are often able to bear children with assisted reproductive techniques (eg, donor oocyte and embryo transfer), but may have high-risk pregnancies owing to co-morbid cardiovascular conditions associated with Turner syndrome.[68,69] Patients with mixed gonadal dysgenesis typically have hyalinized gonads, few Leydig cells (thus necessitating testosterone supplementation for puberty), and very low to absent spermatogenesis, and are generally considered infertile.[70,71]

FERTILITY CONSIDERATIONS IN TRANSGENDER YOUTH

The care of transgender patients, particularly in the adolescent age group, is an emerging focus for primary care and specialty providers. Although diversity of self-described gender is not a new concept, until recently most patients undergoing gender-affirming procedures (medical or surgical) were adults. The emergence of transgender health care in the adolescent age group has underscored the importance of proactively discussing fertility with these patients. As with pediatric oncology patients, both oocyte cryopreservation and sperm banking, as well as ovarian or testicular cryopreservation (both investigational), may be offered.[72] A minority of gender-diverse and sex-diverse adolescents report having conversations regarding fertility preservations with their providers, although at least 25% to 50% of these patients indicate an interest in preserving fertility and most want to know more about fertility preservation.[73,74] In one study, only 12.8% of patients were referred for conversations regarding fertility preservation, of whom 38.5% went on to use fertility preservation techniques.[75] Timely discussion of fertility preservation options is especially important in these patients, as many gender-diverse children experience significant emotional distress at puberty when secondary sex characteristics that are not congruent with the self-identified gender begin to develop; hormonal suppression (eg, histrelin implants) can successfully delay pubertal development both externally and at the gonadal level. Similarly, exogenous hormones administered to promote the development of gender-congruent secondary sexual characteristics will further suppress endogenous gonadotropins, although preservation of ovarian follicles and maturation is seen even after prolonged androgen exposure.[76] As with oncologic therapies, cost, provider knowledge, and desire to promptly initiate therapy have also been identified as reasons that fertility preservation was not pursued.[75] Finally, gender-affirming surgery (including gonadectomy, vaginoplasty, hysterectomy, or phalloplasty) may limit the future reproductive options available to transgender persons.

GONADOTOXIC DRUGS

Successful treatment of many nononcologic medical conditions involving increased immune system activity involves drugs that dampen the immune response and limit cellular division. Notably, liver and kidney failure may result in impaired fertility secondary to influence on the hypothalamic-pituitary-gonadal axis, with fertility restored approximately 1 year after transplantation.[77,78] In particular, pharmaceuticals used for organ transplantation and rheumatologic diseases may have adverse effects on fertility.[79–81] Women with rheumatoid arthritis tend to have prolonged time to conception (only approximately 50%–75% are able to conceive within 1 year of unprotected intercourse), earlier menopause, and elevated levels of anti-Mullerian hormone.[82–84] The effects of the disease and the treatment are difficult to tease apart, because difficulty conceiving and abnormal hormone levels are more prevalent during disease flares, and some investigators have postulated that women with rheumatologic diseases are less likely to be sexually active during periods of more acute disease severity.[82] Regardless of the independent contribution of the disease process, numerous categories of drugs used for treatment of rheumatologic conditions have been associated with impaired fertility. Alkylating agents, such as cyclophosphamide, can cause permanent gonadal damage. The anti-prostaglandin effect of nonsteroidal anti-inflammatories may impair spermatogenesis, although the consistency and reversibility of adverse gonadal effects is not well described.[85,86] Corticosteroids may adversely affect fertility by blocking inflammatory pathways and also by direct feedback on the hypothalamic-pituitary-gonadal axis, but are not consistently associated with decreased sperm counts.[85,87,88] Similarly, methotrexate, chloroquine, and tumor necrosis factor inhibitors all have postulated mechanisms of action that may

impair fertility, but semen analyses in patients on these medications has not shown a consistent negative effect on sperm production.[85,87,88] Interestingly, although stem cell transplantation (particularly after irradiation) has been found to correlate with impaired fertility in oncology patients, patients undergoing stem cell transplantation for autoimmune disease fared better: in one study, 36% of women were able to achieve pregnancy, and no patients suffered premature gonadal failure.[89]

Literature on education regarding fertility preservation in adolescents with rheumatologic diseases undergoing potentially gonadotoxic therapy is lacking. One study found that fewer than half of patients had conversations regarding fertility preservation documented in the medical chart; in this study, fewer than 25% of men were offered sperm banking, and female individuals were offered only hormonal therapy with leuprolide acetate for fertility preservation.[90] These findings support the need for providers to initiate conversations about fertility preservation with adolescent patients in these settings.

VARICOCELES IN PEDIATRIC AND ADOLESCENT BOYS

Varicoceles, or dilated veins in the pampiniform plexus that drains the testicle, are increasingly common in adolescents and even in prepubertal children. Although prevalence estimates are widely variable, approximately 1 in 6 teen boys will be diagnosed with a varicocele.[91,92] The relative venous stasis (**Fig. 4**) associated with varicoceles has been associated with an increase in local temperature in the ipsilateral (and to a lesser degree the contralateral) testis; because optimal spermatogenesis occurs within a narrow temperature window, this excess heat may be associated with decreased sperm production. Oxidative stress and changes in blood flow in and around the testis may be associated with the altered

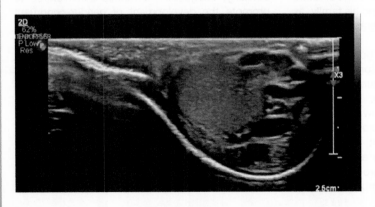

Fig. 4. Grade 3 varicocele in adolescent boy. Note enlarged caliber of pampiniform plexus.

semen parameters and decreased DNA quality observed in the testes of men with varicoceles. Although the precise mechanisms remain unknown, surgical repair has been associated with improvement in semen parameters and DNA fragmentation in some series.[93,94]

Although more than 1000 articles have been published on the topic of adolescent varicoceles, there is ongoing debate regarding whether (and when) to repair varicoceles in pediatric patients. In adults, abnormal semen parameters and a substantial (>15%) variation in testicular size are indications for repair. However, these indications are less clear cut in adolescents who may still be growing (and for whom transient, not permanent, testicular asymmetry may represent a normal pattern of growth) and for whom fertility has not yet been assessed. Published literature on adolescent varicoceles also has few randomized studies, but many meta-analyses; the consistency of data collection in the various studies included in many meta-analyses is variable, with patient Tanner stage, objective testicular measurements, and semen analysis data often limited or missing.[95] The lack of consistent data collection across studies included in meta-analyses makes drawing definitive conclusions difficult and likely contributes to some of the clinical confusion surrounding varicocele management.

Although semen analyses are recommended during the evaluation of adolescents with varicoceles, only approximately 1 in 8 pediatric urologists routinely obtain semen analyses in such patients, with practitioner and family discomfort and lack of patient knowledge cited as the most common reasons that semen analyses were not obtained.[96] Even in patients for whom semen analyses were obtained, there are currently no standard parameters akin to the World Health Organization guidelines for adult semen analyses, making interpretation difficult and limiting the utility of the test for clinical planning. Despite this, at least one meta-analysis suggests that the presence of a varicocele in adolescence is associated with decreased sperm concentration and altered sperm characteristics (motility and morphology), and that surgical intervention is associated with an improvement in sperm concentration and motility on serial semen analyses.[97] However, the relationship between testicular asymmetry and abnormal semen parameters has been well documented. Patients with symmetric testes are less likely to have poorer semen parameters over time, and varicocelectomy appears to have beneficial effects on "catch-up" growth for patients with greater than 10% testicular asymmetry.[98,99]

Although testicular size and semen parameters appear to be correlated, the inconsistent findings in meta-analyses and individual studies suggests that a third factor may modify his relationship. Although this modifying factor has not been identified, one candidate is testosterone production. Meta-analyses assessing serum testosterone levels in men with varicoceles before and after surgical intervention have found decreased testosterone levels preoperatively compared with healthy controls, and often (but not always) improved serum testosterone levels after surgical correction of the varicocele.[100,101] However, these data should be considered in light of the facts that few studies consistently measure serum testosterone, variations in testosterone level do not necessarily correlate with preoperative severity of the varicocele or postoperative improvement in semen parameters, and some men actually had decreased serum testosterone levels following surgical repair. A prospective study[102] assessing hormone levels and fertility in men with varicoceles and a median age of 19 years found no differences in serum testosterone levels, but did find that the men with varicoceles had lower levels of inhibin-B and increasing levels of LH and FSH, as well as more abnormal semen parameters, compared with healthy controls. The severity of the hormonal derangements and abnormal semen parameters increased in higher-grade varicoceles. Again, the variability in clinical results reported in studies included in meta-analyses and in individual prospective studies likely reflects the content and quality of the data collected in each study.

The potentially protracted period between surgical intervention and attempts at fertility further cloud the picture of whether varicocelectomy provides clinical benefits to future fertility in teenagers. One study[103] of more than 400 young men with palpable varicoceles found that, after a mean 16-year follow-up, the fertility rate was 77.3% in those who had undergone repair, compared with 48.4% of those who had not. Mean time to conception was also significantly shorter (11.2 vs 16.9 months) in those men who had undergone surgical repair compared with those who had not. Although this study was performed at a single institution with a single surgeon and had more than 16 years of follow-up, there was no randomization (patients were allowed to choose whether or not to pursue surgical intervention), and nearly two-thirds of patients had bilateral varicoceles, which may have a different natural history than unilateral disease.

FERTILITY CONSIDERATIONS IN PEDIATRIC PATIENTS WITH CRYPTORCHIDISM

Cryptorchidism, or undescended testes, affects approximately 1% to 2% of male individuals after term birth; by the age of 3 months, almost all of these testes will have descended spontaneously into the scrotum.[104] The incidence of cryptorchidism is higher in premature infants.[105] Cryptorchidism has been consistently associated with an adverse effect on fertility parameters, including decreasing number of germ cells and smaller size of the cryptorchid testis in the first several years of life (although these 2 parameters are not necessarily correlated).[106] The decreased number of germ cells is thought to arise from a lower rate of development of Type Ad (dark) spermatogonia from gonocytes.[107] Early orchidopexy (**Fig. 5**), ideally between the ages of 6 months and 1 year, is currently recommended to preserve fertility in these patients.[108] Later age at definitive surgical repair has also been found to correlate with more abnormal hormone (FSH and LH) levels and abnormal semen analyses in adulthood.[109] Importantly, children with syndromes associated with increased risk of cryptorchidism (eg, Prader-Willi syndrome) may be at increased risk of fertility issues despite surgical treatment in keeping with current best practices.[110] In the past, hormonal treatment with hCG or gonadotropin-releasing hormone (GnRH) was offered as a nonsurgical option for treatment of undescended testicles; however, this approach is no longer recommended to facilitate descent,[108] although GnRH has been shown to be associated with changes in the expression of genes within the hypothalamic-pituitary-gonadal axis, which directly influences fertility.[111]

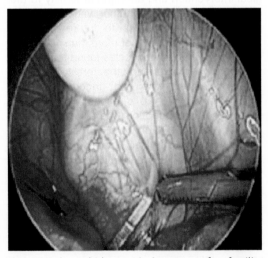

Fig. 5. Early orchidopexy is important for fertility preservation, especially for intra-abdominal testes.

Recent research[112] has demonstrated that the concentration of Type Ad spermatogonia, but not germ cells, in unilateral cryptorchid testes is associated with differences in sperm count and quality on adult semen analysis. Although patients with decreased concentrations of Type Ad spermatogonia continued to have FSH levels and sperm concentrations and motility that were within the normal range, FSH levels were significantly higher and sperm concentrations and motility significantly lower than levels seen in patients with unilateral cryptorchidism but normal concentrations of Type Ad spermatogonia. In patients with bilateral cryptorchidism, hormone levels and sperm characteristics in adulthood were abnormal in patients with decreased concentrations of Type Ad spermatogonia, but these levels were not significantly different from those of patients with bilateral cryptorchidism and normal concentrations of Type Ad spermatogonia. Sperm density was significantly decreased in patients with bilateral undescended testes and decreased concentrations of Type Ad spermatogonia. The investigators concluded that the unilateral and bilateral undescended testes may have differential sensitivity to the development of endocrinopathy, and that the concentration of Type Ad spermatogonia per tubule (at the time of orchidopexy) is a better predictor of adult fertility parameters than the concentration of germ cells per tubule.

HYPOGONADISM IN ADOLESCENTS

Hypogonadism arises when the testicles are unable to produce adequate testosterone for normal endocrinologic and sustentacular function. Hypogonadism may be primary (failure of testosterone production at the testis level), secondary (low levels of gonadotropins secreted by the pituitary), or tertiary (failure of GnRH to be released at the hypothalamic level).[113] In all 3 cases, the end result is low testosterone production by the testis, but the 3 subtypes are distinguished by variations in early-morning of the hypothalamic and pituitary hormones. A diagnosis of hypogonadism should prompt further evaluation for metabolic syndrome and osteoporosis.[114] Hypogonadism in DSD was discussed earlier.

Hypogonadotrophic hypogonadism is associated with decreased levels of hypothalamic hormones (GnRH), pituitary hormones (FSH and LH), and testis-derived androgens (testosterone), and typically arises when there is some type of damage at the hypothalamic level, such as congenital hypogonadotrophic hypogonadism (CHH; known as Kallmann syndrome when it is associated with anosmia).[115] In recent years, significant advances have been made in the identification and sequencing of genes associated with CHH, and many children with CHH can successfully achieve fertility with a combination of GnRH treatment and assisted reproductive technology.[115] Prader-Willi syndrome, in which a child carries 2 copies of the paternally imprinted chromosome 15, has also been associated with hypogonadotrophic hypogonadism and cryptorchidism.[116]

Childhood cancer survivors are at increased risk of developing hypogonadism as well as premature puberty.[117] Precocious puberty, in which the development of secondary sexual characteristics begins before 9 years old, is most common in children who received cranial irradiation at doses exceeding 18 Gy.[118,119] Central hypogonadism is more likely to develop in children who have received cranial irradiation at doses exceeding 30 Gy or who have had cranial surgery with potential damage to either the hypothalamus or the pituitary.[120–122] Primary hypogonadism in cancer survivors can develop secondary to direct chemotherapy-induced or radiation-induced toxicity; the chemotherapeutic effects do not appear to be dose-dependent, whereas those of radiation are, modified by the age of the patient (24 Gy before puberty and 30 Gy after puberty).[123–125]

SUMMARY

Fertility is an important arena for pediatric urologists, as fertility concerns impact our patients and families. Knowledge and ongoing advances in the field will greatly impact the quality of the care we deliver to our pediatric and adolescent patients as well as the quality of life for our patients across their lifetimes.

REFERENCES

1. Nahata L, Ziniel SI, Garvey KC, et al. Fertility and sexual function: a gap in training in pediatric endocrinology. J Pediatr Endocrinol Metab 2017; 30:3–10.
2. Practice Committee of the American Society for Reproductive Medicine. Definitions of infertility and recurrent pregnancy loss. Fertil Steril 2008; 90:S60.
3. Zebrack BJ, Casillas J, Nohr L, et al. Fertility issues for young adult survivors of childhood cancer. Psychooncology 2004;13:689–99.
4. Hammond C, Abrams JR, Syrjala KL. Fertility and risk factors for elevated infertility concern in 10-year hematopoietic cell transplant survivors and case-matched controls. J Clin Oncol 2007;25: 3511–7.
5. Saito K, Suzuki K, Iwasaki A, et al. Sperm cryopreservation before cancer chemotherapy helps in the emotional battle against cancer. Cancer 2005; 104:521–4.
6. Schrader M, Muller M, Straub B, et al. The impact of chemotherapy on male fertility: a survey of the biologic basis and clinical aspects. Reprod Toxicol 2001;15:611–7.
7. Meistrich ML. Male gonadal toxicity. Pediatr Blood Cancer 2009;53:261–6.
8. Howell SJ, Shalet SM. Spermatogenesis after cancer treatment: damage and recovery. J Natl Cancer Inst Monogr 2005;(34):12–7.
9. Isaksson S, Bogefors K, Ståhl O, et al. High risk of hypogonadism in young male cancer survivors. Clin Endocrinol (Oxf) 2018;88:432–41.
10. Meirow D, Nugent D. The effects of radiotherapy and chemotherapy on female reproduction. Hum Reprod Update 2001;7:535–43.
11. Sanders JE, Hawley J, Levy W, et al. Pregnancies following high-dose cyclophosphamide with or without high-dose busulfan or total-body irradiation and bone marrow transplantation. Blood 1996;87: 3045–52.
12. Rivkees SA, Crawford JD. The relationship of gonadal activity and chemotherapy-induced gonadal damage. JAMA 1988;259:2123–5.
13. Meistrich ML, Chawla SP, Da Cunha MF, et al. Recovery of sperm production after chemotherapy for osteosarcoma. Cancer 1989;63:2115–23.
14. Averette HE, Boike GM, Jarrell MA. Effects of cancer chemotherapy on gonadal function and reproductive capacity. CA Cancer J Clin 1990;40:199–209.
15. Pryzant RM, Meistrich ML, Wilson G, et al. Long-term reduction in sperm count after chemotherapy with and without radiation therapy for non-Hodgkin's lymphomas. J Clin Oncol 1993;11:239–47.
16. Brydoy M, Fossa SD, Klepp O, et al. Paternity following treatment for testicular cancer. J Natl Cancer Inst 2005;97:1580–8.
17. Chow EJ, Stratton KL, Leisenring WM, et al. Pregnancy after chemotherapy in male and female survivors of childhood cancer treated between 1970 and 1999: a report from the Childhood Cancer Survivor Study cohort. Lancet Oncol 2016;17:567–76.
18. Longhi A, Macchiagodena M, Vitali G, et al. Fertility in male patients treated with neoadjuvant chemotherapy for osteosarcoma. J Pediatr Hematol Oncol 2003;25:292–6.
19. Williams D, Crofton PM, Levitt G. Does ifosfamide affect gonadal function? Pediatr Blood Cancer 2008;50:347–51.
20. Ridola V, Fawaz O, Aubier F, et al. Testicular function of survivors of childhood cancer: a comparative study between ifosfamide- and cyclophosphamide-based regimens. Eur J Cancer 2009;45:814–8.

21. Wasilewski-Masker K, Seidel KD, Leisenring W, et al. Male infertility in long-term survivors of pediatric cancer: a report from the childhood cancer survivor study. J Cancer Surviv 2014;8:437–47.

22. Webster KE, O'Bryan MK, Fletcher S, et al. Meiotic and epigenetic defects in Dnmt3L-knockout mouse spermatogenesis. Proc Natl Acad Sci U S A 2005; 102:4068–73.

23. Yaman R, Grandjean V. Timing of entry of meiosis depends on a mark generated by DNA methyltransferase 3a in testis. Mol Reprod Dev 2006;73:390–7.

24. Hammoud SS, Purwar J, Pflueger C, et al. Alterations in sperm DNA methylation patterns at imprinted loci in two classes of infertility. Fertil Steril 2010;94:1728–33.

25. Marques CJ, Costa P, Vaz B, et al. Abnormal methylation of imprinted genes in human sperm is associated with oligozoospermia. Mol Hum Reprod 2008;14:67–74.

26. Barton TS, Robaire B, Hales BF. Epigenetic programming in the preimplantation rat embryo is disrupted by chronic paternal cyclophosphamide exposure. Proc Natl Acad Sci U S A 2005;102: 7865–70.

27. Oakes CC, Kelly TL, Robaire B, et al. Adverse effects of 5-aza-2'-deoxycytidine on spermatogenesis include reduced sperm function and selective inhibition of de novo DNA methylation. J Pharmacol Exp Ther 2007;322:1171–80.

28. Shnorhavorian M, Schwartz SM, Stansfeld B, et al. Differential DNA methylation regions in adult human sperm following adolescent chemotherapy: potential for epigenetic inheritance. PLoS One 2017;12:e0170085.

29. Schover LR. Premature ovarian failure and its consequences: vasomotor symptoms, sexuality, and fertility. J Clin Oncol 2008;26:753–8.

30. Wo JY, Viswanathan AN. Impact of radiotherapy on fertility, pregnancy, and neonatal outcomes in female cancer patients. Int J Radiat Oncol Biol Phys 2009;73:1304–12.

31. Dillon KE, Gracia CR. Pediatric and young adult patients and oncofertility. Curr Treat Options Oncol 2012;13:161–73.

32. Koch J, Ledger W. Ovarian stimulation protocols for onco-fertility patients. J Assist Reprod Genet 2013; 30:203–6.

33. Noyes N, Porcu E, Borini A. Over 900 oocyte cryopreservation babies born with no apparent increase in congenital anomalies. Reprod Biomed Online 2009;18:769–76.

34. Dolmans MM, Marinescu C, Saussoy P, et al. Reimplantation of cryopreserved ovarian tissue from patients with acute lymphoblastic leukemia is potentially unsafe. Blood 2010;116:2908–14.

35. Dolmans MM, Marotta ML, Pirard CL, et al. Ovarian tissue cryopreservation followed by controlled ovarian stimulation and pick-up of mature oocytes does not impair the number or quality of retrieved oocytes. J Ovarian Res 2014;7:80.

36. Lawrenz B, Rothmund R, Neunhoeffer E, et al. Fertility preservation in prepubertal girls prior to chemotherapy and radiotherapy–review of the literature. J Pediatr Adolesc Gynecol 2012;25:284–8.

37. Nahata L, Caltabellotta NM, Yeager ND, et al. Fertility perspectives and priorities among male adolescents and young adults in cancer survivorship. Pediatr Blood Cancer 2018;65(7):e27019.

38. Shnorhavorian M, Harlan LC, Smith AW, et al. Fertility preservation knowledge, counseling, and actions among adolescent and young adult patients with cancer: a population-based study. Cancer 2015;121:3499–506.

39. Wallace WH. Fertility preservation for young people treated with cancer: what are the attitudes and knowledge of clinicians. Pediatr Blood Cancer 2007;48:2–3.

40. Klosky JL, Simmons JL, Russell KM, et al. Fertility as a priority among at-risk adolescent males newly diagnosed with cancer and their parents. Support Care Cancer 2015;23:333–41.

41. Stein DM, Victorson DE, Choy JT, et al. Fertility preservation preferences and perspectives among adult male survivors of pediatric cancer and their parents. J Adolesc Young Adult Oncol 2014;3:75–82.

42. Shnorhavorian M, Kroon L, Jeffries H, et al. Creating a standardized process to offer the standard of care: continuous process improvement methodology is associated with increased rates of sperm cryopreservation among adolescent and young adult males with cancer. J Pediatr Hematol Oncol 2012;34:e315–9.

43. Ginsberg JP, Li Y, Carlson CA, et al. Testicular tissue cryopreservation in prepubertal male children: an analysis of parental decision-making. Pediatr Blood Cancer 2014;61:1673–8.

44. Loren AW, Mangu PB, Beck LN, et al. Fertility preservation for patients with cancer: American Society of Clinical Oncology clinical practice guideline update. J Clin Oncol 2013;31:2500–10.

45. Hudson J, Vadaparampil ST, Tamargo C, et al. Fertility preservation in cancer patients with a poor prognosis: the controversy of posthumous reproduction. Future Oncol 2016;12:1675–7.

46. Claahsen-van der Grinten HL, Stikkelbroeck NMML, Sweep CG, et al. Fertility in patients with congenital adrenal hyperplasia. J Pediatr Endocrinol Metab 2006;19:677–85.

47. Nebesio TD, Eugster EA. Growth and reproductive outcomes in congenital adrenal hyperplasia. Int J Pediatr Endocrinol 2010;2010:298937.

48. Conway GS, Casteras A, De Silva P, et al. Reassessing fecundity in women with classical congenital adrenal hyperplasia (CAH): normal pregnancy

rate but reduced fertility rates. Clin Endocrinol 2009;70:833–7.

49. Bidet M, Bellanne-Chantelot C, Galand-Portier MB, et al. Fertility in women with nonclassical congenital adrenal hyperplasia due to 21-hydroxylase deficiency. J Clin Endocrinol Metab 2010;95:1182–90.

50. Sahakitrungruang T. Clinical and molecular review of atypical congenital adrenal hyperplasia. Ann Pediatr Endocrinol Metab 2015;20:1–7.

51. Burckhardt MA, Udhane SS, Marti N, et al. Human 3-beta-hydroxysteroid dehydrogenase deficiency seems to affect fertility but may not harbor a tumor risk: lesson from an experiment in nature. Eur J Endocrinol 2015;173:K1–12.

52. Fukami M, Tsutomu O. Cytochrome P450 oxidoreductase deficiency: rare congenital disorder leading to skeletal malformations and steroidogenic defects. Pediatr Int 2014;56:805–8.

53. Diamond DA, Yu RN. Disorders of sexual development: etiology, evaluation, and medical management. In: Wein AJ, Kavoussi LR, Partin AW, et al, editors. Campbell-Walsh urology. 11th edition. Philadelphia: Elsevier; 2016. p. 3469–97.

54. Guercio G, Costanzo M, Grinspon RP, et al. Fertility issues in disorders of sex development. Endocrinol Metab Clin North Am 2015;44:867–81.

55. Marsh CA, Auchus RJ. Fertility in patients with genetic deficiencies of cytochrome P450c17 (CYP17A1): combined 17-hydroxylase/17,20-lyase deficiency and isolated 17,20-lyase deficiency. Fertil Steril 2014;101:317–22.

56. Rutgers JL, Scully RE. The androgen insensitivity syndrome (testicular feminization): a clinicopathologic study of 43 cases. Int J Gynecol Pathol 1991;10:126–44.

57. Kang HJ, Imperato-McGinley J, Zhu YS, et al. 5-alpha- reductase-2 deficiency's effect on human fertility. Fertil Steril 2014;101:310–6.

58. Wisniewski AB, Hiort O, Holterhus PM. Androgen insensitivity and male infertility. Int J Androl 2003;26:16–20.

59. Mazur T. 46,XY DSD with female or ambiguous external genitalia at birth due to androgen insensitivity syndrome, 5alpha-reductase-2 deficiency, or 17beta-hydroxysteroid dehydrogenase deficiency: a review of quality of life outcomes. Int J Pediatr Endocrinol 2009;2009:567430.

60. Cools M, Drop SL, Wolffenbuttel KP, et al. Germ cell tumors in the intersex gonad: old paths, new directions, moving frontiers. Endocr Rev 2006;27:468–84.

61. Schultz BAH, Roberts S, Rodgers A, et al. Pregnancy in true hermaphrodites and all male offspring to date. Obstet Gynecol 2009;113:534–6.

62. Sugawara N, Kimura Y, Araki Y. A successful second delivery outcome using refrozen thawed testicular sperm from an infertile male true hermaphrodite with a 46,XX/46,XY karyotype: case report. Hum Cell 2012;25:96–9.

63. Vorona E, Zitzmann M, Gromoll J, et al. Clinical, endocrinological, and epigenetic features of the 46,XX male syndrome, compared with 47,XXY Klinefelter patients. J Clin Endocrinol Metab 2007;92:3458–65.

64. Wattendorf DJ, Muenke M. Klinefelter's syndrome. Am Fam Physician 2005;72:2259–62.

65. Aksglaede L, Wikström AM, Rajpert-De Meyts E, et al. Natural history of seminiferous tubule degeneration in Klinefelter syndrome. Hum Reprod Update 2006;12:39–48.

66. Franik S, Hoeijmakers Y, D'Hauwers K, et al. Klinefelter syndrome and fertility: sperm preservation should not be offered to children with Klinefelter syndrome. Hum Reprod 2016;31:1952–9.

67. Gies I, Oates R, De Schepper J, et al. Testicular biopsy and cryopreservation for fertility preservation of prepubertal boys with Klinefelter syndrome: a pro/con debate. Fertil Steril 2016;105:249–55.

68. Hovatta O. Pregnancies in women with Turner's syndrome. Ann Med 1999;31:106–10.

69. Karnis MF. Fertility, pregnancy, and medical management of Turner syndrome in the reproductive years. Fertil Steril 2012;98:787–91.

70. Johansen ML, Hagen CP, Rajpert-De Meyts E, et al. 45,X/46,XY mosaicism: phenotypic characteristics, growth, and reproductive function e a retrospective longitudinal study. J Clin Endocrinol Metab 2012;97:E1540–9.

71. Martinerie L, Morel Y, Gay CL, et al. Impaired puberty, fertility, and final stature in 45,X/46,XY mixed gonadal dysgenetic patients raised as boys. Eur J Endocrinol 2012;166:687–94.

72. Finlayson C, Johnson EK, Chen D, et al. Proceedings of the working group session on fertility preservation for individuals with gender and sex diversity. Transgend Health 2016;1:99–107.

73. Chen D, Matson M, Macapagal K, et al. Attitudes toward fertility and reproductive health among transgender and gender-nonconforming adolescents. J Adolesc Health 2018 [pii:S1054-S1139X(17)30908-4].

74. Strang JF, Jarin J, Call D, et al. Transgender youth fertility attitudes questionnaire: measure development in nonautistic and autistic transgender youth and their parents. J Adolesc Health 2017;62:128–35.

75. Chen D, Simons L, Johnson EK, et al. Fertility preservation for transgender adolescents. J Adolesc Health 2017;61:120–3.

76. De Roo C, Lierman S, Tilleman K, et al. Ovarian tissue cryopreservation in female-to-male transgender people: insights into ovarian histology and physiology after prolonged androgen treatment. Reprod Biomed Online 2017;34:557–66.

77. Eckersten D, Giwercman A, Pihlsgård M, et al. Impact of kidney transplantation on reproductive hormone levels in males: a longitudinal study. Nephron 2018;138:192–201.

78. Sarkar M, Bramham K, Moritz M, et al. Reproductive health in women following abdominal organ transplant. Am J Transplant 2018;18(5):1068–76.

79. de Jong PH, Dolhain RJ. Fertility, pregnancy, and lactation in rheumatoid arthritis. Rheum Dis Clin North Am 2017;43:227–37.

80. Micu MC, Ostensen M, Villiger PM, et al. Paternal exposure to antirheumatic drugs—What physicians should know: review of the literature. Semin Arthritis Rheum 2018 [pii:S0049-0172(17)30747-3].

81. Brouwer J, Hazes JM, Laven JS, et al. Fertility in women with rheumatoid arthritis: influence of disease activity and medication. Ann Rheum Dis 2015;74:1836–41.

82. Provost M, Eaton JL, Clowse ME. Fertility and infertility in rheumatoid arthritis. Curr Opin Rheumatol 2014;26:308–14.

83. Brouwer J, Laven JS, Hazes JM, et al. Levels of serum anti-Mullerian hormone, a marker for ovarian reserve, in women with rheumatoid arthritis. Arthritis Care Res (Hoboken) 2013;65:1534–8.

84. Henes M, Froeschlin J, Taran FA, et al. Ovarian reserve alterations in premenopausal women with chronic inflammatory rheumatic diseases: impact of rheumatoid arthritis, Behcet's disease and spondyloarthritis on anti-Mullerian hormone levels. Rheumatology (Oxford) 2015;54:1709–12.

85. Martini AC, Molina RI, Tissera AD, et al. Analysis of semen from patients chronically treated with low or moderate doses of aspirin-like drugs. Fertil Steril 2003;80:221–2.

86. Østensen M. Sexual and reproductive health in rheumatic disease. Nat Rev Rheumatol 2017;13:485–93.

87. Kokoszko-Bilska A, Sobkiewicz S, Fichna J. Inflammatory bowel diseases and reproductive health. Pharmacol Rep 2016;68:859–64.

88. Dejaco C, Mittermaier C, Reinisch W, et al. Azathioprine treatment and male fertility in inflammatory bowel disease. Gastroenterology 2001;121:1048–53.

89. Massenkeil G, Alexander T, Rosen O, et al. Long-term follow-up of fertility and pregnancy in autoimmune diseases after autologous haematopoietic stem cell transplantation. Rheumatol Int 2016;36:1563–8.

90. Nahata L, Sivaraman V, Quinn GP. Fertility counseling and preservation practices in youth with lupus and vasculitis undergoing gonadotoxic therapy. Fertil Steril 2016;106:1470–4.

91. Akbay E, Cayan S, Doruk E, et al. The prevalence of varicocele and varicocele-related testicular atrophy in Turkish children and adolescents. BJU Int 2000;86:490–3.

92. Meacham RB, Townsend RR, Rademacher D, et al. The incidence of varicoceles in the general population when evaluated by physical examination, gray scale sonography and color Doppler sonography. J Urol 1994;151:1535–8.

93. Bertolla RP, Cedenho AP, Hassun Filho PA, et al. Sperm nuclear DNA fragmentation in adolescents with varicocele. Fertil Steril 2006;85:625–8.

94. Lacerda JI, Del Giudice PT, da Silva BF, et al. Adolescent varicocele: improved sperm function after varicocelectomy. Fertil Steril 2011;95:994–9.

95. Locke JA, Noparast M, Afshar K. Treatment of varicocele in children and adolescents: a systematic review and meta-analysis of randomized controlled trials. J Pediatr Urol 2017;13:437–45.

96. Fine RG, Gitlin J, Reda EF, et al. Barriers to use of semen analysis in the adolescent with a varicocele: survey of patient, parental, and practitioner attitudes. J Pediatr Urol 2016;12:e1–6.

97. Nork JJ, Berger JH, Crain DS, et al. Youth varicocele and varicocele treatment: a meta-analysis of semen outcomes. Fertil Steril 2014;102:381–7.

98. Li F, Chiba K, Yamaguchi K, et al. Effect of varicocelectomy on testicular volume in children and adolescents: a meta-analysis. Urology 2012;79:1340–5.

99. Keene DJ, Fitzgerald CT, Cervellione RM. Sperm concentration and forward motility are not correlated with age in adolescents with an idiopathic varicocele and symmetrical testicular volumes. J Pediatr Surg 2016;51:293–5.

100. Alkaram A, McCullough A. Varicocele and its effect on testosterone: implications for the adolescent. Transl Androl Urol 2014;3:413–7.

101. Li F, Yue H, Yamaguchi K, et al. Effect of surgical repair on testosterone production in infertile men with varicocele: a meta-analysis. Int J Urol 2012;19:149–54.

102. Damsgaard J, Joensen UN, Carlsen E, et al. Varicocele is associated with impaired semen quality and reproductive hormone levels: a study of 7035 healthy young men from six European countries. Eur Urol 2016;70:1019–29.

103. Cayan S, Şahin S, Akbay E. Paternity rates and time to conception in adolescents with varicocele undergoing microsurgical varicocele repair vs observation only: a single institution experience with 408 patients. J Urol 2017;198:195–201.

104. Cortes D, Kjellberg EM, Breddam M, et al. The true incidence of cryptorchidism in Denmark. J Urol 2008;179:314–8.

105. Nah SA, Yeo CS, How GY, et al. Undescended testis: 513 patients' characteristics, age at orchidopexy and patterns of referral. Arch Dis Child 2014;99:401–6.

106. Noh PH, Cooper CS, Snyder HM 3rd, et al. Testicular volume does not predict germ cell count in patients with cryptorchidism. J Urol 2000;163:593–6.

107. Hadziselimovic F, Thommen L, Girard J, et al. The significance of postnatal gonadotropin surge for testicular development in normal and cryptorchid testes. J Urol 1986;136:274–6.

108. Kolon TF, Herndon CDA, Baker LA, et al. Evaluation and treatment of cryptorchidism: AUA guideline. J Urol 2014;192:337–45.

109. Rohayem J, Luberto A, Nieschlag E, et al. Delayed treatment of undescended testes may promote hypogonadism and infertility. Endocrine 2017;55: 914–24.

110. Pacilli M, Heloury Y, O'Brien M, et al. Orchidopexy in children with Prader-Willi syndrome: results of a long-term follow-up study. J Pediatr Urol 2018; 14:e1–6.

111. Hadziselimovic F, Gegenschatz-Schmid K, Verkauskas G, et al. GnRHa treatment of cryptorchid boys affects genes involved in hormonal control of the HPG axis and fertility. Sex Dev 2017;11: 126–36.

112. Kraft KH, Canning DA, Snyder HM 3rd, et al. Undescended testis histology correlation with adult hormone levels and semen analysis. J Urol 2012;188: 1429–35.

113. Dohle GR, Arver S, Bertocchi C, et al. EAU guidelines on male hypogonadism. 2016. Available at: http://www.uroweb.org/guidelines/online-guidelines/. Accessed April 1, 2018.

114. Howell SJ, Radford JA, Adams JE, et al. The impact of mild Leydig cell dysfunction following cytotoxic chemotherapy on bone mineral density (BMD) and body composition. Clin Endocrinol (Oxf) 2000;52:609–16.

115. Maione L, Dwyer AA, Francou B, et al. Genetics in endocrinology: genetic counseling for congenital hypogonadotropic hypogonadism and Kallmann syndrome: new challenges in the era of

oligogenism and next-generation sequencing. Eur J Endocrinol 2018;178:R55–80.

116. Driscoll DJ, Miller JL, Schwartz S, et al. Prader-Willi syndrome. In: Adam MP, Ardinger HH, Pagon RA, et al, editors. GeneReviews®. Seattle (WA): University of Washington, Seattle; 2017. p. 1993–2018.

117. Kenney LB, Cohen LE, Shnorhavorian M, et al. Male reproductive health after childhood, adolescent, and young adult cancers: a report from the Children's Oncology Group. J Clin Oncol 2012;30: 3408–16.

118. Oberfield SE, Soranno D, Nirenberg A, et al. Age at onset of puberty following high-dose central nervous system radiation therapy. Arch Pediatr Adolesc Med 1996;150:589–92.

119. Ogilvy-Stuart AL, Clayton PE, Shalet SM. Cranial irradiation and early puberty. J Clin Endocrinol Metab 1994;78:1282–6.

120. Romerius P, Stahl O, Moell C, et al. Hypogonadism risk in men treated for childhood cancer. J Clin Endocrinol Metab 2009;94:4180–6.

121. Livesey EA, Hindmarsh PC, Brook CG, et al. Endocrine disorders following treatment of childhood brain tumours. Br J Cancer 1990;61:622–5.

122. Darzy KH, Shalet SM. Hypopituitarism following radiotherapy revisited. Endocr Dev 2009;15:1–24.

123. Izard MA. Leydig cell function and radiation: a review of the literature. Radiother Oncol 1995;34:1–8.

124. Shalet SM, Horner A, Ahmed SR, et al. Leydig cell damage after testicular irradiation for lymphoblastic leukaemia. Med Pediatr Oncol 1985;13: 65–8.

125. Blatt J, Sherins RJ, Niebrugge D, et al. Leydig cell function in boys following treatment for testicular relapse of acute lymphoblastic leukemia. J Clin Oncol 1985;3:1227–31.

Transitional Urology

Robert C. Kovell, MD[a],*, Alexander J. Skokan, MD[b], Dan N. Wood, MD, PhD[c]

KEYWORDS

- Transitional urology • Spina bifida • Exstrophy • Posterior urethral valves • Prune belly syndrome
- Disorders of sexual development • Hypospadias

KEY POINTS

- Transitional urology has taken on an increasing importance in recent years, with more individuals with congenital urologic issues living and thriving into adulthood.
- Transition may be a difficult time for patients; families and providers are crucial to successful transition.
- For patients with congenital urologic issues, the urologic goals of management in the adolescent years and beyond include: maintaining function of the upper tracts, achieving continence if possible, minimizing infections, improving sexual function, maximizing fertility potential, and optimizing overall quality of life.
- For many individuals, continued care with an adult urologist beyond the pediatric period is helpful in ensuring lifelong urologic health.
- Much work remains to be done to understand the optimal pathways for transitioning patients to adult providers.

INTRODUCTION

For many individuals living with congenital conditions of the genitourinary tract, lifelong care is essential. Transitional urology, loosely defined as the urologic care provided to these individuals from adolescence onward, has taken on increasing importance in recent years as more individuals are living into adulthood. Making the shift from pediatric to adult care and encouraging a young adult to play a greater part in their own health care remains challenging for patients and providers alike, and there is much to learn about how to optimize the process. The stakes are high for everyone involved.

THE TRANSITION PROCESS

The ultimate aim of the transition process is to ensure optimal care for the individual from adolescence onward, setting them up for excellent health outcomes throughout the rest of their lifetime. To this point, an optimal strategy has yet to be developed; therefore, transition remains a highly individualized process. Although the details may vary by health care system, institution, provider, and patient, the ultimate goal remains the same.

Timing of Transition

The optimal age at which patients should transition into the care of adult providers has not been firmly established and may need to be individualized to the patient based on their unique situation. Although many services set a firm deadline by which the process should be completed (eg, age 18 years), an abrupt and unexpected transition of care seems to be unfavorable for patients and providers. Such factors as the patient's emotional maturity, family support, and current health status

[a] Division of Urology, Department of Surgery, University of Pennsylvania Health System, Children's Hospital of Philadelphia, Perelman Center for Advanced Medicine, 3400 Civic Center Boulevard, 3 West, Philadelphia, PA 19104, USA; [b] Division of Urology, Department of Surgery, University of Pennsylvania Health System, Perelman Center for Advanced Medicine, 3400 Civic Center Boulevard, 3 West, Philadelphia, PA 19104, USA; [c] Department of Urology, University College London Hospitals, 16-18 Westmoreland Street, London W1H 6PL, UK
* Corresponding author.
E-mail address: robert.kovell@uphs.upenn.edu

Urol Clin N Am 45 (2018) 601–610
https://doi.org/10.1016/j.ucl.2018.06.007

may all affect their readiness for a major shift in their care.

A model of gradual introduction of the adult provider into the health care team may facilitate the process of transition for many individuals and families. For patients who require lifelong urologic care, this may start as a simple introduction alongside the pediatric urologist several years before the targeted time of transition. Having the two providers together at visits demonstrates an implicit approval from the long-trusted pediatric urologist. This initial visit also provides an opportunity for information sharing where the patient's history and current urologic issues are relayed by a provider who knows the patient and family well. Over subsequent visits, incorporating the adult urologist further into the team may help to build familiarity and trust over time while easing the individual's trepidation with the new provider. Additionally, if any surgical procedures or diagnostic studies are planned during early adolescence, having the adult provider take part in these procedures can further familiarize the provider with the patient's anatomy and solidify his or her relationship with the patient and family.

When possible, retaining the pediatric provider as part of the care team during the transition process may also be beneficial. Depending on the clinical practice, the pediatric provider may be available to greet the patient and family at the time of their initial visit at the adult facility or may simply be available as needed for ongoing consultation regarding the patient's anatomy and condition. In both ways, the trusted pediatric urologist can continue to play a role in the patient's management and may add valuable information during a critical period of care.

For patients who have been lost to follow-up for some time or who are moving to a new area, a gradual transition may not be possible. Recreating a thorough but succinct medical record for these patients and arranging a telephone conversation between providers to clarify key issues may help to ease an otherwise abrupt transition process.

Factors Affecting Transition

Providers at the Riley Hospital for Children reviewed their experience in an attempt to identify predictors of a successful transition to an integrated urologic clinic.[1] The only factor that showed a trend toward improved transfer was the number of clinic appointments in the pediatric clinic over the 3 years leading up to transition (although this did not reach statistical significance). Other factors evaluated in the study, such as race, age at transition, insurance coverage, distance from home to clinic, and prior medical and surgical history, were not associated with successful transition. It is not clear whether these more frequent appointments were related to higher patient compliance or more active issues around the time of transition.

BARRIERS TO THE TRANSITION PROCESS
Practitioner-Related Factors

Ultimately, the pediatric urologist is the gatekeeper of the transition. A recent study suggests that the long-term relationship between the pediatric urologist and patient may serve as the most important factor and the greatest barrier to successfully establishing adult-focused care.[2] After many years of dedicated work to achieve excellent urologic health for their patient, the pediatric urologist must be ready to entrust the individual and family to a new provider. This requires a certain level of comfort with the adult provider, and possibly with his or her institution, to provide the endorsement necessary to begin a trusting relationship. Over time, some pediatric urologists may wish to remain more involved in the patient's care, and an ongoing discussion about goals and expectations between providers may be helpful.

Identifying an adult provider with the requisite knowledge, ability, and willingness to assume the care of these complex patients is also important for successful transition. Understanding the unique history, anatomy, and social situation of patients with congenital urologic issues often requires an incredible commitment. In some countries, these endeavors are often poorly incentivized for the adult providers and the institution. Additionally, many adult providers lack specialized training in the conditions faced by patients with congenital issues and may not be aware of the subtleties involved in their care. Although many providers have some exposure during training, formal fellowship programs are limited.

Institutional Factors

For many years, transitional care has been an afterthought at most adult hospitals. This has left many adult facilities poorly equipped to handle the needs of patients with congenital issues. Specialized equipment, such as pressure mattresses and specially fitted urodynamics tables, may not be easily accessible. Adult facilities often lack dedicated latex-free environments to accommodate patients with spina bifida (SB) and others with latex allergies or precautions.

Although many patients with congenital conditions involving the genitourinary tract, such as SB or bladder exstrophy, may be accustomed to receiving care in a multidisciplinary clinic, these are often not well coordinated or completely absent in adult facilities. Seeking care from fragmented specialists, often over multiple visits and in multiple locations, is a significant change for these individuals. Dedicated social work and social support teams to help patients navigate the nuances of adult care are also often in short supply.

Many pediatric urology clinics do not have dedicated systems in place to ensure transition of care or appropriate follow-up when social conditions change. At adolescence, patients often move away from pediatric hospitals to pursue employment or college without a plan in place for their next steps in care. Locating and following up with patients after such moves to assess their health status is difficult or impossible.

System Factors

In countries without a universal health system, lack of insurance coverage is a significant detriment to transition of care. Once patients in such systems reach adulthood, coverage via family or government plans may lapse and insurance coverage can quickly become unaffordable. This limits their ability to see providers for preventative health visits, forcing them to delay seeking care until problems progress significantly in severity or acuity.[3]

Patient-Related Factors

For many patients with congenital urologic issues, care has been provided by the same group of providers and their teams since birth (or even before). Strong personal connections may form over years of care, and these cannot easily be replaced with a new provider. Patients may have concern that a new provider cannot understand the complexities of their medical history to the same degree as their pediatric urologist. These patients and their parents have often become experts in their diagnosis and treatment; they are quick to detect teams who do not have an expertise that they are familiar with, and this is a significant barrier.

ISSUES RELATED TO FAILURE OF TRANSITION

Despite best efforts, transition is not always smooth or successful. Some individuals struggle to effectively transition to adult care, necessitating ongoing care at a pediatric facility well into adulthood or foregoing any continuing urologic care.

Some patients are initially be seen at an adult clinic, but for any number of reasons, they may not accept further care in the adult setting and instead return to their pediatric providers.

Although these patients continue to obtain urologic follow-up from their pediatric team, this situation may be suboptimal for any of several important reasons. Pediatric urologists, although immensely capable practitioners, may be less comfortable or capable of managing such issues as erectile function, fertility, and sexual health. With aging, many patients also begin to develop more "adult" nonurologic health problems, such as atherosclerotic disease or complications of diabetes that may be better managed by adult specialists. Additionally, many pediatric specialists, such as anesthesiologists or emergency medicine physicians, are uncomfortable managing patients well outside the age range that they usually see. Ultimately, caring for a large number of adult patients pulls the attention and resources of the pediatric facility away from its primary mission of caring for children.

Although some patients lost to any urologic follow-up may do well, others develop significant issues, such as deterioration of renal function or urinary stone disease. With better follow-up and earlier identification, these issues could be mitigated or even halted before they become major or emergency issues. In a cohort from Indiana, patients who did not successfully transition were significantly more likely to present for emergency department visits than those patients who were able to transition successfully.[1] Additionally, in a report from the University of Michigan, patients who did not successfully transition had a higher usage of outpatient and emergency care and a higher use of inpatient admissions and surgeries.[4] In another study of patients referred to a transitional SB clinic, surgical interventions were performed on one-third of patients after initial referral. This included 10.8% of patients who underwent a major urologic reconstruction.[5] It is unclear whether these procedures could have been avoided with earlier follow-up or transition.

EXPERIENCE WITH TRANSITION TO DATE

Several institutions have reported further on their experiences related to transitioning urologic patients to adult care, primarily in the SB population.

In Halifax, adolescents are considered for transition beginning between the ages of 15 and 16 years.[6] All active medical issues must be managed and stabilized before the transition process is initiated. Exposure to the adult provider is gradually increased with alternating visits to the pediatric and adult practices over the course of the first year. The early years of transition were a high-risk time, with 75% of urologic issues developing within the first 3 years of transition to the adult clinic. Of these issues, 27% were managed with medical therapy, 27% with surgery, and 10% with the initiation of catheterization.

Urologic centers in Phoenix and Dallas reported their combined experience with transitioning patients between 2013 and 2015.[3] In their pathway, patients are referred to an adult transitional clinic at age 18 years and are no longer seen in the pediatric clinic. Overall, 73% of the patients referred established care in adult clinics. Issues with insurance coverage were cited as a primary barrier to establishing or continuing transitional care, reported as a major concern by nearly 50% of those who failed to transition. The programs addressed these concerns by adding social workers and nurse navigators to the team to help navigate insurance issues and social challenges that were hindering transition. Since these cohorts were followed from 2013 to 2015, further implementation of US government initiatives targeting insurance eligibility and maintenance of coverage could further address issues related to health care access.

In University of Minnesota and University of Utah transitional SB cohorts, patients tended to be older (30.6 years) with a high prevalence of active urologic issues (85%) at initial referral.[5] More than 10% of this cohort required major abdominal reconstruction after initial transition, highlighting the importance of continued care for these patients. The authors theorized that a shared transitional clinic involving adult and pediatric providers could ameliorate the high rate of surgical interventions implemented early after transition. Adult providers can offer earlier insight into the issues patients face in young adulthood, allowing their pediatric colleagues to consider earlier intervention for previously conservatively managed chronic issues.

UROLOGIC ISSUES AT TRANSITION AND BEYOND

Although most patients seen by the pediatric urologist do not require long-term follow-up, those with issues persisting into adulthood may benefit from lifelong care. Patients with exstrophy/epispadias complex, SB, posterior urethral valves (PUV), prune belly syndrome, disorders of sexual development (DSD), renal anomalies, and prior major urinary reconstructions require follow-up well into adulthood to monitor genitourinary function. The need for follow-up is less clear in other populations, such as those who have undergone hypospadias repair without complication in childhood, patients with ureteropelvic junction obstruction

after successful pyeloplasty, and individuals with varicoceles that have not required surgical or radiographic intervention.

For many patients transitioning to adulthood with congenital urologic issues, the primary urologic management goals focus on maintaining function of the upper urinary tracts, achieving continence, minimizing urinary tract infections, improving sexual function, maximizing fertility potential, and optimizing overall quality of life. Unfortunately, quality long-term outcome data are sparse given the length of follow-up necessary and the significant patient- and care-related changes that occur over time.

SELECTED CONDITIONS AND CONSIDERATIONS

Although a comprehensive overview of all conditions that may benefit from transitional urologic care is beyond the scope of this article, the following presents some of the pertinent issues faced by many patients in adolescence and adulthood.

Spina Bifida

Renal and urinary issues

Historically, renal failure was the most common cause of mortality for these patients, making urologic monitoring throughout life especially important.[7,8] Upper tract issues are often attributable at least in part to neurogenic pathology of the lower urinary tract. Detrusor-sphincter dyssynergia can contribute to chronically elevated intravesical pressures resulting in remodeling of the bladder wall.[9,10] Changes to the bladder dynamics can also occur as a result of chronic infections, inflammation, or lower urinary tract stones. These changes may cause worsening lower tract compliance, leading to transmission of elevated pressures to the upper tracts or worsening urinary incontinence (UI).[10] Recent data suggest this can improve with careful management.[11]

Adolescence is a critical time for urologic monitoring in many of these patients because multiple changes occur in the bladder, including an increase in detrusor leak point pressure, bladder capacity, and maximum detrusor pressure. These changes can lead to hydronephrosis and worsening renal function if left unchecked.[10] Urodynamics studies are helpful in defining a "safe zone" in these patients: a storage volume range over which low intravesical pressure is maintained and the risk for upper tract damage should be low. Many patients with poor bladder compliance may need aggressive management with catheterization; antimuscarinic agents; intradetrusor botulinum toxin injections; or even surgical interventions, such as augmentation cystoplasty. Although no guidelines exist regarding when to obtain urodynamics testing in patients at risk for lower tract deterioration, a practical approach involves considering repeat evaluation with any significant change in urinary issues. Such changes can include increasing frequency of urinary tract infections, worsening incontinence, worsening renal function, or increasing hydronephrosis. In adult patients with stable symptoms, baseline urodynamic testing should be considered once every 5 to 10 years. Patients also require lifelong monitoring for hypertension, urinary stone disease, and urinary tract infections.

UI has major ramifications for patients living with SB in terms of health and quality of life. The stigmata of UI are major concerns for many patients, and those who achieve and maintain better continence report higher levels of independence and greater opportunities for social participation.[12] An analysis of the National Spina Bifida Patient Registry from 2009 to 2015 with a mean follow-up of 16.6 years identified that 22.4% of participants in the registry had undergone bladder continence procedures, and 92.6% of patients in the cohort were using at least some mode of bladder management (eg, medications or clean intermittent catheterization).[13] Overall, 45.8% of participants reported they had achieved continence, and analysis revealed that previous continence surgery and current bladder management routines were associated with successful continence.

Significant ongoing UI is a prevalent issue among a large number of patients who establish care with adult providers, and many of these individuals elect for procedures to improve continence following transition.[14] Procedures often aim to increase capacity (augmentation cystoplasty) and/or increase bladder outlet resistance (bladder neck reconstruction/closure, urethral/bladder neck slings, or artificial urinary sphincter placement). The type of procedure chosen must be selected carefully in accordance with the patient's individual goals and physiology, balancing the risks and benefits inherent to each procedure.

For those patients who previously underwent bladder augmentation, ongoing care and surveillance is also essential. These individuals are at risk of catheterizable channel stenosis, bladder stones, augment perforation, metabolic abnormalities, vitamin B_{12} deficiency, and bone demineralization. With a median follow-up of 10.8 years, the Indiana group reported their results from 369 patients with SB who had undergone bladder reconstruction with an overall mortality rate of 7.6%.[15] The leading causes of death were nonurologic (ventriculoperitoneal shunt complications, sacral decubitus ulcers, and pulmonary disease). Only two patients in the cohort died of renal failure, and no patients died of urologic malignancies or augment-related complications during their follow-up period. These patients seem to become more challenging to manage as they age, and their risk of surgical complications is significant.[16]

Sexual health and fertility issues

Although most young adults with SB express interest in addressing sexual health issues with their providers, only one-third report they have actually discussed sexual wellness with a physician.[17] In a South Korean study using the International Index of Erectile Function questionnaire in 47 men with SB, only 51% of patients were sexually active compared with 98.8% in the general population. Interestingly, the lower participation rate in sexual activity reported had little effect on self-reported overall quality of life.[18] In other studies, an even smaller proportion of men with SB had ever been sexually active (around 40%) with nearly 10% experiencing some degree of sexual dysfunction.[6,17]

The spinal cord level of a patient's defect may be predictive of several elements of sexual function, including independent erectile function and genital sensation. Most patients with low spinal cord lesions (below L3) are capable of achieving spontaneous erections, whereas fewer than one in four patients with higher lesions have independent erectile function. SB patients with erectile dysfunction (ED) frequently have a good response to oral phosphodiesterase-5 inhibitors.[19] There are also lower rates of intact penile sensation reported among patients with spinal cord lesions above the mid-lumbar spine.[20] Although at least some patients have difficulty with orgasm or ejaculation, the relationship between climactic function and the level of spinal cord lesions is not yet entirely clear. Male fertility also may be related to the patient's spinal cord lesion level, and it is also important to discuss with patients that they may have an increased risk of having a child with SB.[17]

Sexuality among females with SB is also understudied at the current time. Females with lower spinal lesions are more frequently able to achieve orgasm (40% of those below L3 vs 12.5% of patients at or above L3), paralleling the sexual dysfunction seen in the male population.[20] It is thought that the incidence of pregnancy-related complications may be higher for mothers with SB and their children. The rate of delivery in patients with SB is rising, with slightly more than half of patients undergoing cesarean sections (52.4%) over vaginal deliveries, compared with 31.9% of deliveries via cesarean section for those without SB.[21] Mothers with SB have a higher risk of intensive care unit admission and respiratory morbidity than the general population, and their infants have a higher risk of hemorrhage, birth hypoxia, and prolonged length of hospital stay.[22]

Exstrophy/Epispadias Complex

The exstrophy/epispadias complex includes a broad spectrum of urologic conditions ranging from mild distal epispadias (which may require no long-term management) to classic bladder exstrophy and even cloacal exstrophy (discussed separately later). Although some of these patients may have fewer long-term issues requiring multidisciplinary care than those with SB, their urologic conditions require lifelong follow-up.

Whether initially managed by a single-stage or multi-stage repair in infancy, many patients with exstrophy ultimately require additional surgical intervention. It is estimated that 40% of these patients require a secondary continence procedure at some point in their lifetime. About 19% of women report UI in adulthood, noting that the cited group had undergone a mean eight total reconstructive procedures by adulthood.[23]

UI becomes a significant issue for many women during pregnancy, but patients tend to return to baseline function after delivery. At some centers, artificial urinary sphincter placement was once a common component in the algorithm for the management of UI in exstrophy patients; although urinary sphincter implantation today is far less common than it used to be in these patients, transitional providers may still take care of patients who previously had a sphincter implanted. Providers should be aware of the risk of device erosion and potential need for future bladder augmentation.

Patients with a history of bladder exstrophy also require long-term monitoring for their potentially increased risk of pelvic malignancies. Although the actual risk is unknown and depends on many factors, exstrophy patients may face a 65-fold increased risk of death from cancer when compared with the general population. There is a 3.3% to 7.5% reported incidence of bladder cancer (32 times higher than that in the general population), although the studied populations were highly heterogeneous with respect to bladder closure and subsequent reconstructive procedures.[24,25] Although this incidence has not shown a change over the past 70 to 80 years, the risk of malignancy among patients treated with modern-era infant closure remains to be seen. The median age at diagnosis of bladder cancer is 39 years, and up to 75% of patients who develop bladder malignancies have previously undergone cystectomy; this indicates that any bladder remnant left in situ is at risk for developing malignancy. The prevalence of metastatic disease at or shortly after diagnosis of pelvic malignancy is markedly higher than that seen in the general population. The historical cohort of patients who underwent ureterosigmoidostomy in childhood deserves special mention, because providers continue to encounter these patients in adult practice today. Diversion of the urine into the fecal stream is associated with more than a 1700-fold increase in the risk of developing bladder or bowel adenocarcinoma.[24] The significant risk of malignancy in this group mandates close surveillance with annual colonoscopy, and since initiating routine surveillance there have been no reported deaths from colon cancer in the ureterosigmoidostomy population.[25]

Sexual function and fertility are variable in the exstrophy population, and these patients can face unique anatomic issues related to their sexual health. Male patients with exstrophy have a foreshortened phallus at birth; although some of the shortened length is related to patients' pubic diastasis, the average corporeal body in patients with exstrophy is also shorter and has a greater diameter than that of the general population. This yields a shorter phallus with a greater girth than the average male even after exstrophy closure. In the adult patient dissatisfied with penile length, it is important to determine if correctable residual defects, such as dorsal curvature, are present. Some patients may benefit from phalloplasty, but this is generally a select population. To date, no safe, reliable penile lengthening procedures have been demonstrated.

Up to 94% of male patients report normal erections after reconstruction, but half report dissatisfaction related to reduced phallic length.[26] Rarely, injury to the erectile nerves during the pelvic dissection in a patient's initial reconstruction can contribute to lifelong ED. About 58% of patients with exstrophy surveyed with the International Index of Erectile Function-15 report ED, primarily related to difficulty maintaining erections.[27] The rare patient who requires intracavernosal injection therapy for ED should be taught to inject into both corporal bodies, because patients with exstrophy do not develop normal cross-circulation between their erectile bodies. About 75% of men with bladder exstrophy report satisfactory orgasmic function.[26]

In patient-reported quality of life studies among women with bladder exstrophy, quality of life is comparable with that of the general population in all domains except for body image, urinary continence, and sexual function. Females with exstrophy tend to have a shortened vagina with the vaginal long axis lying parallel to the ground when standing, and the introitus is narrowed; many patients require vaginal dilation, episiotomy, or vaginoplasty to allow for penetrative intercourse.[23] Among adult female patients, 81% to 89% report they have been sexually active, and most report good satisfaction with intercourse.[23,26] Notably, patients do score worse than the general population in measures of female sexual function, and these scores tend to correlate with patients' lower self-reported psychological well-being.[28]

Pelvic organ prolapse remains highly prevalent in females with exstrophy and is attributable to the anatomic pelvic anomalies present since prenatal development. The configuration of the levator ani is altered by patients' congenital pelvic skeletal anomalies, resulting in a more posteriorly positioned and laterally deviated muscle complex that yields limited central pelvic support. Osteotomy does not actually seem to impact the risk of subsequent pelvic organ prolapse, and only the width of patients' initial pubic diastasis predicts subsequent risk of pelvic organ prolapse, suggesting that these prenatal changes to the anatomic structure of the pelvic floor cannot be corrected with early intervention.[29] By a median age of 23 years the incidence of pelvic organ prolapse reaches 30%, and may subsequently rise up to 52%.[27,30] During pregnancy, 42% of patients develop *de novo* prolapse that is usually manageable with conservative measurements including a ring pessary.[23]

Fertility includes several unique issues related to the intrinsic development of the pelvis and to prior surgical repairs. Retrograde ejaculation or anejaculation are prevalent in male patients.[26,31] The bulbocavernosus muscle is typically absent or hypoplastic, resulting in impaired antegrade propulsion of the ejaculate. About 60% of men conceive during their lifetime, although the actual fertility rate among men who have attempted conception is not clear.[30] Females are thought to have a lower fertility rate than in the general population, and in one cohort 68% of those who had attempted were able to conceive. Only one in five patients were able to conceive within 1 year of attempting.[28] One in four patients may require or seek infertility treatments. During pregnancy, patients have an increased risk of preterm birth (29%), spontaneous abortion (22%–35%), and major obstetric hemorrhage, and potential neonatal complications.[32] Patients may have undergone several complex pelvic surgeries including bladder augmentation or urinary diversion that make safe subsequent abdominal surgeries more challenging, which should be taken into account for delivery planning. It is recommended that these patients deliver by elective cesarean section at 37 weeks with a urologist involved in or available for their delivery.

Disorders of Sexual Development and Cloacal Malformations

Children with DSD require continued multidisciplinary follow-up that includes urologists and endocrinologists.

Cloacal anomalies are rare and occur over a broad spectrum, with a reported incidence of 1 in 50,000 live births.[27] Reconstruction is a complex process that involves at minimum urologic and general surgery specialists. Data on long-term outcomes are limited and primarily constrained to small retrospective cohorts. Vaginoplasty is necessary to achieve future sexual function. Whether using adjacent tissue, bowel, or oral mucosal grafts, vaginoplasty yields a satisfactory result with 70% of women able to have penetrative intercourse after reconstruction.[27] More than half of patients who undergo vaginoplasty as part of their primary reconstruction still require a second vaginal reconstruction later in life.[33] Based on the high incidence of subsequent vaginal stenosis and the need for additional interventions, some pediatric urologists advocate delaying vaginoplasty until patients are old enough to make decisions about their own care. In some cases, vaginal reconstruction is necessary as a component of the primary reconstruction or may be mandated by obstructed menstruation when patients begin puberty. It is estimated that 42% to 71% of patients are sexually active later in life, and 38% have normal menstruation beginning at puberty.[27] There are cases of patients achieving fertility, with most deliveries performed via cesarean section; however, the data on fertility in patients with cloacal anomalies are exceedingly sparse.

Cancer formation has been reported in the remnant müllerian structures, gonads, adrenal glands, and neovagina. Surveillance should be considered throughout the patient's lifetime. Optimal surveillance regimens have not been defined, but any bloody discharge or postcoital bleeding should prompt further evaluation.

Patients with DSD and cloacal anomalies should be aware of potential difficulties with fertility. Fertility is widely variable and depends on a patient's underlying disorder. Females with congenital adrenal hyperplasia may have decreased fertility when compared with the general population. Patients with Klinefelter syndrome generally demonstrate azoospermia on semen analyses, but paternity is achieved with testicular sperm extraction. Some patients with ovotesticular DSD may achieve pregnancy from functional ovarian tissue, although they generally first require removal of any existing testicular tissue. Many females with cloacal anomalies are fertile but require caesarean delivery.

Posterior Urethral Valves

The incidence of PUV has been variably estimated at between 1 in 3000 and 8000 live male births and is the most common congenital cause of lower urinary tract obstruction.[34] Even with early ablation or prenatal intervention, many patients continue to manifest the classic valve bladder syndrome later in life with progressive bladder and renal functional deterioration.[35] Valve bladders are characteristically small, thick walled, poorly compliant bladders with chronic overdistension caused by incomplete emptying. Incomplete emptying is attributable to detrusor function and drainage from dilated upper tracts. Renal concentrating abnormalities contribute to polyuria, and patients demonstrate decreased bladder sensation. Patients' function is improved by overnight catheter drainage, with or without daytime catheterization.

Patients with PUV require long-term monitoring of their renal function with urologists and nephrologists, and they demonstrate a lifetime cumulative risk of progression to end-stage renal disease. Up to one-third of patients develop renal failure by early adulthood, and still more develop renal failure later in adult life. The incidence of renal failure by early adulthood has actually risen to at least 36.6% in the cohort of patients born after 1982 (the implementation of prenatal ultrasound); this rise is thought to be related to the improved survival of more critically ill patients that previously died of comorbid neonatal disease. In the Helsinki cohort, 22.8% progressed to end-stage renal disease with 32% of these patients progressing later in life, demonstrating a need to follow and optimize renal function in these patients closely in adulthood.[34]

UI and other bothersome lower urinary tract symptoms are common in patients with a history of PUVs. Approximately 36% of patients continue to have issues with UI beyond 5 years of age.[34]

There is a suggestion that erectile function, libido, and paternity rates in patients with PUVs are comparable with those of the general population.[36] However, chronic kidney disease is associated with a higher incidence of ED and may place these patients at risk for issues with sexual function as they age. Ejaculation may also be impaired, in part because of the dilated posterior urethra and bladder neck anomalies. Semen analyses in this population demonstrate some abnormal semen parameters, including an increased incidence of immotile sperm, longer liquefaction times, and variably low or normal sperm counts.[37,38]

With limited follow-up data, quality of life in adulthood seems to be comparable with the normal population in most domains, although those with renal impairment score lower overall.[39]

Prune Belly Syndrome

Prune belly syndrome is a rare disorder that encompasses bilateral undescended testes, abnormalities of the urinary tract, and absent anterior abdominal wall musculature. Although the bladders of patients with prune belly syndrome are normal or enlarged in size, they may empty poorly.[40] Ureters tend to be dilated and may have peristaltic abnormalities. The urethra may be narrowed or stenotic in some patients. Care must be taken with catheterization because these patients may be susceptible to urinary tract infections.

Patients are at significant risk for renal failure over the course of their lifetimes. Most who develop renal failure later in life show evidence of reflux and infection.[41] Whenever possible, abnormalities of the lower tract should be corrected before considering transplantation. Renal transplantation also requires surgical fixation of the kidney, because there is a risk for vascular pedicle torsion given the diminished abdominal wall support.[42]

In general, fertility potential is limited given the poor quality of testicular sperm production likely related to patients' history of cryptorchidism. Some patient who underwent early orchiopexy may be able to achieve paternity.[43,44] Libido tends to be normal, and patients are capable of normal orgasmic function. Ejaculation may be inhibited or retrograde.

Hypospadias

Hypospadias includes a spectrum of congenital anatomic defects related to inadequate development of the urethra and ventral compartment of the penis. Determining appropriate follow-up for patients with hypospadias long-term remains controversial, because most patients with hypospadias do well with minimal further urologic issues after initial repair. About one in four patients with hypospadias require one or more subsequent surgical revisions later in life, including a large proportion of those with complex proximal defects.[27] Most complications requiring revision occur more than 1 year after initial reconstruction, and patients requiring complex revisions can present with recurrent issues well into adulthood.[45]

Even after successful initial repair, individuals may report several bothersome urinary symptoms including spraying (40%–50% incidence), post-void dribbling (20%–40%), and downward deflection of the urinary stream (25%) later in life. Long-term, 37% of patients report dissatisfaction with their urinary function. Symptoms can sometimes be the first sign of a urethral complication, but they can also occur in the absence of new pathology.

Patients can also present with concerns regarding sexual function and fertility. Recurrent penile curvature can occur later in life, especially around the time of puberty when an increase in systemic testosterone spurs increases in penile length. Management is guided by the degree of bother and may be complicated by the need to manage the urethra in such cases as recurrent curvature.

Erectile function has not been studied in a rigorous manner, but there is suggestion that up to one in four patients may have perceived or objective abnormal erectile function in adolescence and adulthood. Up to 37% of patients report an issue with ejaculation, some of which may be attributable to a congenital deficiency in the corpus spongiosum or to a lack of corpus spongiosum surrounding the neourethra.[27]

Infertility is prevalent, and 13% of men with isolated hypospadias have previously used infertility treatments. There have not been consistently demonstrated abnormalities in semen analysis parameters among patients with isolated hypospadias, suggesting that one must have a heightened index of suspicion for urethral complications, such as stricture disease in patients presenting with infertility.[46] Further study of fertility and sexual function in patients with a history of hypospadias is necessary to help with counseling and managing these patients well into adulthood.

SUMMARY

Patients with congenital urologic anomalies have often had complex care that requires coordinated lifelong management. The move from pediatric to adult care is difficult for a variety of reasons. Transitional urology seeks to improve the care of these patients as they enter adulthood. It also offers the opportunity to further investigate the long-term outcomes of pediatric interventions. Much work lies ahead to define optimal pathways of care to improve the process of transitioning patient care and to optimize patient outcomes over time.

REFERENCES

1. Szymanski KM, Cain MP, Hardacker TJ, et al. How successful is the transition to adult urology care in spina bifida? A single center 7-year experience. J Pediatr Urol 2017;13:40.e1–6.
2. Van Der Toorn M, Cobussen-Boekhorst H, Kwak K, et al. Needs of children with a chronic bladder in preparation for transfer to adult care. J Pediatr Urol 2013;9:509–15.
3. Grimsby GM, Burgess R, Culver S, et al. Barriers to transition in young adults with neurogenic bladder. J Pediatr Urol 2016;12:258.e1–5.
4. Shepard CL, Doerge EJ, Eickmeyer AB, et al. Ambulatory care use among patients with spina bifida: change in care from childhood to adulthood. J Urol 2018;1050–5. https://doi.org/10.1016/j.juro.2017.10.040.
5. Summers SJ, Elliott S, McAdams S, et al. Urologic problems in spina bifida patients transitioning to adult care. Urology 2014;84:440–4.
6. Duplisea JJ, Romao RLP, MacLellan DL, et al. Urological follow-up in adult spina bifida patients: is there an ideal interval? Urology 2016;97:269–72.
7. Oakeshott P, Hunt GM. Long-term outcome in open spina bifida. Br J Gen Pract 2003;53:632–6.
8. Woodhouse CRJ. Myelomeningocele in young adults. BJU Int 2005;95:223–30.
9. Mundy AR, Shah PJR, Borzyskowski M, et al. Sphincter behaviour in myelomeningocele. Br J Urol 1985;57:647–51.
10. McGuire EJ, Woodside JR, Borden TA, et al. Prognostic value of urodynamic testing in myelodysplastic patients. J Urol 1981;126:205–9.
11. Malakounides G, Lee F, Murphy F, et al. Single centre experience: long term outcomes in spina bifida patients. J Pediatr Urol 2013;9:585–9.
12. Fischer N, Church P, Lyons J, et al. A qualitative exploration of the experiences of children with spina bifida and their parents around incontinence and social participation. Child Care Health Dev 2015;41:954–62.
13. Liu T, Ouyang L, Thibadeau J, et al. Longitudinal study of bladder continence in patients with spina bifida in the national spina bifida patient registry. J Urol 2018;199:837–43.
14. Chan R, Scovell J, Jeng Z, et al. The fate of transitional urology patients referred to a tertiary transitional care center. Urology 2014;84:1544–8.
15. Szymanski KM, Misseri R, Whittam B, et al. Mortality after bladder augmentation in children with spina bifida. J Urol 2015;193:643–8.
16. Loftus CJ, Moore DC, Cohn JA, et al. Postoperative complications of patients with spina bifida

undergoing urologic laparotomy: a multi-institutional analysis. Urology 2017;108:233–6.

17. Bong GW, Rovner ES. Sexual health in adult men with spina bifida. ScientificWorldJournal 2007;7: 1466–9.

18. Choi EK, Ji Y, Han SW. Sexual function and quality of life in young men with spina bifida: could it be neglected aspects in clinical practice? Urology 2017; 108:225–32.

19. Palmer JS, Kaplan WE, Firlit CF. Erectile dysfunction in spina bifida is treatable. Lancet 1999;354:125–6.

20. Cass AS, Bloom BA, Luxenberg M. Sexual function in adults with myelomeningocele. J Urol 1986;136: 425–6.

21. Shepard CL, Yan PL, Hollingsworth JM, et al. Pregnancy among mothers with spina bifida. J Pediatr Urol 2017;14:11.e1–6.

22. Auger N, Arbour L, Schnitzer ME, et al. Pregnancy outcomes of women with spina bifida. Disabil Rehabil 2018;1–7. https://doi.org/10.1080/09638288. 2018.1425920.

23. Deans R, Banks F, Liao LM, et al. Reproductive outcomes in women with classic bladder exstrophy: an observational cross-sectional study. Am J Obstet Gynecol 2012;206:496.e1–6.

24. Strachan JR, Woodhouse CRJ. Malignancy following ureterosigmoidostomy in patients with exstrophy. Br J Surg 1991;78:1216–8.

25. Smeulders N, Woodhouse CRJ. Neoplasia in adult exstrophy patients. BJU Int 2002;87:623–8.

26. Ben-Chaim J, Jeffs RD, Reiner WG, et al. The outcome of patients with classic bladder exstrophy in adult life. J Urol 1996;155:1251–2.

27. Higuchi T, Holmdahl G, Kaefer M, et al. International consultation on urological diseases: congenital anomalies of the genitalia in adolescence. Urology 2016;94:288–310.

28. Deans R, Liao L-M, Wood D, et al. Sexual function and health-related quality of life in women with classic bladder exstrophy. BJU Int 2015;115:633–8.

29. Anusionwu I, Baradaran N, Trock BJ, et al. Is pelvic osteotomy associated with lower risk of pelvic organ prolapse in postpubertal females with classic bladder exstrophy? J Urol 2012;188:2343–6.

30. Creighton SM, Wood D. Complex gynaecological and urological problems in adolescents: challenges and transition. Postgrad Med J 2013;89:34–8.

31. Gargollo PC, Borer JG. Contemporary outcomes in bladder exstrophy. Curr Opin Urol 2007;17:272–80.

32. Dy GW, Willihnganz-Lawson KH, Shnorhavorian M, et al. Successful pregnancy in patients with

exstrophy–epispadias complex: a University of Washington experience. J Pediatr Urol 2015;11: 213.e1–6.

33. Couchman A, Creighton SM, Wood D. Adolescent and adult outcomes in women following childhood vaginal reconstruction for cloacal anomaly. J Urol 2015;193:1819–23.

34. Heikkilä J, Holmberg C, Kyllönen L, et al. Long-term risk of end stage renal disease in patients with posterior urethral valves. J Urol 2011;186:2392–6.

35. Lambert SM. Transitional care in pediatric urology. Semin Pediatr Surg 2015;24:73–8.

36. Taskinen S, Heikkilä J, Santtila P, et al. Posterior urethral valves and adult sexual function. BJU Int 2012;1–5. https://doi.org/10.1111/j.1464-410X. 2012.11091.x.

37. Puri A, Gaur KK, Kumar A, et al. Semen analysis in post-pubertal patients with posterior urethral valves: a pilot study. Pediatr Surg Int 2002;18(2–3):140–1.

38. López Pereira P, Miguel M, Martínez Urrutia MJ, et al. Long-term bladder function, fertility and sexual function in patients with posterior urethral valves treated in infancy. J Pediatr Urol 2013;9:38–41.

39. Jalkanen J, Mattila AK, Heikkilä J, et al. The impact of posterior urethral valves on adult quality of life. J Pediatr Urol 2013;579–84. https://doi.org/10. 1016/j.jpurol.2012.07.006.

40. Perlmutter AD, Retik AB. Prune-belly syndrome. Am J Dis Child 1970;119:191.

41. Reinberg Y, Manivel JC, Pettinato G, et al. Development of renal failure in children with the prune belly syndrome. J Urol 1991;145:1017–9.

42. Fusaro F, Zanon GF, Ferreli AM, et al. Renal transplantation in prune-belly syndrome. Transpl Int 2004;17:549–52.

43. Woodhouse CR, Snyder HM 3rd. Testicular and sexual function in adults with prune belly syndrome. J Urol 1985;133:607–9.

44. Massad CA, Cohen MB, Kogan BA, et al. Morphology and histochemistry of infant testes in the prune belly syndrome. J Urol 1991;146: 1598–600.

45. Barbagli G, Sansalone S, Djinovic R, et al. Surgical repair of late complications in patients having undergone primary hypospadias repair during childhood: a new perspective. Adv Urol 2012;2012:1–5.

46. Asklund C, Jensen TK, Main KM, et al. Semen quality, reproductive hormones and fertility of men operated for hypospadias. Int J Androl 2010;33:80–7.

Minimally Invasive Surgery in Pediatric Urology
Adaptations and New Frontiers

Kunj R. Sheth, MD[a], Jason P. Van Batavia, MD[b],
Diana K. Bowen, MD[b], Chester J. Koh, MD[a],
Arun K. Srinivasan, MD[b],*

KEYWORDS

- Pediatric urology • Laparoscopy • Robotic surgery • Minimally invasive surgery

KEY POINTS

- Laparoscopy is becoming the gold standard, replacing open surgery in some cases of pediatric urology.
- The new technologic advances in laparoscopy, such as single-site systems, 3-D visualization, and natural orifice surgery, are beginning to have established roles in pediatric urology.
- The use of robotic surgery in reconstructive pediatric urologic procedures is expanding, but there are still limitations.
- As newer robotic platforms and technology develop, there is promise for better pediatric directed options, such as minimally invasive surgical advances like scarless and digital surgery.

LAPAROSCOPIC SURGERY IN PEDIATRIC UROLOGY

Background and History

Since the first use of laparoscopy in pediatric urology in the 1960s for children with nonpalpable testicles, laparoscopic surgery has become an integral part of pediatric urologic practice and has replaced open surgery in some cases to become the gold standard approach.[1] Most of the early literature on minimally invasive surgery (MIS) in pediatric urology included descriptions of new techniques and single-institution feasibility studies that attempted to bring these techniques to the greater urologic community. These initial studies led to a wider expansion and adaptation in pediatric urology in part due to the improved optics and development of laparoscopic instruments specifically for pediatric patients with smaller diameters and shorter lengths, allowing for improved safety and ergonomics.[1,2] Over the past several years, studies have begun to focus on the generalizability of these techniques, ideal patient factors for success, and comparative studies between available modalities to define the associated costs and benefits. In addition, new frontiers in laparoscopy include single-site systems, 3-D visualization, and natural orifice surgery. Herein, the most recent innovations in laparoscopy relevant to pediatric urology are discussed.

Recent Major Innovations

Single-site laparoscopy

Laparoscopic techniques have evolved tremendously from the conventional approach of multiple

Disclosures: C.J. Koh is a course director and consultant for Intuitive Surgical.
[a] Pediatric Urology, Baylor College of Medicine, Texas Children's Hospital, 6621 Fannin Street, Houston, Texas 77030, USA; [b] Pediatric Urology, Children's Hospital of Philadelphia, Civic Center Boulevard, Philadelphia, PA 19104, USA
* Corresponding author. 3401 Civic Center Boulevard, Philadelphia, PA 19104-4399.
E-mail address: srinivasana3@email.chop.edu

Urol Clin N Am 45 (2018) 611–621
https://doi.org/10.1016/j.ucl.2018.06.008

3-mm to 5-mm port sites for camera and each instruments-like endoshears, Maryland forceps etc. Over the past decade, laparoendoscopic single-site surgery (LESS) has been reported for many pediatric urology procedures, including initially varicocelectomy and nephrectomy.[3,4] Several single-institution series have recently been published focused on varicocelectomy, orchiopexy, and extirpative procedures, such as simple nephrectomy, to demonstrate equivalency of LESS with open and traditional laparoscopy in operative time, efficacy, and safety.[5–7] In general, the advantages of LESS over conventional laparoscopy include better cosmesis and decreased risk of port site related complications (ie, bowel or vascular injury, injury during closure, or port site hernia). Several single-port platforms are available commercially, ranging in size from 12 mm to 25 mm, including the TriPort+ (Olympus), GelPOINT advanced access platform (Applied Medical, Rando Santa Margarita, California), and the SILS port (Medtronic).[1]

For transperitoneal LESS, the most common site for port placement is the umbilicus with an incision between 1 cm and 2.5 cm within the inferior portion of the umbilicus, depending on the port that is used.[8–11] An experience at the Children's Hospital of Philadelphia demonstrated that a 1.5-cm incision is sufficient for use with the GelPOINT and can accommodate 5-mm to 12-mm instruments. The single incision can be hidden completely within the umbilicus for improved cosmesis, although objective assessments and patient-centered outcomes have yet to be reported.[9] Patient selection factors for the LESS technique are similar to the established principles used for conventional laparoscopic surgery. Although some investigators have proposed 3 years of age as the lower limit for safely performing LESS due to the port system size, there have been numerous reports in the literature of patients as young as 2.5 months safely undergoing LESS procedures.[7,10,12]

In terms of specific surgical procedures, LESS has been used for the gamut of pediatric urology procedures, with published reports most commonly describing inguinal hernia repair, varicocelectomy, gonadectomy, orchiopexy, nephrectomy, and pyeloplasty. Multiple approaches for inguinal hernia repair with LESS have been proposed, including percutaneous extraperitoneal closure and transperitoneal closures. Intrapertioneal LESS inguinal hernia repairs with slight variations have been described based on simply closing the internal inguinal ring with a purse-string suture versus division of the patent processus vaginalis (ie, hernia sac) and closing the peritoneum.[13] In 2010, Giseke and associates[14] described a conventional laparoscopic peritoneal leaflet method with a 1% recurrence rate. Recently, a modification of this peritoneal leaflet procedure was described, using a single-site transperitoneal approach with division of the patent processus and closure of the peritoneal leaflets with a V-loc suture.[15]

The past decade has also seen an increase in the use of LESS for renal extirpative surgery. A recent systematic review of LESS by Symeonidis and colleagues[16] included 169 patients who underwent transperitoneal LESS nephrectomy or nephroureterectomies. Incision size ranged from 1.0 cm to 2.5 cm and operative time was highly variable, with a range of 6 minutes to 370 minutes. Conversion to open rate was low (1.7%) and postoperative complication rate was 2.9% with the majority Clavien-Dindo grade II.[16] Despite promising results, the high variability in operative time likely reflects the fact that the majority of studies analyzed included fewer than 10 patients and only 1 study included more than 25 patients. Another systematic review was undertaken by Till and associates[17] to determine the best MIS approach to pediatric nephrectomy and heminephrectomy. The investigators identified 11 studies that compared conventional laparoscopy to LESS or robotic-assisted surgery. Although minimal descriptive statistics were presented, the investigators concluded that LESS requires more operative time and has lack of patient benefits compared with conventional laparoscopy.[17]

Intuitively, LESS seems to offer several benefits over conventional laparoscopic, including use of a single larger incision for specimen extraction in extirpative procedure and improved cosmesis. Its expansion to reconstructive procedures in pediatric urology, however, has been more controversial given the current lack of comparative studies versus traditional laparoscopy and robotics. One of the most important factors limiting the adoption of LESS more generally in pediatric urology is the learning curve involved for LESS procedures. Various studies of LESS in adult urologic surgeries have noted a steep learning curve and this is even noted in the 2013 European Association of Urology guidelines for LESS, which recommend that LESS only be performed by expert laparoscopic surgeons.[18] In 1 recent study, Abdel-Karim and associates[6] found that even in experienced hands, the number of LESS procedures required to obtain professional competence in adult patients was at least 30. Unfortunately, there are no similar reports that have been published to date in the pediatric urologic literature on the LESS learning curve. Regardless, despite the paucity of rigorous comparative studies, the experienced laparoscopic surgeon may consider LESS a viable and safe option for several pediatric urology interventions, including hernia repair, gonadectomy, varicocelectomy, orchiopexy, urachal cyst excision, renal cyst ablation, nephrectomy/nephroureterectomy, and heminephrectomy.

Alternative access: extraperitoneal/retroperitoneal

Although transperitoneal or intraperitoneal laparoscopy has been the most commonly used approach for laparoscopic surgery in pediatric urology, the retroperitoneal or extraperitoneal approach has been described for various indications, including inguinal herniorrhaphy, varicocelectomy, pyeloplasty, and nephrectomy. The first use of retroperitoneal access for a laparoscopic pyeloplasty (LP) in children was reported in 2001.[19] Use of this approach for organs, such as the kidney, renal pelvis, and ureter, located in the retroperitoneal space seems ideal; however, 1 major concern with retroperitoneal laparoscopy in children is the limited retroperitoneal space available in pediatric patients and possible limitations of this small working space, including increased instrument clashes and longer operative times. Although age and size limitations for retroperitoneal approach vary based on surgeon and institution, many publications cite an approximately 2 years of age minimum for retroperitoneal surgery.[20,21] Badawy and associates[20] have recently challenged this lower age limit and presented their results on retroperitoneal LP in 15 children aged less than 2 years of age. The investigators found that although the approach was feasible, safe, and successful, there was a high conversion rate to open in children aged less than 3 months (43% or 3 of 7 children).[20]

One of the most common uses of the extraperitoneal access in the literature is for inguinal herniorrhaphy. In a recent systematic review and meta-analysis, Chen and colleagues[21] reviewed 37 studies comprising 11,815 pediatric patients who underwent single-site laparoscopic percutaneous extraperitoneal closure and noted overall recurrence and hydrocele formation rates of 0.7% (range 0%–15.5%) and 0.23% (range 0%–3.6%), respectively. The investigators noted that intraoperative and postoperative complications can be reduced by increased surgeon experience, performing hydrodissection, and use of nonabsorbable sutures.

Few studies compare the transperitoneal versus the retroperitoneal approach in children, and only 1 prospective, randomized trial has compared the 2 directly for pyeloplasty. Badawy and partners[22] randomized 38 children greater than 2 years of age to LP via a transperitoneal or retroperitoneal approach. Although both approaches had high success rates, the retroperitoneal approach was associated with a shorter operative time, shorter hospital stay, quicker recovery of intestinal movement, and earlier resumption of oral feeding compared with the transperitoneal approach.[22] In a separate single-surgeon experience, Liu and colleagues[23] compared outcomes using different laparoscopic approaches to pyeloplasty in 1750 children. Although not randomized, the investigators found that retroperitoneal LP had similar safety and efficacy compared with conventional transperitoneal and single-site transperitoneal LP. When comparing the groups, retroperitoneal LP was associated with shorter return to oral feeding and shorter hospital stay but longer operative time.[23] The results of these studies, although promising, require additional studies to support the generalizability of these findings to other surgeons/institutions and to other laparoscopic procedures.

3-D vision laparoscopy

An inherent limitation of laparoscopy is the 2-D image obtained from traditional laparoscopic cameras. The conversion of a 3-D operative field to a 2-D image leads to a loss of depth perception, which can potentially impact operative time and learning curve. Despite the availability of 3-D imaging in laparoscopy for well over 20 years, its permeability across the field has been slow perhaps due to limitation of early technology (ie, heavy instruments and head gear for displays and lack of high definition [HD]) and equipment costs.[24] Obtaining 3-D imaging requires use of a special camera that uses either a single-lens or dual-lens system. In the dual-lens system, 2 separate lenses sit side-by-side in a single laparoscope and each is attached to its own camera. By displaying the images from each camera onto a video screen and viewing the images with special polarized glasses, a 3-D image is rendered in a process called stereoscopy.[25]

Early studies resulted in conflicting results with some suggesting benefits of 3-D versus 2-D laparoscopy on performance of surgical tasks and other showing no difference between the 2 groups.[26,27] This lack of clear efficacy and safety benefit and the older often bulky equipment with poorer image quality for 3-D led to limited expansion of the technology. Modern innovations in technology, however, have allowed for easier-to-use HD 3-D laparoscopic systems, which seem to offer several potential benefits, including depth perception, tactile feedback, improved accuracy and safety, increased surgical precision with decreased operative times, and ideally a shorter learning curve compared with conventional 2-D laparoscopy.[25] In a recent systematic review, Fergo and associates[24] reviewed 13 randomized controlled trials comparing 3-D and 2-D laparoscopy (only 2 trials were clinical and remaining 11 were ex vivo studies of tasks). A majority of studies reviewed found a significant reduction in performance time and errors with use of 3-D compared with 2-D laparoscopy. Furthermore, all trials with subjective evaluation found 3-D laparoscopy superior to 2-D laparoscopy.[25]

To date, there is only 1 published study on the use of 3-D laparoscopy in pediatric urology. In their study, Abou-Haidar[28] and associates compare outcomes of children undergoing LP using the 3-D system versus a 2-D system. The investigators found that although complication rate and length of hospital stay were identical between the groups, the mean operative time was 48 minutes lower in the 3-D laparoscopic group compared with the 2-D group.[28] Similar results were obtained by Kozlov and colleagues when comparing a variety of 3-D and 2-D laparoscopic surgeries in 110 neonates and infants—decreased operative time with 3-D compared with 2-D laparoscopy but similar postoperative outcomes and length of stay between the groups.[29] Limited availability of data on the use of 3-D laparoscopy in the pediatric population is likely due to the size of the current 3D H-D laparoscopy systems, which includes laparoscope with at minimal a 10-mm diameter.[29] If 1 goal is to minimize scarring and risk for port site hernia formation, keeping fascial incisions smaller with use of a 3-mm or 5-mm camera may limit desire to move toward a more expensive 3-D system with the required larger 10-mm scope. It is likely that innovations in technology will lead to smaller and smaller diameters needs for 3-D HD laparoscopes; thus, at some point in the near future, the benefits of 3-D laparoscopy will outweigh the risks or drawbacks in the eyes of many pediatric urologists.

Recent studies have suggested that 3-D vision laparoscopy may have a role to play in laparoscopy training. Sørensen and partners[30] performed a randomized controlled trial in surgical residents using a laparoscopic simulator trainer under 3-D or 2-D conditions. The investigators showed that 3-D vision reduced the time to proficiency on the laparoscopic simulator and that these skills learned under 3-D vision were transferrable to 2-D laparoscopic conditions.[30] These results are encouraging and suggest that even if 3-D laparoscopy in its current state does not find a more standard use in pediatric urology, it may have a use in training of residents and practicing urologists.

Pushing the Envelope: New Frontiers

As a natural extension of the push toward even less MIS, natural orifice transluminal endoscopic surgery (NOTES) was first described in pig models in 2004.[31] NOTES involves using natural body orifices, such as the stomach, rectum, or vagina, to gain access to the peritoneal cavity, thus avoiding skin incisions and scars altogether. Several feasibility case reports have been published over the past decade using NOTES for mostly general surgery procedures, such as appendectomy, cholecystectomy, fallopian tube ligation, and splenectomy. Despite initial interest and public appeal, several barriers have led to minimal adoption of NOTES in general surgery and urology, including closure of the enterotomy or vaginotomy, lack of instrument triangulation, and steep learning curve.[32] In the urologic field, there have been no reports of pure NOTES cases, although hybrid NOTES (ie, combination of transvaginal NOTES with transabdominal laparoscopic trocars) has been described for radical nephrectomy in adult women.[33,34] To the authors' knowledge, no pediatric urologic procedures have been reported using pure or hybrid NOTES. Whether this approach has any role in the pediatric urology armamentarium in the future remains to be seen and likely will depend on technologic innovation and development of new instruments or alternative strategies to overcome current limitations.

ROBOTIC SURGERY IN PEDIATRIC UROLOGY
Background and History

Although the smaller surgical scars and decreased hospital stays with laparoscopic surgery have been advantageous, the limitations on surgeon dexterity, visualization, and sensory feedback still limited widespread use for complex reconstructive cases. In 1999, the da Vinci Surgical System (Intuitive Surgical, Sunnyvale, California) addressed many of these limitations and marked the start of a revolutionary transition to robot-assisted laparoscopic surgery, enabling more surgeons to perform minimally invasive procedures.[35] The 3-D visualization via 2 endoscopic cameras, tremor elimination, fourth arm for retraction, and 7° range of motion eliminated many of the compromises in laparoscopy. Over the past 20 years as the device has progressed to S, Si, Xi, and the cheaper X editions, the instrumentation has advanced along with visualization and adaptability to resident teaching with skills simulators and a dual console.

Adaptation of Robotic Surgery in Pediatric Urology

Initial adaptation of the robot within adult urology started with robotic prostatectomy,[36] and, in the world of pediatric urology, robotic pyeloplasty became the first index surgery to be performed robotically.[37] LP was first reported in adults in 1993,[38,39] and the pediatric correlate soon followed in 1995,[40] with decreased length of stay and improved postoperative pain control.[41] The learning curve was steep, however, specifically due to the need for significant intracorporeal suturing. Therefore, widespread use of the laparoscopic procedure was limited. Introduction of the da Vinci Surgical System opened the door to reconstructive pediatric urology procedures, starting with pyeloplasty, allowing for the better technical dexterity and surgical precision needed for such cases. Recently a meta-analysis of 17 studies comparing robotic-assisted pyeloplasty (RAP) and LP, found that RAP resulted in a 27-minute shorter operative time ($P = .003$), a 1.2-day shorter length of stay ($P = .003$), lower complication rate (odds ratio [OR] 0.56; 95% CI, 0.37–0.84; $P = .005$) and higher success rate (OR 2.76; 95% CI, 1.30–5.88; $P = .008$).[42] Although the increased costs of robotic surgery have always been a criticism, the rate of robotic pyeloplasty has continued to grow. A recent report of US national trends found an overall 7% annual decrease in pyeloplasty but a 29% increase in robotic pyeloplasty, accounting for 40% of cases in 2015.[43] Although the utility in infants continues to be debated, reports have shown similar success rates between robotic and laparoscopic cases,[44] and the authors anticipate that the use of robotic pyeloplasty will continue to grow and become the standard.

In addition to pyeloplasty procedures, the introduction of robotic surgery has also opened the door to other reconstructive pediatric urologic cases, such as ureteral reimplantation,[45] appendicovesicostomy,[46] and even bladder augmentation procedures at some institutions.[47] Debate remains about the utility of robotic versus open ureteral reimplantation, but a recent multi-institutional study demonstrated no differences in success rates or complications when compared with historical open series, although the learning curve for proficiency was estimated at approximately 30 cases.[45] Other reconstructive procedures, although reported, have not yet become widespread and clear benefits to open surgery are debatable.

Access and Port Sites

In the pediatric population, new techniques for optimal port position have been necessary to optimize the small amount of intra-abdominal space available and the higher sensitivity of pediatric patients to high intra-abdominal insufflation pressures.[48] Furthermore, development of the hidden incision endoscopic surgery technique has offered better cosmesis without compromising surgical outcomes.[49,50] LESS has furthered the progression toward smaller and fewer incisions. By organizing all instruments to enter through a single incision, this technique, which showed similar success in laparoscopic models, is now being adapted to robotic platforms. Although Intuitive surgical has developed its own single-site port, other port platforms, such as GelPOINT, can be used with the da Vinci surgical robot as well.[51] Use of the da Vinci single-site platform for donor nephrectomy cases found that the approach was safe, but the added cost and complexity did not seem to have a tangible benefit.[52] The need for better articulating instruments and energy sources is key for allowing adaptation of single-site surgery on a larger scale.

Limitations of the da Vinci Robot System

Although the da Vinci surgical robot has dominated the international market with more than 750,000 procedures performed worldwide over the past year,[53] there are many shortcomings and limitations, especially when it comes to the pediatric patients. Overall, the instrument sizes are designed for 8-mm ports, which is ideal for the adult patient but considered by some investigators too large for pediatric patients. A few small 5-mm instruments have been developed and can be used successfully in pediatric robotic pyeloplasty,[54] but there is still significant room for progress. Unfortunately, due to a smaller market on the pediatric site, the monetary benefit of developing more 5-mm instruments serves as a great limitation. In the future, there is increasing hope that further pediatric-friendly smaller instruments can be developed to better accommodate smaller pediatric patients, either from Intuitive Surgical or from one of the many newly developing robotic platforms (**Table 1**), because many of the original patents for the da Vinci robot will be expiring in 2019.[55]

New Robotic Platforms—Food and Drug Administration Approved

Senhance surgical robotic system

The Senhance robotic system was originally developed by an Italian company known as Sofar and called the ALF-X. Thereafter it was bought by a US-based company and renamed Senhance Surgical Robotic System (TransEnterix, Morrisville,

Table 1
New robotic systems

Robotic System	Company and Location	Novel Features
Senhance	TransEnterix (Morrisville, NC)	Haptic feedback, eye-tracking camera control system, individual robotic carts
Flex	Medrobotics (Raynham, MA)	Core flexible, steerable scope that becomes rigid once positioned
SPORT	Titan Medical (Toronto, ON, Canada)	Singe incisions, multiarticulated instruments, single-arm mobile cart
Hominis	Memic Innovative Surgery (Israel)	Humanoid-shaped robotics arms with 360° of articulation, miniature motor unit
MIVR	Virtual Incision (Pleasanton, California) and CAST (Omaha, NE)	Robotic flex tip laparoscope + 2 arms, artificial intelligence + machine learning
Versius	Cambridge Medical Robotics (Cambridge, UK)	Force and position measurements >1000×/second, up to 5 arms, lightweight
Verb Surgical	Johnson & Johnson/Ethicon/Getinge/Verily (Mountain View, CA)	Surgery 4.0—digital surgery combining robotics with data-driven machine learning

North Carolina). The system recently received Food and Drug Administration (FDA) approval in October 2017 for gynecologic and colorectal procedures.[56] At present the only urologic studies have been in porcine models,[57] but Senhance has shown safe and successful outcomes in hysterectomy cases[58–61] and colorectal surgery.[62]

The system is comprised of a remote-control station unit, referred to as the cockpit, manipulator arms, and a connection node. There can be up to 4 robotic arms, each on its own individual cart as opposed to the single cart used in the da Vinci setup. The laparoscopic instruments are attached via magnets, allowing for quicker exchanges during the case. They all require 5-mm ports, except for the articulating needle holder and camera, which require a 10-mm port.[63] At present, there is no articulating cutting tool for the system, but it is in development.[64] The robotic arms provide the same 7° of freedom but in addition have haptic feedback to better facilitate dissection and suturing. The haptic sensing allows for both 1:1 scaled force feedback as well as perception of tissue consistency and instrument stress. At the cockpit, the surgeon has comfortable ergonomic positioning and control of a remote HD 3-D technology display through an eye-tracking camera control system.[63] The camera centers the image automatically to the point the surgeon is looking at, and the zoom can be controlled by the surgeon's head movements forward or backward relative to the display monitor. Furthermore, the entire room shares the same screen as the surgeon, allowing optimal visualization for all. The system seems to have some significant disadvantages, however, starting from the bulky equipment size, lack of articulating instruments, and need for polarizing glasses for the 3D-monitor eye tracking.[55,65]

Flex robotic system

The Flex Robotic System (Medrobotics, Raynham, Massachusetts) is a single-port operator-controlled flexible endoscope specifically developed for transoral robotic surgery and was given FDA approval in July 2015.[66] Initial patient experiences with the new system have shown safe and effective results in visualization and excision of lesions of the oropharynx, hypopharynx, and supraglottic larynx.[67–69]

The surgeon steers an outer robotic joystick with a touchscreen and magnified HD 2-D visual display to guide the core flexible endoscope inside the oral cavity. The flexible scope consists of an inner and outer segment with a single articulation point between the 2 segments, allowing each to be semirigid or flexible, to allow a stable platform through which flexible instruments can be deployed. Two lumens can be found within the scope, opening a path for irrigation fluid or electrical wiring. Furthermore, the 2 flexible guide tubes, referred to as external accessory channels, provide a pathway to use different compatible flexible instruments as small as 3 mm in size with almost 180° articulation.

In January 2018, the FDA extended the use of Flex Robotic System to include general, gynecologic, and thoracic procedure involving the transabdominal and transthoracic cavities through incisions rather than only natural cavities.[70] This has opened the door to further adaptation of the Medrobotics device to MIS with its smaller surgical footprint as well as easy transport and setup.

New Robotic Platforms—Non–Food and Drug Administration Approved

SPORT surgical system
The Single Port Orifice Robotic Technology (SPORT) Surgical System (Titan Medical, Toronto, Canada) uses the LESS approach, with a console-based platform. The single-port design offers multiarticulated instruments with single-use replaceable tips. A collapsible system can be inserted into the body through a small 2.5-cm incision and then controlled remotely via an ergonomic open work station operated with a combination of hand controllers, foot pedals and a 3-D HD flat touchscreen monitor.[71] A single-arm mobile patient cart further facilitates its use. Thus far, the system has demonstrated successful single-port nephrectomy in animal models[55] and is tentatively planned to apply for FDA approval in 2019.[72]

Hominis surgical system
The Hominis surgical system (Memic Innovative Surgery, Tel Aviv, Israel) is currently working on usability review for FDA submission. The system consists of small humanoid-shaped robotic arms that mimic human dexterity with novel 360° articulation and various minimally invasive access configurations for seamless robotic surgery. The system is designed to potentially open doors to more surgical applications with a combination of improved ergonomics, low cost, and small footprint. The robotic system allows for both single-port or multiport approaches and is the first to allow a transvaginal approach for hysterectomy.[73,74] At present, animal and human studies of this platform have not yet been reported.

Miniature in vivo robot
A joint collaboration between Virtual Incision Pleasanton, California and the Center for Advanced Surgical Technology at the University of Nebraska Medical Center in Omaha, Nebraska, has led to the development of a miniaturized in vivo robot (MIVR). Initial porcine studies have shown successful colectomy with insertion and removal via a single port.[75] Furthermore, human trials in South Africa have shown feasibility and safety of a robotic colectomy.[76] Additional development of the robotic platform is planned, including small

inexpensive robots for cholecystectomy and hernia repair. The company is finalizing the design and applying for FDA clearance soon.[77]

The goals of this robotic platform are to reduce size with easy maneuverability within the peritoneum, allowing for quick repositioning and access to all 4 quadrants from an umbilical incision entry point.[77] The 2 robotic arms are composed of multiple joints with interchangeable end effectors to provide different instrumental needs. The robotic platform uses artificial intelligence and machine learning technologies to track and guide instruments.[75,78] Furthermore, the miniaturized robot features the first robotic flexible tip laparoscope controlled by the surgeon. The drive technology is completely localized within the small robotic arms themselves, removing the need for larger platforms, and thus improving its ease of use in the operating room.[78] Lastly, the use of multiple miniaturized robots simultaneously could be possible as needed based on the complexity of the procedure with no change in incision size.[78]

Versius robotic system
Cambridge Medical Robotics (Cambridge, United Kingdom) has created Versius, a lightweight robotic system geared toward a variety of transabdominal surgeries, including upper gastrointestinal, colorectal, gynecologic, and renal procedures. Initial cadaveric trials in Cambridge have shown successful use of electrocautery, needle driving, suturing and tissue handling, and FDA approval and Europe's CE mark are anticipated for early 2018.[79]

The system's modular design provides flexibility and versatility with respect to operating room positioning of up to 5 different robotic arms that can connect to a wide variety of 5-mm instruments—electrocautery electrodes, needle drivers, scissors, and graspers.[80] The surgeon controls the modular wristed robotics arms via joystick controllers at the robotic console. HD 3-D glasses are required to view the console monitor. The arms also transmit haptic feedback from the instrument to the surgeon measuring their position and force 1000 times per second.[65]

Verb surgical
Verb Surgical (Mountain View, California) is another joint venture company between the Johnson & Johnson medical device company, Ethicon Endo-Surgery, Getinge, and Verily Life Sciences (Alphabet/Google).[81] The company's goal is to create a true surgical robot for the digital age that is more than just an extension of the surgeon.[82] The company delivered its first demonstration to collaborative partners in January

2017,[81] but limited information has been released about anticipated plans.

The device was described as "democratizing surgery" by increasing available information to the surgeon through incorporation of data analytics and machine learning in addition to the usual goals of advanced instrumentations, connectivity, robotics, and visualization.[83] The goal is not to simply create another robotic platform but rather advance from open (1.0), minimally invasive (2.0), and initial robotic surgery (3.0) to truly digital surgery (4.0) of the future.[84] The prototype reportedly combines robotics and data-driven machine learning to both remove increased costs and enable open access to more surgeons.[83]

FUTURE DIRECTIONS

As the world of MIS continues to evolve with new competitors, the trend is moving toward single-port surgery with smaller incisions and possibly even no incisions as natural orifice entry becomes more feasible. Eventually with the integration of virtual technology and the digital age, a new era of autonomous robotic surgery may become the way of the future.

REFERENCES

1. Gobbi D, Midrio P, Gamba P. Instrumentation for minimally invasive surgery in pediatric urology. Transl Pediatr 2016;5(4):186–204.

2. Kim C, Docimo SG. Use of laparoscopy in pediatric urology. Rev Urol 2005;7(4):215–23.

3. Bayazit Y, Aridogan IA, Abat D, et al. Pediatric transumbilical laparoendoscopic single-site nephroureterectomy: initial report. Urology 2009;74(5):1116–9.

4. Kaouk JH, Palmer JS. Single-port laparoscopic surgery: initial experience in children for varicocelectomy. BJU Int 2008;102(1):97–9.

5. Kawauchi A, Naitoh Y, Miki T. Laparoendoscopic single-site surgery for pediatric patients in urology. Curr Opin Urol 2011;21(4):303–8.

6. Abdel-Karim AM, Fahmy A, Moussa A, et al. Laparoscopic pyeloplasty versus open pyeloplasty for recurrent ureteropelvic junction obstruction in children. J Pediatr Urol 2016;12(6):401.e1–6.

7. Luithle T, Szavay P, Fuchs J. Single-incision laparoscopic nephroureterectomy in children of all age groups. J Pediatr Surg 2013;48(5):1142–6.

8. Khambati A, Wehbi E, Farhat WA. Laparo-endoscopic single site surgery in pediatrics: feasibility and surgical outcomes from a preliminary prospective Canadian experience. Can Urol Assoc J 2015; 9(1–2):48–52.

9. Gor RA, Long CJ, Shukla AR, et al. Multi-institutional experience in laparoendoscopic single-site surgery

10. Bansal D, Cost NG, Bean CM, et al. Pediatric laparoendoscopic single site partial nephrectomy: feasibility in infants and small children for upper urinary tract duplication anomalies. J Pediatr Urol 2014; 10(5):859–63.

11. Bowlin PR, Farhat WA. Laparoscopic nephrectomy and partial nephrectomy: intraperitoneal, retroperitoneal, single site. Urol Clin North Am 2015;42(1): 31–42.

12. Aneiros Castro B, Cabezali Barbancho D, Tordable Ojeda C, et al. Laparoendoscopic single-site nephrectomy in children: is it a good alternative to conventional laparoscopic approach? J Pediatr Urol 2018;14(1):49.e1–4.

13. Wang F, Shou T, Zhong H. Is two-port laparoendoscopic single-site surgery (T-LESS) feasible for pediatric hydroceles? Single-center experience with the initial 59 cases. J Pediatr Urol 2018;14(1):67.e1–6.

14. Giseke S, Glass M, Tapadar P, et al. A true laparoscopic herniotomy in children: evaluation of long-term outcome. J Laparoendosc Adv Surg Tech A 2010;20(2):191–4.

15. Van Batavia JP, Tong C, Chu DI, et al. Laparoscopic inguinal hernia repair by primary peritoneal flap repair: description of technique and initial results in children. J Pediatr Urol 2018;14(3):272.e1–6.

16. Symeonidis EN, Nasioudis D, Economopoulos KP. Laparoendoscopic single-site surgery (LESS) for major urological procedures in the pediatric population: a systematic review. Int J Surg 2016;29:53–61.

17. Till H, Basharkhah A, Hock A. What's the best minimal invasive approach to pediatric nephrectomy and heminephrectomy: conventional laparoscopy (CL), single-site (LESS) or robotics (RAS)? Transl Pediatr 2016;5(4):240–4.

18. Merseburger AS, Herrmann TR, Shariat SF, et al. EAU guidelines on robotic and single-site surgery in urology. Eur Urol 2013;64(2):277–91.

19. Yeung CK, Tam YH, Sihoe JD, et al. Retroperitoneoscopic dismembered pyeloplasty for pelvi-ureteric junction obstruction in infants and children. BJU Int 2001;87(6):509–13.

20. Badawy H, Saad A, Fahmy A, et al. Prospective evaluation of retroperitoneal laparoscopic pyeloplasty in children in the first 2 years of life: is age a risk factor for conversion? J Pediatr Urol 2017; 13(5):511.e1–4.

21. Chen Y, Wang F, Zhong H, et al. A systematic review and meta-analysis concerning single-site laparoscopic percutaneous extraperitoneal closure for pediatric inguinal hernia and hydrocele. Surg Endosc 2017;31(12):4888–901.

22. Badawy H, Zoaier A, Ghoneim T, et al. Transperitoneal versus retroperitoneal laparoscopic pyeloplasty

in children: randomized clinical trial. J Pediatr Urol 2015;11(3):122.e1-6.

23. Liu D, Zhou H, Ma L, et al. Comparison of laparoscopic approaches for dismembered pyeloplasty in children with ureteropelvic junction obstruction: critical analysis of 11-year experiences in a single surgeon. Urology 2017;101:50–5.

24. Fergo C, Burcharth J, Pommergaard HC, et al. Three-dimensional laparoscopy vs 2-dimensional laparoscopy with high-definition technology for abdominal surgery: a systematic review. Am J Surg 2017;213(1):159–70.

25. Sinha RY, Raje SR, Rao GA. Three-dimensional laparoscopy: principles and practice. J Minim Access Surg 2017;13(3):165–9.

26. van Bergen P, Kunert W, Bessell J, et al. Comparative study of two-dimensional and three-dimensional vision systems for minimally invasive surgery. Surg Endosc 1998;12(7):948–54.

27. McDougall EM, Soble JJ, Wolf JS Jr, et al. Comparison of three-dimensional and two-dimensional laparoscopic video systems. J Endourol 1996;10(4):371–4.

28. Abou-Haidar H, Al-Qaoud T, Jednak R, et al. Laparoscopic pyeloplasty: initial experience with 3D vision laparoscopy and articulating shears. J Pediatr Urol 2016;12(6):426.e1–5.

29. Kozlov Y, Kovalkov K, Nowogilov V. 3D laparoscopy in neonates and infants. J Laparoendosc Adv Surg Tech A 2016;26(12):1021–7.

30. Sørensen SMD, Konge L, Bjerrum F. 3D vision accelerates laparoscopic proficiency and skills are transferable to 2D conditions: a randomized trial. Am J Surg 2017;214(1):63–8.

31. Kalloo AN, Singh VK, Jagannath SB, et al. Flexible transgastric peritoneoscopy: a novel approach to diagnostic and therapeutic interventions in the peritoneal cavity. Gastrointest Endosc 2004;60(1):114–7.

32. Siddaiah-Subramanya M, Tiang KW, Nyandowe M. A new era of minimally invasive surgery: progress and development of major technical innovations in general surgery over the last decade. Surg J (N Y) 2017;3(4):e163–6.

33. Alcaraz A, Peri L, Molina A, et al. Feasibility of transvaginal NOTES-assisted laparoscopic nephrectomy. Eur Urol 2010;57(2):233–7.

34. Buttice S, Sener TE, Lucan VC, et al. Hybrid transvaginal NOTES nephrectomy: postoperative sexual outcomes. A three-center matched study. Urology 2017;99:131–5.

35. Rassweiler JJ, Teber D. Advances in laparoscopic surgery in urology. Nature reviews. Urology 2016;13(7):387–99.

36. Rassweiler J, Binder J, Frede T. Robotic and telesurgery: will they change our future? Curr Opin Urol 2001;11(3):309–20.

37. Atug F, Woods M, Burgess SV, et al. Robotic assisted laparoscopic pyeloplasty in children. J Urol 2005;174(4 Pt 1):1440–2.

38. Kavoussi LR, Peters CA. Laparoscopic pyeloplasty. J Urol 1993;150(6):1891–4.

39. Schuessler WW, Grune MT, Tecuanhuey LV, et al. Laparoscopic dismembered pyeloplasty. J Urol 1993;150(6):1795–9.

40. Peters CA, Schlussel RN, Retik AB. Pediatric laparoscopic dismembered pyeloplasty. J Urol 1995;153(6):1962–5.

41. Klingler HC, Remzi M, Janetschek G, et al. Comparison of open versus laparoscopic pyeloplasty techniques in treatment of uretero-pelvic junction obstruction. Eur Urol 2003;44(3):340–5.

42. Light A, Karthikeyan S, Maruthan S, et al. Perioperative outcomes and complications after laparoscopic vs robot-assisted dismembered pyeloplasty: a systematic review and meta-analysis. BJU Int 2018. https://doi.org/10.1111/bju.14170.

43. Varda BK, Wang Y, Chung BI, et al. Has the robot caught up? National trends in utilization, perioperative outcomes, and cost for open, laparoscopic, and robotic pediatric pyeloplasty in the United States from 2003 to 2015. J Pediatr Urol 2018. https://doi.org/10.1016/j.jpurol.2017.12.010.

44. Baek M, Au J, Huang GO, et al. Robot-assisted laparoscopic pyeloureterostomy in infants with duplex systems and upper pole hydronephrosis: variations in double-J ureteral stenting techniques. J Pediatr Urol 2017;13(2):219–20.

45. Boysen WR, Akhavan A, Ko J, et al. Prospective multicenter study on robot-assisted laparoscopic extravesical ureteral reimplantation (RALUR-EV): outcomes and complications. J Pediatr Urol 2018. https://doi.org/10.1016/j.jpurol.2018.01.020.

46. Gundeti MS, Petravick ME, Pariser JJ, et al. A multi-institutional study of perioperative and functional outcomes for pediatric robotic-assisted laparoscopic Mitrofanoff appendicovesicostomy. J Pediatr Urol 2016;12(6):386.e1–5.

47. Murthy P, Cohn JA, Selig RB, et al. Robot-assisted laparoscopic augmentation ileocystoplasty and mitrofanoff appendicovesicostomy in children: updated interim results. Eur Urol 2015;68(6):1069–75.

48. Chang C, Steinberg Z, Shah A, et al. Patient positioning and port placement for robot-assisted surgery. J Endourol 2014;28(6):631–8.

49. Gargollo PC. Hidden incision endoscopic surgery: description of technique, parental satisfaction and applications. J Urol 2011;185(4):1425–31.

50. Hong YH, DeFoor WR Jr, Reddy PP, et al. Hidden incision endoscopic surgery (HIdES) trocar placement for pediatric robotic pyeloplasty: comparison to traditional port placement. J Robot Surg 2018;12(1):43–7.

51. Kan HC, Pang ST, Wu CT, et al. Robot-assisted laparoendoscopic single site adrenalectomy: a comparison of 3 different port platforms with 3 case reports. Medicine 2017;96(51):e9479.

52. LaMattina JC, Alvarez-Casas J, Lu I, et al. Robotic-assisted single-port donor nephrectomy using the da Vinci single-site platform. J Surg Res 2018;222: 34–8.

53. Cole AP, Trinh QD, Sood A, et al. The rise of robotic surgery in the new millennium. J Urol 2017;197(2S): S213–5.

54. Paradise HJ, Huang GO, Elizondo Saenz RA, et al. Robot-assisted laparoscopic pyeloplasty in infants using 5-mm instruments. J Pediatr Urol 2017;13(2): 221–2.

55. Rassweiler JJ, Autorino R, Klein J, et al. Future of robotic surgery in urology. BJU Int 2017;120(6): 822–41.

56. U.S. Food & Drug. FDA clears new robotically-assisted surgical device for adult patients. Secondary FDA clears new robotically-assisted surgical device for adult patients 2017. Available at: http://news.doximity.com/entries/9699292?authenticated=false.

57. Bozzini G, Gidaro S, Taverna G. Robot-assisted laparoscopic partial nephrectomy with the ALF-X robot on pig models. Eur Urol 2016;69(2):376–7.

58. Fanfani F, Monterossi G, Fagotti A, et al. The new robotic TELELAP ALF-X in gynecological surgery: single-center experience. Surg Endosc 2016;30(1): 215–21.

59. Fanfani F, Restaino S, Gueli Alletti S, et al. TELELAP ALF-X robotic-assisted laparoscopic hysterectomy: feasibility and perioperative outcomes. J Minim Invasive Gynecol 2015;22(6):1011–7.

60. Fanfani F, Restaino S, Rossitto C, et al. Total laparoscopic (S-LPS) versus TELELAP ALF-X robotic-assisted hysterectomy: a case-control study. J Minim Invasive Gynecol 2016;23(6):933–8.

61. Gueli Alletti S, Rossitto C, Cianci S, et al. Telelap ALF-X vs Standard laparoscopy for the treatment of early-stage endometrial cancer: a single-institution retrospective cohort study. J Minim Invasive Gynecol 2016;23(3):378–83.

62. Spinelli A, David G, Gidaro S, et al. First experience in colorectal surgery with a new robotic platform with haptic feedback. Colorectal Dis 2018;20(3):228–35.

63. TranEnterix. Senhance™. Secondary Senhance™ 2018. Available at: https://www.transenterix.com/overview/.

64. Rao PP. Robotic surgery: new robots and finally some real competition! World J Urol 2018. https://doi.org/10.1007/s00345-018-2213-y.

65. Peters BS, Armijo PR, Krause C, et al. Review of emerging surgical robotic technology. Surg Endosc 2018;32(4):1636–55.

66. Medrobotics. Flex® Robotic System: Expanding the reach of surgery®. Secondary Flex® Robotic System: Expanding the reach of surgery® 2018. Available at: https://medrobotics.com/gateway/flex-system-int/.

67. Lang S, Mattheis S, Hasskamp P, et al. A european multicenter study evaluating the flex robotic system in transoral robotic surgery. Laryngoscope 2017; 127(2):391–5.

68. Mattheis S, Hasskamp P, Holtmann L, et al. Flex Robotic System in transoral robotic surgery: the first 40 patients. Head Neck 2017;39(3):471–5.

69. Tan Wen Sheng B, Wong P, Teo Ee Hoon C. Transoral robotic excision of laryngeal papillomas with Flex(R) Robotic System - A novel surgical approach. Am J Otolaryngol 2018. https://doi.org/10.1016/j.amjoto.2018.03.011.

70. Taylor NP. FDA clears Medrobotics' robotic surgical platform for expanded use. Secondary FDA clears Medrobotics' robotic surgical platform for expanded use 2018. Available at: https://www.fiercebiotech.com/medtech/fda-clears-medrobotics-robotic-surgical-platform-for-expanded-use.

71. Titan Medical Inc. SPORT™ Surgical System. Secondary SPORT™ Surgical System 2018. Available at: https://titanmedicalinc.com/technology/.

72. Idrus AA. On track for 2019 launch, Titan Medical installs its first surgical robot in Florida. Secondary On track for 2019 launch, Titan Medical installs its first surgical robot in Florida 2017. Available at: https://www.fiercebiotech.com/medtech/track-for-2019-launch-titan-medical-installs-its-first-surgical-robot-florida.

73. Memic. Hominis™- the smallest, farthest reaching surgical robot. Secondary Hominis™- the smallest, farthest reaching surgical robot 2018. Available at: https://www.memicmed.com/.

74. Memic Innovation Surgery. Hominis - Robotic Surgery Made Natural. Secondary Hominis - Robotic Surgery Made Natural 2017. Available at: kenes-exhibitions.com/old/biomed2016/wp-content/uploads/2016/05/MEMIC.docx.

75. Wortman TD. Design, analysis, and testing of in vivo surgical robots. Secondary Design, analysis, and testing of in vivo surgical robots 2011. Available at: https://digitalcommons.unl.edu/mechengdiss/28/.

76. Bedem LJMvd. Realization of a demonstrator slave for robotic minimally invasive surgery. Eindhoven: Technische Universiteit Eindhoven 2010. Available at: https://doi-org.ezproxyhost.library.tmc.edu/10.6100/IR684835.

77. Keenan J. Virtual Incision reels in $18M in series B round to support its surgical robotics. Secondary Virtual Incision reels in $18M in series B round to support its surgical robotics 2017. Available at: https://www.fiercebiotech.com/medtech/virtual-incision-reels-18m-series-b-round-to-support-its-surgical-robotics.

78. Virtual Incision. World;s First Use of Miniaturized Robot in Human Surgery. Secondary World;s First Use of Miniaturized Robot in Human Surgery 2016. Available at: https://www.virtualincision.com/fim-surgery/.

79. CMR Surgical. CMR reveals Versius robotic surgery system. Secondary CMR reveals Versius robotic surgery system 2016. Available at: https://cmrsurgical.com/cmr-reveals-versius-robotic-surgery-system/.

80. Ellis R. UK scientists create world's smallest surgical robot to start a hospital revolution. Secondary UK scientists create world's smallest surgical robot to start a hospital revolution 2017. Available at: https://www.theguardian.com/society/2017/aug/19/worlds-smallest-surgical-robot-versius-keyhole-hospital-revolution?CMP=share_btn_link.

81. Verb Surgical Inc. Verb Surgical Delivers Digital Surgery Prototype Demonstration to Collaboration Partners. Secondary Verb Surgical Delivers Digital Surgery Prototype Demonstration to Collaboration Partners 2017. Available at: https://www.prnewswire.com/news-releases/verb-surgical-delivers-digital-surgery-prototype-demonstration-to-collaboration-partners-300397192.html.

82. Simonite T. The Recipe for the Perfect Robot Surgeon. Secondary The Recipe for the Perfect Robot Surgeon 2016. Available at: https://www.technologyreview.com/s/602595/the-recipe-for-the-perfect-robot-surgeon/.

83. Thibault M. Here's the Latest from Verb Surgical. Secondary Here's the Latest from Verb Surgical 2016. Available at: https://www.mddionline.com/heres-latest-verb-surgical.

84. Khateeb OM. Democratizing Surgery Part 1: What Verb Surgical is Creating. Secondary Democratizing Surgery Part 1: What Verb Surgical is Creating 2016. Available at: https://www.linkedin.com/pulse/democratizing-surgery-how-verb-surgical-invented-new-category.

Pediatric Urology and Global Health
Why Now and How to Build a Successful Global Outreach Program

Jason P. Van Batavia, MD[a],*, Aseem R. Shukla, MD[a],
Rakesh S. Joshi, MCh[b], Pramod P. Reddy, MD[c]

KEYWORDS

- Bladder exstrophy • Global medicine • Collaboration • Regionalization • Surgical coaching

KEY POINTS

- Pediatric urology is an ideal field for global health programs because genitourinary diseases account for a large proportion of congenital diseases.
- Pediatric urologists interested in global health outreach can volunteer through established programs or build de novo collaboration.
- By following several key guidelines with particular emphasis on a long-term commitment and surgical training of the local team, global health partnerships can lead to a sustainable model for increased surgical capacity.

INTRODUCTION: WHAT IS GLOBAL HEALTH?

Global health is a term that has many definitions in the literature and is often used interchangeably with international health and global public health. In 2010, Beaglehole and Bonita proposed the following definition for global health: "collaborative trans-national research and action for promoting health for all."[1] The health in global health can refer to overall health or any of the full gamut of medical conditions (ie, hypertension, diabetes, and infectious diseases) or congenital anomalies. Although some congenital anomalies can be managed medically, many will require "action" such as surgical correction, which can range from commonly performed surgeries to complex reconstructions.

Unfortunately, most severe congenital anomalies, up to 94% as estimated by the World Health Organization (WHO), occur in low- and middle-income countries (LMIC), where families and governments are often resource-constrained and where surgical access may be difficult.[2]

In order to alleviate this large burden of disease on LMIC, the Sixty-Third World Health Assembly in 2010 recommended that member countries not only "build capacity" to prevent and treat children with birth defects but also "promote international cooperation" to combat these disorders.[3] Despite this call to action, the WHO and World Health Assembly (WHA) do not give any guideline on how best to form these international collaborations or

---

Disclosures: None.
[a] Division of Pediatric Urology, Department of Surgery, The Children's Hospital of Philadelphia, University of Pennsylvania Perelman School of Medicine, 3rd Floor Wood Building, 3401 Civic Center Boulevard, Philadelphia PA 19104, USA; [b] Division of Paediatric Surgery, B.J. Medical College and Civil Hospital, Civil Hospital Road, Haripura, Asarwa, Ahmedabad, Gujarat 380016, India; [c] Division of Pediatric Urology, Department of Pediatrics, Cincinnati Children's, University of Cincinnati College of Medicine, University of Cincinnati, 3333 Burnet Avenue #450, Cincinnati, OH 45229, USA
* Corresponding author.
E-mail address: vanbatavij@email.chop.edu

Urol Clin N Am 45 (2018) 623–631
https://doi.org/10.1016/j.ucl.2018.06.009

how to monitor success. In this article, the authors discuss strategies with which to optimize care for complex surgical diseases on the international scale, including ways to enhance regionalization, collaboration, and surgical education to accelerate learning curve limits with rare diseases. By using bladder exstrophy as a model disease and highlighting the work of the International Bladder Exstrophy Consortium (IBEC) as a case report, the importance of these key elements as well as team building, long-term invested commitment, surgical coaching, and mentorship are emphasized.

THE SURGICAL BURDEN OF GLOBAL HEALTH

Despite decades of being underappreciated, in part due to the lack of accurate estimation, the surgical burden of disease as a component of global health has recently garnered focus.[4,5] In 2007 it was estimated that almost half of the world's population lacked access to basic surgical care, and recent estimates are as high as 5 billion people worldwide.[6,7] Weiser and colleagues[8] analyzed surgical volume in more than 50 WHO member states from 2004 to 2012. Although the investigators note that surgical volume growth rate was highest in the most resource poor countries, less than 30% of all surgeries worldwide take place in these countries, which account for more than 70% of the global population.[8,9] Furthermore, the costs of surgical disease on lost economic output are highest in LMIC and are estimated to reach more than 1% of the total gross domestic product for these countries by 2020.[10] Given these staggering statistics and the inequitable distribution of surgical diseases, the need for a global health focus on surgery[11,12] is well justified and has the potential to not only decrease morbidity and mortality but also improve the economic situation and development of LMIC.

THE CASE FOR PEDIATRIC UROLOGY AS A GLOBAL HEALTH PRIORITY

Global health surgical initiatives can provide general surgical care for common conditions or offer disease/condition-specific (ie, cleft lip and palate) surgical intervention, often by subspecialists. Pediatric urology with its variety of congenital malformations represents an ideal field for both types of global health surgical initiatives, especially given that genitourinary (GU) tract anomalies are 5 to 10 times more common than cleft lip and palate.[11,12] In fact, congenital anomalies of the GU tract are the third most common group of nonchromosomal congenital anomalies behind congenital heart defects and limb defects.[13]

When considering specific pediatric urologic conditions, the number of affected infants and children worldwide are even more staggering. Hypospadias itself is one of the most common birth defects and occurs in 1 of every 150 to 300 live male births; the number of new hypospadias cases in sub-Saharan Africa alone with an estimated 40 million live births per year dwarfs the number of new cases in the United States.[14–16] Likewise, in India, where the pediatric population is almost 500 million, there is estimated to be more than 58,000 new congenital GU malformations each year with at least 15,000 of these new cases being hypospadias.[17] Although several other pediatric urology conditions, such as inguinal hernias and cryptorchidism, are similar to hypospadias in having higher prevalence rates, some specific GU anomalies, including bladder exstrophy-epispadias complex (BE) and cloacal malformations, are rarer and often require complex surgical reconstruction.

Despite the lower incidence rates, even these rare GU conditions can account for a substantial number of new cases annually given the higher birth rates globally, especially in LMIC. For example, the incidence of BE is estimated to be 1 in 50,000 live births; although this would lead to only ~80 new cases of BE in the United States per year, based on live birth rates, India would have greater than 500 new infants born with BE per year.[17–19] Furthermore, prenatal care is often limited in LMICs, and few pregnancies are electively terminated for medical reasons, leading to higher birth rate of neonates with undiagnosed congenital malformations. Despite these numbers, the availability of trained pediatric urologists globally is critically low, especially in sub-Saharan Africa where there are less than a handful of pediatric urologists for a population of nearly 500 million children.[14,20]

Thus, the variety of congenital anomalies in pediatric urology, mixed with the sheer prevalence of these conditions worldwide and the lack of access to trained specialists in most LMIC, underscores the critical need to consider pediatric urology as a surgical global health priority. As mentioned earlier, despite recognizing the need for international collaborations to prevent and treat congenital anomalies, the WHO and WHA provide no guideline for how best to accomplish these goals.

TYPES OF SURGICAL GLOBAL HEALTH PROGRAMS

In practice, there are several different surgical "medical missions" or outreach program models that have been implemented or have evolved over time to meet various global health needs. These various programs vary widely in organizational structure, overall goals or mission, ability or desire to establish a sustainable local infrastructure, frequency of contact and follow up, and commitment to surgical education and training. Given these differences, especially in overall philosophy and resources, the ability of each program to have a lasting impact on the local health care system also varies dramatically.

One useful way to categorize surgical global health programs is offered by Dr Ofer Merin in a chapter on the evolution of surgical humanitarian missions.[21] Dr Merin describes 3 types of international surgical health projects: clinical, relief, and developmental projects.[21]

Clinical projects are "preplanned delegations" that focus on chronic diseases or target specific diseases. These programs either go to various underserved locations across the globe with the goal to provide care for surgical conditions or send patients to centralized care centers to receive the care they need. Common examples include missions to provide general surgical care, repair facial deformities, cataracts, and even congenital heart disease.[21–24] The primary focus of these projects are to provide quality care to at-need patients and not on building capacity or training local physicians. Oftentimes, these projects function as a "one-off" with limited to no follow-up, and location may rotate. These projects can be sponsored by medical or academic institutions, international organizations (ie, the United Nations, WHO, and International Committee of the Red Cross), governmental organizations, or nongovernmental (often not-for-profit [NFP]) organizations.[21]

Relief projects are those that focus on rapidly responding to natural disasters or violence from wars.[21] These projects are often short term and involve assembling surgical teams quickly after the inciting event. The goals of these projects can be to either fill in for or supplement a local medical system and are often situational dependent.

Developmental projects are based around a long-term framework with the primary aim to build local surgical capacity by collaborating and partnering with local medical personnel to provide surgical training and education.[21] The emphasis of these projects is on sustainability through the strengthening of the local infrastructure and teaching of local surgeons such that they become self-sufficient and adept at treating the surgical condition or conditions of focus. These programs, like clinical projects, can provide general surgical skills for a variety of conditions or have a specific disease

as the primary focus with expertise provided by subspecialists. Importantly, these projects are based on repeated visits, often over years, which allows for long-term follow-up of surgical patients, increased accountability, and monitoring of outcomes. This last point cannot be overemphasized because one critique of "one-off" clinical outreach projects is the lack of follow-up, and thus, the inability to ensure surgical success and proper treatment of postoperative complications. By committing to the long-term sustainability of the program, humanitarian surgeons engaged in developmental projects can overcome this limitation and continue to honor the "Do no harm" pillar of the Hippocratic Oath.[21] These projects also enable ongoing coaching or mentoring of the local surgeons by the international team members.

The number of surgical global health programs that have embraced the "teach a man to fish" philosophy of the developmental model has grown steadily over the past couple of decades. Examples of these types of programs exist in many pediatric surgical subspecialties, including cardiovascular surgery, plastic surgery, otorhinolaryngology (ENT), ophthalmology, orthopedics, neurosurgery, and urology. Combination programs between plastics and ENT include Smile-Train and Operation Smile, both of which strive to provide a sustainable model to "empower local doctors…in their own communities."[25–27] Many congenital heart disease global initiatives have also moved away from the clinical model and toward a developmental one, including Save a Child's Heart and Heart to Heart Global Cardiac Care, whose mission is to "develop self-sustaining medical programs in areas of need."[22,28]

In pediatric urology, surgical global health projects range from one-time clinical missions to formal developmental model programs. According to a recent survey by the Global Philanthropic Committee, more than 90% of urologists in the American Urological Association, European Association of Urology, and International Society of Urology were interested in global volunteer services with more than 50% performing some form of voluntary philanthropic activity in the past 10 years.[29,30] Interestingly, most of the volunteering urologists participated in short-term clinical projects and not with a formally established group such as IVUmed (formerly International Volunteers in Urology), the WHO, or Doctors Without Borders.[29] In fact, most volunteers were unaware of the services provided by these organizations for surgical global outreach.[29] Given the high level of interest in international volunteerism, yet lack of knowledge about how to get involved, there is need to publicize available opportunities as well as share information on how to successfully implement a global health program.

GLOBAL HEALTH PROGRAMS IN PEDIATRIC UROLOGY

There are several programs available for the pediatric urologist interested in global health outreach. One of the most well-established programs is IVUmed, which was founded in 1995 by Dr Catherine deVries.[12,31] IVUmed has a long track record of excellence and serves as a prime example of an organization that can be used by urologists interested in medical volunteerism for a 1- or 2-week commitment.[31] A quick search of IVUmed's Web site provides a list of upcoming international missions with locations, dates, focused urologic area, and needed personnel for each trip.[31] These positions for the most part are not recurring, and one can sign up via an online application. Although volunteers may go to a specific international location only once, IVUmed as an organization provides a long-term commitment to each location with an overall mission to "make quality urologic care available worldwide."[31]

IVUmed provides global urologic care in multiple areas, including reconstructive, oncology, female urology, and pediatrics. In pediatric urology, IVUmed international outreach programs provide the breadth of surgical care with some workshops focused on a specific condition or type of case. By starting with a common condition, such as hypospadias, and providing more advanced training over time through continued interaction, IVUmed helps build surgical capacity at each location.[12] Although the same volunteer surgeons do not necessarily return each time, the framework and overall program plan are anchored by IVUmed to ensure long-term success.

An alternative approach for global health outreach to the programs currently available, such as those offered by IVUmed, is to establish a de novo collaboration between an academic research center (ARC) in a high-income country (HIC) and a hospital/local surgical team in an LMIC. Although starting such a collaboration from scratch may seem daunting, these programs, when based on the solid foundation of a mutual, shared vision of local surgical training, can be fruitful and lead to marked increases in surgical capacity and surgical learning in both directions. These programs must be based on continued interaction between the HIC ARC surgical team and the same local LMIC team, and as such, are dependent on strong team-building and long-term personal commitments by each member. Although these types of programs can offer general surgical

care, they are particularly useful for the care of complex conditions because they allow the same surgical teams to provide care and monitor outcomes over time.

One example of a program that fits into this category is the IBEC, which was founded by Drs Richard Grady and a coauthor (ARS) from 2 ARCs in the United States in collaboration with the Department of Pediatric Surgery at the Civil Hospital and B.J. Medical College in Ahmedabad, India in 2009.[18] IBEC currently includes a multidisciplinary team from 3 ARCs in both the United States and Qatar (Seattle Children's Hospital, Seattle, Washington; Children' Hospital of Philadelphia, Philadelphia, Pennsylvania; Cincinnati Children's Hospital, Cincinnati, Ohio; and Sidra Medicine, Doha, Qatar) that travels to Ahmedabad for 8 days annually to provide continued hands-on surgical training of the local pediatric surgery team as well as long-term follow-up of treated patients. A recent publication by Joshi and colleagues[18] evaluated the IBEC program and determined that not only was long-term follow up and retention feasible within the infrastructure of the collaborative model, but also the outcomes of these complex reconstructive procedures for BE and epispadias were comparable to those at ARCs in HIC.

KEY PRINCIPLES FOR SUCCESS

Based on a review of the missions and structures of several surgical global health projects that fit into the developmental model framework, including the personal experiences of 3 of the current authors with IBEC, the authors propose a set of key principles that they believe are critical for success of surgical outreach programs.

Collaboration/Partnership with Local Team

The most important first step in developing a global health surgical outreach program is selecting an appropriate site and establishing a local team with which to partner. The key is not just in collaborating with, but in partnering with, the local team: surgeons (often pediatric general surgeons), anesthesiologists, and nurses. These surgical partnerships allow staff and resources from ARCs in HIC to combine with the high-volume and local surgical team in a LMICs. The partner site (ie, hospital) must have appropriate surgical equipment, staff, capacity for postoperative care, and ability to provide long-term follow-up. The local surgical team must be included in the global health program as equal partners from the start because this will allow for the eventual self-sustainability of the local surgical program and for building of surgical capacity. After all, much of the postoperative care, including near-term complications, will be managed by the local team and thus both the international and local groups must be devoted to the overall mission. Without a true sense of partnership, one or both sides may feel less invested and thus less dedicated to the long-term success of the program. Another key point to improve the outcomes of the global health program is early commitment or buy-in from the local hospital administration. If the local hospital administration is committed to the program and provides the necessary infrastructure to support the program, then the probability of success will only increase.

For IBEC, the partnership between the American ARCs and Civil Hospital has allowed for consistency of the team, which makes possible the long-term investment in both surgical training and delivering of high-quality patient care. The ultimate goal must be to build surgical capacity in LMICs with limited access to surgical subspecialists, and IBEC is one approach to comprehensively address complex conditions in pediatric urology through collaboration between a committed traveling team and a strong local team.[18]

Building a Multidisciplinary Team

Perhaps equally as important as finding a committed international site and local team, is building a strong traveling team. The components of the team must ensure appropriate care for the patient through the surgical care pathway from preoperative evaluation to postoperative management. For pediatric urology in general, the multidisciplinary team at minimum should include personnel specialized in pediatric urology, pediatric anesthesiologist, and pediatric nursing. The focus on team building is also emphasized by IVUmed, which describes a typical team as consisting of 2 to 3 surgeons, 2 anesthesia staff, 2 to 3 nurses, and 1 to 2 support personnel for research.[12]

As a part of IBEC, given the focus on BE, the team also includes a local pediatric orthopedic surgeon and health care advocates from patient advocacy organizations (specifically from the Association for Bladder Exstrophy Community [A-BE-C]).[32] The team has also included pediatric urology fellows and research fellows who have helped record and monitor outcomes. Two years ago, a nurse specialized in the postoperative care of pediatric patients from one of the ARCs joined the IBEC team and added tremendous value for education of local nursing

teams as well as patient families. A well-built multidisciplinary team is based on mutual respect by each member toward the important roles played by all other members. This congeniality among team members cannot be overstressed especially when building a team across different ARCs because the coordination will become more complex and need for frequent communication will be essential for success. All team members must have enthusiasm or "buy-in" for the overall mission of the program and be committed in the long term in order for the program to have sustainability and achieve the predefined goals.

Defining the Mission: A Shared Vision

The importance of defining the mission or goals of the global health surgical program early serves multiple purposes. As suggested in the previous 2 sections, building a lasting partnership and forming both the traveling and the local surgical teams is in large part dependent on having a common mission or goal. If the traveling team and local team have different ideas for how the program will function or what the long-term goals are, then this can lead to not only failure of the program but also poor outcomes for patients. A shared vision will ensure that all team members are working toward the same outcome and committed to the success of the program.

As mentioned previously, IVUmed clearly defines its mission as providing access to high-level urologic care for all people worldwide. The motto of IVUmed is "Teach One, Reach Many," and the goal of surgical training and education of local physicians is front and center on the group's Web site.[31] Likewise, the mission of IBEC is to provide quality care for a complex pediatric urology condition while engaging in surgical training of the collaborating pediatric surgeons at Civil Hospital. In addition to surgical training and education of the local team, other goals, such as monitoring of patient outcomes and other research endeavors, should also be defined early on and preferably before the program starts.

Emphasis on Surgical Education, Training, and Coaching

A central tenant of any global health surgical program that aims to increase local surgical capacity must include surgical training and education of the local team. Without this commitment to training, the program will not be sustainable, and the ability to provide quality care in underserved areas will end with the conclusion of the global health project. By using all of the key principles already mentioned, the collaboration between ARCs from HIC and local hospitals in LMIC can result in the development of a high-quality center with an experienced local surgical team that can treat complex surgical conditions. Although this transformation may take years, this investment in surgical education and training is what leads to building surgical capacity and regionalization of the care of complex conditions. Regionalization of surgery by limiting high-risk surgeries to centers with high volumes has been suggested as a quality improvement (QI) strategy in HICs based on lower mortalities at high-volume centers.[33,34] In essence, the ultimate outcome of a successful global health surgical program devoted to surgical training is the regionalization of the surgical care of complex or specialized conditions in LMIC such that the outcomes rival those of the ARCs in HIC. Through regionalization of care, the local team is often exposed to a high volume of complex cases, which allows for not only more rapid accumulation of experience but also the ability to report outcomes of larger patient series than even the sponsoring ARCs.[18]

Even after the local surgical team becomes adept at performing the specialized surgical procedures, there is a role for continued surgical coaching or mentoring in the operating room. The idea of surgical coaching has gained some traction recently in the literature, as some have questioned why surgeons do not have coaches, whereas professionals in other disciplines (including music and sports) that also emphasize performance do.[35,36] To provide context, when using the term surgical coaching, the authors are not referring to teaching or mentoring of residents and fellows by faculty, but the actual coaching of attending surgeons by peers or more senior faculty members. The goal of surgical coaching and teaching is to provide continuous professional development of surgeons,[36] and this mentality can also be thought of as part of a component of a successful global health program. By providing coaching, the surgical technique and procedures can be further standardized and outcomes can be measured. This Coaching allows for the local surgical team to not only become experts but also provide valuable research results to the international community.

Furthermore, the international community can also directly benefit from the surgical education at the global health site via expanded access to the surgical training program. Once the global surgical health program has become well established, the program can be opened up to host surgeons from other nations. Allowing other international surgeons to witness and experience the program is particularly beneficial for rare, complex diseases, such as BE, where exposure even in HICs can be limited because of regionalization and from, possibly, early termination. Over the past several years, the IBEC program has hosted more than 20 surgeons from nations as diverse as the United States, Canada, Germany, Spain, Brazil, Qatar, Iran, Turkey, Uganda, and Kenya. These international surgeons benefit from observing a high concentration of BE surgical cases over a short period of time and are able to directly interact with the surgeons who are actively teaching. Impressively, these surgeons in just 1 week will be exposed via IBEC to more BE surgeries than almost all graduating pediatric urology fellows in the United States participate in during their entire fellowships. Interactions between the global health program and international surgeons also offer additional benefits. In partnership with A-BE-C, Ugandan surgeons have traveled to India in consecutive years with their BE patients to observe surgery and participate in postoperative care. These surgeons are now actively planning on creating a center of excellence following the IBEC model in Africa.

Interaction with Local Policy Makers and Government Officials

The traveling health care team is in a unique position to engage with local policy-makers and government officials to ensure adequate funding and resources to the hospitals in the LMICs that participate in the global health surgical program. Although funding for global health projects vary in origin and amount depending on the nature of the project, goals, and long-term commitment, the local hospital and government also have resources that can often be used to create a working partnership with equal investment in the program. Although this may not seem obvious initially, this partnership will be critical for continuation of the program and building relationships based on trust. By monitoring patient outcomes and successes from the global health program and reporting these data to local officials, both the impact of the program and the dedication of the traveling and local surgical teams will be emphasized and likely foster further interest and support for continued or additional resources.

The importance of this key principle is clear in the work done by both IVUmed and IBEC. IVUmed recognized the need for a "long-term memorandum of understanding" between the traveling team and both the hospital administration and the country's ministry of health.[12] Likewise, IBEC has actively engaged with the hospital administration at Civil Hospital, including the superintendent and other local government officers in the Indian state of Gujarat.

Commitment to Quality Improvement

In addition to providing surgical care to patients, an essential component of a high-impact global surgical health program is the ability to monitor patient outcomes, report these outcomes, and initiate QI projects. The ability to implement QI projects is dependent on many of the principles already described and should not be overlooked when developing the global health partnership. These projects have the potential to impact the care of local patients as well as provide important research data that can impact health care abroad. QI projects often take the form of small, incremental changes to care and are based on previously collected data and research from the global health program. In fact, the ability to implement QI projects depends on having a strong commitment to research and monitoring surgical outcomes. As part of IBEC, research personnel have traveled with the international team to record and collect outcome data. Prospective collection and analysis allows reporting of the data and assessment of program success as well as identification of areas for improvement. For example, after the initiation of IBEC, the host team began a process of nutritional status assessments preoperatively and a program to ensure adequate caloric intake and nutritional goals assessments postoperatively. Similarly, an institutional database was created to ensure that comprehensive patient data from surgical procedure performed, to radiological studies, to urodynamics assessments were properly scored and tabulated.

Dedication to a Long-Term Commitment

Finally, the ultimate success of a global health surgical program depends on the dedication from both the traveling and the local teams to a long-term commitment. This commitment allows for sustainability through surgical training and coaching, and for improvements in surgical technique and innovation through research and reporting of outcomes. Both in IVUmed and in IBEC, emphasis on the importance of repeat visits to the host site and the long-term investment required to build surgical capacity and decrease the burden of global disease remain hallmarks of the model. Currently, IBEC is in its 10th year with almost all members having participated in at least 6 trips, and the collaboration is entering a phase of expanding the surgical armamentarium related to long-term exstrophy care, and also fulfilling a global education role with the unique opportunity of exposing surgeons from HIC and LMIC to a high volume of exstrophy, diagnosis, treatment, and follow-up care over an accelerated time continuum.

Securing Financial Support

Global health surgical programs are expensive to initiate and to continue; thus, one must consider from the beginning the costs involved and the financial options that exist. In addition to travel expenses (ie, flights, lodging, food, and local transportation) for the ARC team, other costs include surgical supplies (ie, sutures, sterile gloves, special instruments if needed, catheters, and bandages/dressings), operating room space and time, hospital space for preoperatiave and postoperative care, and time requirement for local health care personnel from administration to nurses to surgeons. Furthermore, each traveling ARC team member must consider the loss of revenue involved with leaving their home institution and not participating in clinic or operating during the time abroad. To support the finances involved in a global health program and the loss of revenue, several options are available. Hospital administrative support and commitment to global health programming may be leveraged depending on institutional priorities; philanthropic outreach may serve to bolster divisional or departmental travel allotments, and/or efforts may be expended to endow a chair for international global health that will reliably generate revenue. At a national level, government support or grant support from foundations such as the Gates Foundation or foundations with specific interests relevant to the global work (ie, A-Be-C), are possible sources for financial support, including federal bodies if research is relevant. In addition, NFP organizations may offer support for specific components of the global health outreach. For instance, some NFP organizations gather surgical supplies or clothing that may be useful during global health program visits. Interacting with these groups can decrease the financial burdens/costs to the traveling ARC team.

SUMMARY

Global health programs are needed in multiple areas of medicine and surgery to help ease the burden of global disease. Pediatric urology is an ideal field for global health programs because GU diseases account for a large proportion of congenital diseases, and access to surgical subspecialists is lacking in most LMICs. Pediatric urologists interested in global health outreach can volunteer through established programs or build de novo collaborations. By following several key guidelines with particular emphasis on a long-term commitment and surgical training of the local surgical team, global health partnerships between ARCs from HIC and hospitals from LMICs can lead to a sustainable model for increased surgical capacity.

REFERENCES

1. Beaglehole R, Bonita R. What is global health? Glob Health Action 2010;3.
2. World Health Organization. Congenital anomalies: 2012 fact sheet No. 370. Available at: http://www.who.int/mediacentre/factsheets/fs370/en/. Accessed March 20, 2018.
3. World Health Assembly. WHA resolution WHA63.17 on birth defects. Available at: http://apps.who.int/gb/ebwha/pdf_files/WHA63/A63_R17-en.pdf?ua=1&ua=1. Accessed March 20, 2018.
4. Tollefson TT, Larrabee WF Jr. Global surgical initiatives to reduce the surgical burden of disease. JAMA 2012;307(7):667–8.
5. Taira BR, Kelly McQueen KA, Burkle FM Jr. Burden of surgical disease: does the literature reflect the scope of the international crisis? World J Surg 2009;33(5):893–8.
6. Contini S. Surgery in developing countries: why and how to meet surgical needs worldwide. Acta Biomed 2007;78(1):4–5.
7. Meara JG, Leather AJ, Hagander L, et al. Global Surgery 2030: evidence and solutions for achieving health, welfare, and economic development. Lancet 2015;386(9993):569–624.
8. Weiser TG, Haynes AB, Molina G, et al. Size and distribution of the global volume of surgery in 2012. Bull World Health Organ 2016;94(3):201–209f.
9. Weiser TG, Regenbogen SE, Thompson KD, et al. An estimation of the global volume of surgery: a modelling strategy based on available data. Lancet 2008;372(9633):139–44.
10. Alkire BC, Shrime MG, Dare AJ, et al. Global economic consequences of selected surgical diseases: a modelling study. Lancet Glob Health 2015;3(Suppl 2):S21–7.
11. Centers for Disease Control and Prevention. Data and statistics: birth defects. 2017. Available at: https://www.cdc.gov/ncbddd/birthdefects/data.html. Accessed April 5, 2018.
12. Jalloh M, Wood JP, Fredley M, et al. IVUmed: a nonprofit model for surgical training in low-resource countries. Ann Glob Health 2015;81(2):260–4.
13. Dolk H, Loane M, Garne E. The prevalence of congenital anomalies in Europe. Adv Exp Med Biol 2010;686:349–64.
14. UNICEF. "Children in Africa: key statistics on child survival, protection, and development.". 2015. Available at: https://data.unicef.org/wp-content/uploads/2015/12/Children-in-Africa-Brochure-Nov-23-HR_245.pdf. Accessed April 5, 2018.
15. Snodgrass WT, Bush NC. Chapter 147: hypospadias. In: Wein A, Kavoussi L, Partin A, et al, editors. Campbell-Walsh urology. 11th edition. Philadelphia: Elsevier; 2016. p. 3399–429.
16. Springer A, van den Heijkant M, Baumann S. Worldwide prevalence of hypospadias. J Pediatr Urol 2016;12(3):152.e1-7.
17. World Health Organization - Regional Office for South-East Asia. Birth defects in south-east Asia a public health challenge: situation analysis. 2013. Available at: http://apps.searo.who.int/PDS_DOCS/B4962.pdf. Accessed March 20, 2018.
18. Joshi RS, Shrivastava D, Grady R, et al. A model for sustained collaboration to address the unmet global burden of bladder exstrophy-epispadis complex and penopubic epispadis: the international bladder exstrophy consortium. JAMA Surg 2018. https://doi.org/10.1001/jamasurg.2018.0067.
19. Siffel C, Correa A, Amar E, et al. Bladder exstrophy: an epidemiologic study from the international clearinghouse for birth defects surveillance and research, and an overview of the literature. Am J Med Genet C Semin Med Genet 2011;0(4):321–32.
20. Wilmshurst JM, Morrow B, du Preez A, et al. The African pediatric fellowship program: training in Africa for Africans. Pediatrics 2016;137(1). https://doi.org/10.1542/peds.2015-2741.
21. Merin O. Chapter 2: the evolution of surgical humanitarian missions. In: Roth R, Frost EAM, Gevirtz C, et al, editors. The role of anesthesiology in global health, vol. 1. Switzerland: Springer International Publishing; 2015. p. 9–30.
22. Cohen AJ, Tamir A, Houri S, et al. Save a child's heart: we can and we should. Ann Thorac Surg 2001;71(2):462–8.
23. Butler MW. Fragmented international volunteerism: need for a global pediatric surgery network. J Pediatr Surg 2010;45(2):303–9.
24. Pezzella AT. International aspects of cardiac surgery. Ann Thorac Surg 1998;65(4):903–4.
25. SmileTrain. 2018. Available at: https://www.smiletrain.org/our-cause. Accessed March 25, 2018.
26. Abenavoli FM. Operation smile humanitarian missions. Plast Reconstr Surg 2005;115(1):356–7.
27. Operation smile. "Medical programs - operation smile.". 2018. Available at: https://www.operationsmile.org/approach/medical-programs. Accessed March 25, 2018.
28. Heart to heart global cardiac care. 2018. Available at: https://www.heart-2-heart.org/who-we-are/about-us/. Accessed March 28, 2018.

29. Badlani G. International volunteerism and global responsibility. Transl Androl Urol 2017;6(2): 258–63.

30. Erickson BA. International surgical missions: how to approach, what to avoid. Urology Times; Oct 3, 2013.

31. IVUmed. "What we do". Available at: https://www. ivumed.org/what-we-do/. Accessed February 22, 2018.

32. Association for the Bladder Exstrophy Communitiy (A-BE-C). A-BE-C: You are not alone. 2018. Available at: https://www.bladderexstrophy.com/. Accessed March 20, 2018.

33. Chhabra KR, Dimick JB. Strategies for improving surgical care: when is regionalization the right choice? JAMA Surg 2016;151(11):1001–2.

34. Reames BN, Ghaferi AA, Birkmeyer JD, et al. Hospital volume and operative mortality in the modern era. Ann Surg 2014;260(2):244–51.

35. Beasley HL, Ghousseini HN, Wiegmann DA, et al. Strategies for building peer surgical coaching relationships. JAMA Surg 2017;152(4):e165540.

36. Greenberg CC, Ghousseini HN, Pavuluri Quamme SR, et al. A statewide surgical coaching program provides opportunity for continuous professional development. Ann Surg 2018;267(5):868–73.

Bladder Bowel Dysfunction

Liza M. Aguiar, MD*, Israel Franco, MD

KEYWORDS

- Bladder bowel dysfunction • Dysfunctional elimination syndrome • Lower urinary tract symptoms
- Pediatric urinary consultations

KEY POINTS

- Bladder bowel dysfunction (BBD) was previously known as dysfunctional elimination syndrome.
- BBD describes a spectrum of lower urinary tract symptoms associated with bowel complaints.
- The true incidence of BBD is unknown.
- Given the close interaction between the bladder and bowel due to their common innervation, as well as associated pelvic floor muscles, patients often also present with bowel complaints.
- Increasing awareness of BBD over the past 30 years has led to better diagnostic criteria and treatment methods.

INTRODUCTION

Bladder bowel dysfunction (BBD), previously known as dysfunctional elimination syndrome, describes a spectrum of lower urinary tract symptoms associated with bowel complaints. The true incidence of BBD is unknown; however, it is estimated that BBD symptoms represent approximately 40% of pediatric urology consultations.[1] The connection between lower urinary tract symptoms and bowel symptoms is well described in the literature.[2–4] Given the close interaction between the bladder and bowel due to their common innervation as well as associated pelvic floor muscles, patients often present with bowel complaints as well.

Over the past 30 years, there has been an increasing understanding of BBD. This awareness has led to better diagnostic criteria and treatment methods. In this article, we review the clinical presentation, diagnostic approach, pathophysiology, and treatment options for children with BBD.

TERMINOLOGY AND CLINICAL PRESENTATION

To standardize terminology used for diagnosis and management of BBD, the International Children's Continence Society (ICCS) created a list of urinary symptoms and their definitions to improve communication, research, and treatment across the various disciplines that are involved in diagnosing and treating BBD. The ICCS categorized symptoms into those associated with urine storage and those associated with voiding (**Table 1**).

Other symptoms at presentation can include voiding postponement or holding maneuvers, feeling of incomplete emptying, and postvoid dribbling.[5]

PATHOPHYSIOLOGY OF BLADDER BOWEL DYSFUNCTION

To void normally and completely, the detrusor muscle of the bladder contracts in coordination with the pelvic floor muscles' relaxation. Dysfunctional voiding is defined as failure of the pelvic floor muscles to relax during voiding. This can be due to the external sphincter or the bladder neck (internal sphincter). Dysfunctional voiding can lead to incomplete bladder emptying, suprapubic discomfort, dysuria, and terminal hematuria. Incomplete emptying and/or stasis of urine can increase the risk of urinary tract infection and urinary leakage if associated

Disclosure: The authors have nothing to disclose.
2 Dudley Street, Providence, RI 02905, USA
* Corresponding author.
E-mail address: Liza_Aguiar@brown.edu

Urol Clin N Am 45 (2018) 633–640
https://doi.org/10.1016/j.ucl.2018.06.010

urologic.theclinics.com

Table 1
International Children's Continence Society (ICCS) voiding symptoms

Storage Symptoms	Voiding Symptoms
Increased frequency of urination: ≥8 times per day	Hesitancy: difficulty in initiating voiding
Decreased frequency of urination: ≤3 times per day	Straining: increased effort of abdominal pressure to initiate voiding
Incontinence: involuntary leakage of urine	Weak stream: observed or uroflowmetry demonstrating weak stream
Nocturia: waking at night to void	Dysuria: burning or discomfort with urination
Urinary urgency: sudden need to void	Intermittency: voiding that is not continuous

Data from Austin P, Bauer S, Neveus T. The standardization of terminology of lower urinary tract function in children and adolescents: update report from the Standardization Committee of the International Children's Continence Society. J Urol 2014;191:1863–5.

with overflow incontinence.[3,6] Colonic contractions mediated by the gastrocolic reflex may also trigger bladder spasms, leading to urge incontinence. This cross-talk has been investigated in both animal and human models.[7,8]

Although the pathophysiology behind BBD is not completely understood, some theorize that it stems from a dysfunction in cortical control of the bladder efferent signals going to the brain. There appears to be inadequate suppression of bladder activity, which allows for uninhibited detrusor contractions to occur and in some cases incontinence with or without urgency. Continued detrusor overactivity and urgency can lead to a pattern of learned behavior that in some cases will cause bladder-sphincter incoordination during voiding. In other instances, we know that children with attention-deficit disorder/attention-deficit hyperactivity disorder (ADHD) have dyspraxia and this pattern of incoordination can be associated with external sphincter dyssynergia. Furthermore, we know that dysfunction in the frontal lobes, especially the anterior cingulate gyrus, has been associated with autonomic dysfunction, and a recent publication by Franco and colleagues[9] has shown that there is an association with bladder neck dysfunction as evidenced by prolonged lag times and autonomic dysfunction.

There are several studies identifying a higher incidence of BBD in children with neuropsychiatric disorders. It is estimated that 20% to 40% of children with daytime urinary incontinence have a behavioral disorder as well.[10,11] von Gontard and colleagues[12] found that ADHD symptoms were more common in children with urinary incontinence compared with dry children (16.8% vs 3.4%). These symptoms, in the setting of ADHD, can be more challenging to treat.[13] Children with encopresis have the highest rates of comorbid behavioral disorders with up to 50% exhibiting behavioral disturbances.[10] Most of the neuropsychiatric disorders that are seen in children center around the executive functioning centers, and work by Fowler and Griffiths[14] indicate that most of the control of the sensation of bladder filling and the processing of when and where to urinate is processed in the frontal lobes. These are the same areas that are involved in executive functioning disorders. Thereby linking these seemingly unrelated problems and explaining these comorbidities.[14]

DIAGNOSIS
Terminology

In addition to standardizing the terminology used to describe BBD symptoms, the ICCS aimed to also standardize the nomenclature used for conditions or diagnoses associated with BBD (**Table 2**).[3]

It is important to take a complete history in the setting of a possible BBD diagnosis. This will help differentiate between a functional problem and, less commonly, a structural/anatomic or neurologic problem that may present similarly. A history should include the following:

- Voiding frequency
- Urinary incontinence
- Voiding postponement
- Retentive posturing
- Symptoms of urgency, hesitation, and dysuria
- History of urinary tract infections
- Penile or scrotal pain in boys
- Abdominal pain or cramps, suggestive of constipation, irritable bowel syndrome, or inflammatory bowel disease
- Frequency of bowel movements, including consistency, shape, and size
- Encopresis

Symptoms of muscle weakness, difficulty walking/running, lower extremity tingling or numbness, and lower back pain should prompt a neurologic evaluation to rule out cause for a neuropathic bladder. A history of a febrile urinary tract infection

Table 2
International Children's Continence Society
(ICCS) bowel bladder dysfunction conditions

Condition	Description
Dysfunctional voiding	Contraction of the urethral sphincter during voiding
Overactive bladder (OAB) and urge incontinence	Urgency, incontinence in the setting of urgency
Voiding postponement	Habitual postponement of voiding
Underactive bladder	Low voiding frequency with the need to increase intra-abdominal pressure to void
Obstruction	Increased detrusor pressure and decreased urinary flow, often due to dysfunctional voiding or, less commonly, anatomic obstruction
Stress incontinence	Incontinence in the setting of increased intra-abdominal pressure
Giggle incontinence	Complete void during or after laughter
Extraordinary daytime urinary frequency	Small volume voids (<50% estimated bladder capacity) at least every hour

Data from Yazbeck S, Schick E, O'Regan S. Relevance of constipation to enuresis, urinary tract infection and reflux. Eur Urol 1987;13:318–21.

Table 3
Voiding diary example

Time	Oral Intake	Voided Urine	Urine Leakage (+/−)
10:00 AM	8 oz of juice		
11:00 AM		200 mL	

There are multiple validated voiding scales that are useful as well, including The Dysfunctional Voiding Scoring System created by Farhat and colleagues,[15] the Vancouver Symptom Score for Dysfunctional Elimination Syndrome (VSSDDES),[16] and the Pediatric Urinary Incontinence Quality of Life Questionnaire (PinQ).[17] These tools are helpful in obtaining more objective evidence to support the diagnosis of BBD. In addition, they aid in creating individualized treatment plans for patients.

PHYSICAL EXAMINATION

Physical examination should include examining the abdomen as well as a thorough genital examination. Inspection of the patient's underwear can reveal urine staining due to urge incontinence, vaginal voiding, or postvoid dribbling. This is in

should prompt an ultrasound ± a voiding cystourethrogram (VCUG) to rule out vesicoureteral reflux or any other structural abnormality of the urinary tract that can increase the risk of pyelonephritis. The VCUG can be part of a video urodynamic study, if indicated.

Obtaining voiding and stooling pattern information from the patient and family can be difficult at times, especially after potty training, when the parents are not regularly following these habits. A voiding diary (**Table 3**) can be useful in obtaining objective data, especially regarding the patient's functional bladder capacity, frequency of urinating, and timing of accidents/leakage. The Bristol Stool Chart (**Fig. 1**) is another useful tool in gathering information regarding the appearance and consistency of the patient's stool.

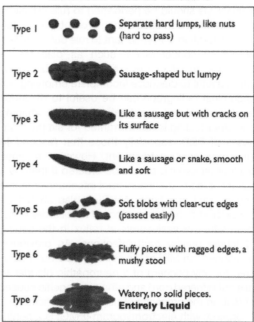

Bristol Stool Chart

Type 1		Separate hard lumps, like nuts (hard to pass)
Type 2		Sausage-shaped but lumpy
Type 3		Like a sausage but with cracks on its surface
Type 4		Like a sausage or snake, smooth and soft
Type 5		Soft blobs with clear-cut edges (passed easily)
Type 6		Fluffy pieces with ragged edges, a mushy stool
Type 7		Watery, no solid pieces. **Entirely Liquid**

Fig. 1. Stool chart example. (*From* Lewis SJ, Heaton KW. Stool form scale as a useful guide to intestinal transit time. Scand J Gastroenterol 1997;32(9):920–4; with permission.)

contrast to full incontinence, in which the underwear is soaked. Stool soiling is also important to note. Stool streaking can be an indicator of stool hoarding. Abdominal examination can reveal palpable stool in the left lower and upper quadrant or a palpable bladder. Genitourinary examination should include looking for any urine pooling in the vaginal vault, suggesting vaginal voiding or an ectopic ureter. Inspection for any evidence of abuse should be included. Ellsworth and colleagues[18] reported that 6% of patients evaluated for voiding dysfunction had a history of sexual abuse. Most of these patients (89%) were female. Any history or evidence of abuse on examination should be addressed appropriately.

A neurologic examination is necessary to rule out potential cause for a neuropathic bladder. This includes testing lower extremity strength, sensation, and looking for any presacral abnormalities, including flattening of the buttocks and abnormal gluteal creases. Low-lying sacral dimples are usually not of concern, but those that are high, without an obvious base, or associated with a tuft of hair should prompt an MRI of the lumbar and sacral spine to rule out any underlying spinal abnormality. Observing the child walk can also help identify an underlying neurologic diagnosis if the child has an abnormal gait or toe walks.

IMAGING AND OTHER TESTING

A urinalysis should be performed to rule out signs of infection, which should then prompt a urine culture. In addition, it is important to rule out disorders of urinary concentration, such as diabetes. A bladder scan, which measures the postvoid residual, is useful to diagnose incomplete emptying. An abdominal radiograph can be useful to diagnose fecal loading and constipation. Routine imaging and other testing is not warranted for simple diagnoses of BBD, especially those that respond to initial conservative treatment. However, a renal/bladder ultrasound should be ordered if there is a history of recurrent urinary tract infections or febrile urinary tract infections. A VCUG also should be considered if there is a concern for bladder outlet obstruction or vesicoureteral reflux in the setting of febrile urinary tract infections. As previously mentioned, an MRI of the spine should be considered for any concern of a neuropathic bladder to rule out tethered cord and other neurogenic causes of BBD in the presence of neurologic deficits.

Uroflow with electromyogram (EMG) is a noninvasive way to assess the coordination of bladder contract/flow of urine and relaxation of the pelvic floor muscles. It should be considered de rigor in patients with elevated postvoid residuals to evaluate for bladder neck or external sphincter issues. The uroflowmetry should be done after a bowel program and timed voiding have been initiated, because fecal retention can lead to an increase in pelvic floor activity and thereby create a false-positive result for dyssynergia. Evaluation of a uroflowmetry curve without EMG cannot rule out abnormal sphincter activity, because one can see evidence of bladder neck dysfunction with smooth curves that are not fractionated (staccato or interrupted), as well as tower voids without fractionated curves in patients with external sphincter dyssynergia. Evaluation of the flow curves is a very subjective process and should not be used as a sole means of making a diagnosis, as this has been shown by numerous investigators as indicating poor interobserver and intraobserver reliability. More recent work by Franco and colleagues[19,20] indicates that the flow index, which is a measure of voiding efficiency, can be a better means of evaluating intrapatient voids and assessing treatment outcomes than by relying on flow shapes and isolated flow rates.

Urodynamics and video urodynamics (VUD) are invasive studies requiring catheterization and should be reserved for recalcitrant patients. A multicenter prospective controlled trial reported by Bael and colleagues[21] revealed that VUD for urge syndrome has little to offer in the way of additional value. This study found that urodynamic findings of detrusor overactivity and increased pelvic floor activity during voiding did not correlate with treatment outcome. In addition, neither maximum detrusor pressure during voiding, cystometric bladder capacity, and bladder compliance, nor free flow patterns correlated with treatment outcome. Performing VUD, therefore, offers little additional data that a good history or voiding calendar could not add.[12]

TREATMENT
Educating the Patient and the Family

It is important to first manage the family's expectations. Typically, there is no quick fix when it comes to treatment of BBD, which frustrated parents usually want. Educating the patient and family about what normal voiding habits are is essential. This includes educating them about normal voiding frequency, adequate hydration, comfort and relaxation while voiding, and education regarding normal stooling habits. Furthermore, it is important to let parents know that in children with known neuropsychiatric problems, it can be more difficult to correct incontinence and in some instances it is not possible unless the underlying neuropsychiatric problem is corrected.

Behavioral

Behavioral modification and treatment of constipation is the first step in treating BBD. It is estimated that 50% of patients will improve with just constipation management and behavioral changes.[1]

Timed voiding

Children should be encouraged to void every 2 to 3 hours while the child is awake. This requires a shift from relying on when the child says they need to urinate to a routine schedule, and often urinating when the child does not want to. Of course, this requires parents to obtain control over their child's habits, which can be difficult for some. Motivational star charts can be helpful in that it diffuses the parental control perception. Implementing a timed voiding schedule in school may require a note from the physician to the teacher and school nurse, as some schools have strict rules regarding bathroom breaks.

Adequate hydration

To comply with timed voiding, it is necessary to maintain adequate hydration throughout the day. Adequate hydration varies according to the child's weight; however, a general recommendation of 48 to 64 oz is typically sufficient. This may require a note for school to carry around a water bottle.

Comfort and relaxation during voiding

Pelvic floor muscle awareness is important to focus on while educating patients and families about normal voiding habits. To adequately relax the pelvic floor muscles, children should be comfortable in the bathroom. This may require a foot stool to prop their legs up in addition to fully lowering the pants and underwear. Spreading of the legs can help encourage pelvic floor relaxation. Girls can be taught to sit backward on the toilet to force spreading of the legs.

Pelvic floor muscle physical therapy and biofeedback has been proven to be an effective treatment for dysfunctional voiding.[22–24] Biofeedback provides real-time monitoring of how well the patient is relaxing their pelvic floor muscles, often improving their voluntary control over those muscles.

Bowel management

A regular, ideally daily, soft bowel movement should be the goal for any patient. Loening-Baucke[25] reported that treatment of chronic constipation resulted in resolution of daytime urinary incontinence and nighttime incontinence in 89% and 63% of patients, respectively. Simple constipation can be treated by increasing hydration and adding juices high in sorbitol, such as prune and pear juice. Corn syrup and barley malt extract also can be used to soften the stools and can be used for small infants by mixing with water in their bottle or cups. Should dietary interventions fail, other treatment options include osmotic laxatives, such as polyethylene glycol, lactulose, sorbitol, or milk of magnesia. The addition of senna laxatives or bisacodyl also may be necessary. There is no evidence to support that these cathartics are habit forming or detrimental to the bowel, thereby they can be used liberally as needed. No evidence currently exists supporting the use of prebiotic or probiotic dietary supplements for treatment of constipation.[26,27] If the patient has a significant amount of hard stool in the rectum, manual fecal disimpaction may be necessary.

Medications

For symptoms of an overactive bladder (OAB), urgency, and urinary frequency that are persistent after an adequate trial of behavioral modification, one can consider an anticholinergic. Currently, the only Food and Drug Administration (FDA)-approved anticholinergic in children is oxybutynin, which is dosed at 0.1 to 0.2 mg/kg 2 to 3 times a day. A postvoid residual should be documented soon after starting an anticholinergic, as there is a risk of urinary retention, likely due to the constipation effect rather than the actual medication effect on the bladder. Constipation should be carefully monitored, as it can worsen with an anticholinergic. Other adverse effects include dry mouth, facial flushing, headaches, cognitive impairment, and visual disturbances. There are other anticholinergics, such as tolterodine, fesoterodine, and solifenacin, darifenacin, and propiverine that can be used off-label. Solifenacin and darifenacin have been touted to have fewer effects on cognition due to the reduced ability to cross the blood-brain barrier in this group.

More recently, mirabegron, a beta-3 agonist, has been approved for OAB in adults. There are few data on the use of this drug in children; however, Blais and colleagues,[28] in a prospective, open-label study, reported a statistically significant improvement in bladder capacity and continence. Clinical trials are presently going on worldwide in patients with neurogenic detrusor overactivity.

Imipramine, a tricyclic antidepressant, can be used in children with refractory non-neurogenic daytime incontinence. In a retrospective review, Franco and colleagues[29] demonstrated up to two-thirds of their study population experienced treatment response.

For children with dysfunctional voiding, selective alpha-blockers, such as tamsulosin, alfuzosin, and silodosin, can be used to relax the external sphincter due to the increased alpha 1A activity in these drugs. Cain and colleagues[30] found that alpha-blockers can be useful in improving bladder emptying and decreasing postvoid residual volume. Nonselective alpha-blockers (terazosin and doxazosin) have been noted to have significant effects on irritative voiding symptoms in adults, and in the senior author's experience, it can be useful in ameliorating irritative symptoms in children as well. The mechanism of action for its success is the predominant alpha 1D activity that these drugs exhibit. Because there are alpha 1D receptors in the bladder muscle and submucosa binding to these receptors alters the signaling from the bladder, thereby reducing irritative symptoms.

Surgical Treatment

The use of onabotulinumtoxinA (BoNTA), injected into the detrusor muscles, can be offered as an off-label treatment option in cases of refractory OAB. Studies have mostly been centered around patients with spinal cord injury or myelodysplasia. However, Hoebeke and colleagues[31] found that there can be relief of OAB symptoms after a single injection, lasting more than 12 months in more than 50% of their study population (15 pediatric patients with non-neuropathic bladder with long-term follow-up). Up to 9% of patients will experience urinary retention after injection of BoNTA, so it is necessary to counsel parents appropriately about the possible need for intermittent catheterization after treatment.[32]

BoNTA also can be injected into the external sphincter for dyssynergic voiding. The toxin acts at the neuromuscular junction at the external sphincter to block vesicle transport of acetylcholine. Effects are reversible due to terminal resprouting within 6 months. Franco and colleagues[33] and Vricella and colleagues[34] demonstrated efficacy and durability of intrasphincteric botulinum toxin A injection in children with refractory dysfunctional voiding.

Neuromodulation has been proven to be effective in children with OAB. It is typically used for refractory cases that have not responded to more conservative therapies. It is not FDA approved, and therefore can be offered only off-label. Neuromodulation can be performed with percutaneous tibial nerve stimulation (PTNS), transcutaneous electrical nerve stimulation (TENS), and sacral nerve stimulation devices. For PTNS, a cure rate of OAB and incontinence symptoms of up to 67%, and an improvement rate of 24% have been reported by Patidar and colleagues.[35] Boudaoud and colleagues[36] also reported similar

efficacy. Although prior studies have shown efficacy of up to 56% to 100% for TENS,[37,38] more recent studies, comparing TENS with treatment with anticholinergic medication, demonstrated similar efficacy between the two.[39,40] Sacral nerve modulation is more invasive, and should be reserved for severe, intractable OAB in children. Dwyer and colleagues[41] published a 10-year single-center experience with sacral neuromodulation in pediatric patients with dysfunctional voiding and found that urinary incontinence, constipation, frequency and/or urgency, and nocturnal enuresis improved in 88% of their study population. Nearly all children (94%) experienced improvement of at least 1 symptom. Schober and colleagues[42] also demonstrated statistically significant improvement in voiding dysfunction scores. It has been proven to be successful in adults, but limited research exists regarding its use in the pediatric population.

For intractable constipation, an antegrade continence enema or a cecostomy tube can be considered. This procedure should be offered only when the patient has failed maximal conservative therapy, including maximum doses of medications for constipation.

PSYCHOSOCIAL BURDEN

It is important to keep in mind that the stigma associated with wetting and bowel accidents can significantly impact the patient. This can lead to problems with isolation and shame. Children may exhibit other behavioral changes as well. In addition, it can have an effect on the family.[43] It is important to ask about patient distress associated with BBD symptoms, and to offer psychological counseling when appropriate.

SUMMARY

Pediatric BBD is a common problem that should be addressed early, as it may continue throughout adulthood, leading to significant morbidity. The primary method of treatment should include behavioral modification with timed voiding and pelvic floor relaxation. There are other treatment options for those who fail conservative treatment, including pharmacologic and surgical.

REFERENCES

1. Dos Santos J, Varghese A, Koyle M. Recommendations for the management of bladder bowel dysfunction in children. Pediatr Therapeut 2014;4:1.
2. Halachmi S, Farhat W. Interactions of constipation, dysfunctional elimination syndrome, and vesicoureteral reflux. Adv Urol 2008;828275.

3. Yazbeck S, Schick E, O'Regan S. Relevance of constipation to enuresis, urinary tract infection and reflux. Eur Urol 1987;13:318–21.

4. O'Regan S, Yazbeck S, Schick E. Constipation, bladder instability, urinary tract infection syndrome. Clin Nephrol 1985;23:152–4.

5. Austin P, Bauer S, Neveus T. The standardization of terminology of lower urinary tract function in children and adolescents: update report from the Standardization Committee of the International Children's Continence Society. J Urol 2014;191:1863–5.

6. De Paepe H, Renson C, Hoebeke P, et al. The role of pelvic floor therapy in the treatment of lower urinary tract dysfunctions in children. Scand J Urol Nephrol 2002;36:260–7.

7. Pezzone MA, Liang R, Fraser MO. A model of neural cross-talk and irritation in the pelvis: implications for the overlap of chronic pelvic pain disorders. Gastroenterology 2005;128:1953–64.

8. Ustinova EE, Fraser MO, Pezzone MA. Colonic irritation in the rat sensitizes urinary bladder afferents to mechanical and chemical stimuli: an afferent origin of pelvic organ cross-sensitization. Am J Physiol Renal Physiol 2006;290:F1478–87.

9. Franco I, C Grantham E, Cubillos J, et al. Dizziness as a predictor of bladder neck dysfunction in children with lower urinary tract symptoms. J Pediatr Urol 2016;12(3):157.e1-8.

10. Von Gontard AV, Nevéus T. Management of disorders of bladder and bowel control in childhood. London: Mac Keith Press; 2006.

11. Joinson C, Heron J, von Gontard A. Early childhood risk factors associated with daytime wetting and soiling in school-age children. J Pediatr Psychol 2008;33:739–50.

12. Von Gontard A, Moritz AM, Thome-Granz S, et al. Association of attention deficit and elimination disorders at school entry: a population based study. J Urol 2011;186(5):2027–32.

13. Duel BP, Steinberg-Epstein R, Hill M, et al. A survey of voiding dysfunction in children with attention deficit-hyperactivity disorder. J Urol 2003;170(4 Pt 2):1521–3.

14. Fowler CJ, Griffiths DJ. A decade of functional brain imaging applied to bladder control. Neurourol Urodyn 2010;29:49–55.

15. Farhat W, Bägli DJ, Capolicchio G, et al. The dysfunctional voiding scoring system: quantitative standardization of dysfunctional voiding symptoms in children. J Urol 2000;164:1011–5.

16. Ashfar K, Mirbagheri A, Scott H, et al. Development of a symptom score for dysfunctional elimination syndrome. J Urol 2009;182:1939–43.

17. Bower WF, Sit FK, Bluyssen N, et al. PinQ: a valid, reliable and reproducible quality-of-life measure in children with bladder dysfunction. J Pediatr Urol 2006;2:185–9.

18. Ellsworth PE, Merguerian PA, Copening ME. Sexual abuse: another causative factor in dysfunctional voiding. J Urol 2002;168:2184–7.

19. Franco I, Shei-Dei Yang S, Chang SJ, et al. A quantitative approach to the interpretation of uroflowmetry in children. Neurourol Urodyn 2016; 35(7):836–46.

20. Franco I, Franco J, Lee YS, et al. Can a quantitative means be used to predict flow patterns: agreement between visual inspection vs. flow index derived flow patterns. J Pediatr Urol 2016;12(4):218.e1-8.

21. Bael A, Lax H, de Jong TP, et al. European Bladder Dysfunction Study (European Union BMH1-CT94-1006). J Urol 2008 Oct;180(4):1486–93.

22. Vesna Z, Milica L, Marina V. Correlation between uroflowmetry parameters and treatment outcome in children with dysfunctional voiding. J Pediatr Urol 2010;6:396–402.

23. Kajbafzadeh A, Sharifi-Rad L, Ghahestani S. Animated biofeedback: an ideal treatment for children with dysfunctional elimination syndrome. J Urol 2011;186:2379–85.

24. Zivkovic V, Lazovic M, Vlajkovic M. Diaphragmatic breathing exercises and pelvic floor retraining in children with dysfunctional voiding. Eur J Phys Rehabil Med 2012;48:413–21.

25. Loening-Baucke V. Urinary incontinence and urinary tract infection and their resolution with treatment of chronic constipation of childhood. Pediatrics 1997; 100:228–32.

26. Wald A. Constipation: advances in diagnosis and treatment. JAMA 2016;315(2):185–91.

27. Tabbers MM, Boluyt N, Berger MY, et al. Nonpharmacologic treatments for childhood constipation: systematic review. Pediatrics 2011;128(4):753–61.

28. Blais A, Nadeau G, Moore K, et al. Prospective pilot study of mirabegron in pediatric patients with overactive bladder. Eur Urol 2016;70:9–13.

29. Franco I, Arien AM, Collett-Gardere T, et al. Imipramine for refractory daytime incontinence in pediatric population. J Pediatr Urol 2018;14(1):58.e1-58.

30. Cain M, Wu S, Rink R. Alpha blocker therapy for children with dysfunctional voiding and urinary retention. J Urol 2003;170:1514–5.

31. Hoebeke P, De Caestecker K, Vande Walle J, et al. The effect of botulinum-A toxin in incontinent children with therapy resistant overactive detrusor. J Urol 2006;176:328–30.

32. Greer T, Abbott J, Breytenbach W, et al. Ten years of experience with intravesical and intrasphincteric onabotulinumtoxinA in children. J Pediatr Urol 2016;12:94.e1-6.

33. Franco I, Landau-Dyer L, Isom-Batz G, et al. The use of botulinum toxin A injection for the management of external sphincter dyssenergia in neurologically normal children. J Urol 2007;178:1775–9.

34. Vricella GJ, Campigotto M, Coplen DE, et al. Long-term efficacy and durability of botulinim-A toxin for refractory dysfunctional voiding in children. J Urol 2014;191:1586–91.

35. Patidar N, Mittal V, Kumar M, et al. Transcutaneous posterior tibial nerve stimulation in pediatric overactive bladder: a preliminary report. J Pediatr Urol 2015;11:351.e1-6.

36. Boudaoud N, Binet A, Line A, et al. Management of refractory overactive bladder in children by transcutaneous posterior tibial nerve stimulation: a controlled study. J Pediatr Urol 2015;11:138.e1-10.

37. Hoebeke P, Van Laecke E, Everaert K, et al. Transcutaneous neuromodulation for the urge syndrome in children: a pilot study. J Urol 2001;166:2416–9.

38. Malm-Buatsi E, Nepple KG, Boyt MA, et al. Efficacy of transcutaneous electrical nerve stimulation in children with overactive bladder refractory to pharmacotherapy. Urology 2007;70:980–3.

39. Sillen U, Arwidsson C, Doroszkiewicz M, et al. Effects of transcutaneous neuromodulation (TENS) on overactive bladder symptoms in children: a randomized, controlled trial. J Pediatr Urol 2014; 10:1100–5.

40. Quintiliano F, Veiga ML, Moraes M, et al. Transcutaneous parasacral electrical stimulation vs. oxybutynin for the treatment of overactive bladder in children: a randomized clinical trial. J Urol 2015; 193:1749–53.

41. Dwyer ME, Vandersteen DR, Hollatz P, et al. Sacral neuromodulation for the dysfunctional elimination syndrome: a 10-year single-center experience with 105 consecutive children. Urology 2014;84(4):911–7.

42. Schober MS, Sulkowski JP, Lu PL, et al. Sacral nerve stimulation for pediatric lower urinary tract dysfunction: development of a standardized pathway with objective urodynamic outcomes. J Urol 2015;194: 1721–7.

43. Landgraf JM, Abidari J, Cilento BG Jr, et al. Coping, commitment, and attitude: quantifying the everyday burden of enuresis on children and their families. Pediatrics 2004;113:334–44.

Prenatal Urinary Tract Dilatation

Andrea Balthazar, MD[a], C.D. Anthony Herndon, MD[b],*

KEYWORDS

- Prenatal diagnosis • Urinary tract dilatation • Hydronephrosis • Urinary tract infection • Radiology
- Vesicoureteral reflux

KEY POINTS

- Prenatal urinary tract dilatation (UTD) is a common diagnosis encountered on antenatal ultrasonography imaging.
- Indications for fetal intervention for lower urinary tract obstruction are rare.
- Fetal intervention in the form of vesicoamniotic shunting or fetal cystoscopy increase neonatal survival but have no predictable impact on long-term renal function.
- P1, P2, and P3 UTD are considered low, intermediate, and high risk, respectively. Postnatal imaging and prophylactic antibiotics are dictated by risk stratification.
- It is important to separate benign UTD from clinically significant disorder in the fetus and infant to minimize unnecessary testing and exposures.

INTRODUCTION

Prenatal urinary tract dilatation (UTD) is one of the most common findings encountered on antenatal ultrasonography (US) and occurs in 1% to 3% of all pregnancies.[1] Approximately 40,000 to 80,000 children are diagnosed annually with this condition.[1] In most patients, UTD is transient and represents a physiologic state that is clinically insignificant; however, prenatal identification of UTD may equally represent an obstructive condition or vesicoureteral reflux (VUR) that may have adverse effects on renal development/function and cause significant morbidity. Prenatal identification of UTD represents a variety of possible causes and uropathies that affect the kidney, ureter, and/or bladder, known collectively as congenital abnormalities of the kidney and urinary tract.[2]

The causes of prenatal UTD include transient dilatation, upper tract obstructive uropathies, lower tract obstructive uropathies, and nonobstructive conditions (**Table 1**). The ultimate goal is to separate benign, transient UTD from clinically significant urologic disorder in the fetus in an effort to minimize unnecessary testing in infants while detecting the patients of UTD that may require further prenatal and postnatal evaluation. The aim of this article is to aid clinicians in understanding the grading systems used for evaluating UTD, risk stratification for prenatal and postnatal UTD, and management of postnatal UTD.

DEFINING AND CLASSIFYING URINARY TRACT DILATATION

Multiple classification systems have been developed to classify and grade the severity of antenatal

Disclosure: No authors of this work have any direct or indirect conflicts of interest associated with this article. The work was not funded.
[a] Division of Urology, Department of Surgery, Virginia Commonwealth University School of Medicine, VCU Medical Center, PO Box 980118, Richmond, VA 23298-0118, USA; [b] Pediatric Urology, Division of Urology, Department of Surgery, Children's Hospital of Richmond, Virginia Commonwealth University School of Medicine, VCU Medical Center, PO Box 980118, Richmond, VA 23298-0118, USA
* Corresponding author.
E-mail address: claude.herndon@vcuhealth.org

Urol Clin N Am 45 (2018) 641–657
https://doi.org/10.1016/j.ucl.2018.06.011
0094-0143/18/© 2018 Elsevier Inc. All rights reserved.

Table 1
Cause of prenatal urinary tract dilatation detected on ultrasonography

Cause	Incidence (%)
Transient UTD/physiologic	41–88
Ureteropelvic junction obstruction	10–30
Vesicoureteral reflux	10–40
Ureterovesical junction obstruction/megaureter	5–15
Multicystic dysplastic kidney	2–5
Posterior urethral valves	1–5
Ureterocele, ectopic ureter, duplex system, urethral atresia, prune-belly syndrome, polycystic kidney disease, fetal cysts	Uncommon

Adapted from Nguyen HT, Herndon CD, Cooper C. The Society for Fetal Urology consensus statement on the evaluation and management of antenatal hydronephrosis. J Pediatr Urol 2010;6(3):212–31; with permission.

and postnatal UTD. Navigating and understanding the different grading systems and terminologies used by providers creates a challenge in managing these patients because of a lack of uniformity in defining and grading UTD. There is no consensus on the most appropriate grading system for diagnosing and managing prenatal UTD.[3] In addition, the lack of consensus in defining and grading UTD makes it difficult to appropriately correlate prenatal and postnatal US findings with the eventual diagnosis. Furthermore, meaningful outcomes data are equally difficult to obtain with this lack of uniformity in grading UTD.

Certain grading systems have been used to describe the prenatal evaluation, whereas others are preferred in the postnatal evaluation. Obstetricians prefer using the objective anterior-posterior renal pelvic diameter (APRPD), compared with pediatric urologists who are divided between the APRPD and the Society of Fetal Urology (SFU) grading systems.[3] Furthermore, postnatally, pediatric radiologists prefer a subjective/descriptive (mild, moderate, severe) grading system, whereas urologists use a combination of the APRPD and SFU systems to grade UTD. The recent movement toward a uniform grading system, as described in multidisciplinary consensus statement on UTD, should be beneficial in promoting communication between different specialists involved in the care of the patients, evaluation, and further research efforts.[2] This system is discussed later in the article.

Anterior-Posterior Pelvic Diameter

APRPD or anterior-posterior diameter (APD) is the measurement used to characterize the severity of renal pelvis dilatation.[3] It is the maximum APD of the renal pelvis in the transverse plane measured within the confines of the renal parenchyma. The APD measurement should be reliable, reproducible, and objective; however, in the case of more significant disease, it is operator dependent. To establish normative values, several studies have evaluated the renal pelvis size based on gestational age (GA) of the fetus.[4,5] The diagnosis of UTD using the APD measurement varies depending on GA of the fetus, with the most common use of 2 GA groups, second trimester (16–27 weeks) and third trimester (28–32 weeks).[4,5] These studies established that APD cutoffs are effective measures to aid in predicting both urologic disease and the possible need for surgical intervention. However, there remains a lack of consistency across studies with various cutoff values and no consensus on the threshold APD to define clinically significant prenatal UTD, which reflects a high risk of renal disorder and the degree that necessitates postnatal evaluation.[5–7] Classically, APD greater than 4 mm during the second trimester and greater than 7 mm during the third trimester are the lowest cutoff values for diagnosis of potentially significant UTD in the fetus.[6–8]

Society of Fetal Urology Grading System

The SFU system is the most common system used by pediatric urologists.[3] It is a subjective 5-point (0–4) system based on the assessment of the degree of renal pelvis dilatation, the number of calyces involved (major and minor), and the parenchymal integrity of the kidney[9] (**Fig. 1**). Grade III and grade IV are differentiated based on the presence or absence of parenchymal thinning. The SFU system is simple and has been shown to be predictive of both renal preservation and the need for surgical intervention.[10,11] The SFU grading system was designed and has been used primarily for assessment of postnatal hydronephrosis.

- Grade 0: normal, no dilatation of the collecting system
- Grade I: mild dilatation of the renal pelvis (urine barely splits the renal pelvis), no calyces involved
- Grade II: mild to moderate dilatation of the renal pelvis, major calyces involved
- Grade III: dilatation of the renal pelvis, uniform dilatation of the major and minor calyces, normal renal parenchyma

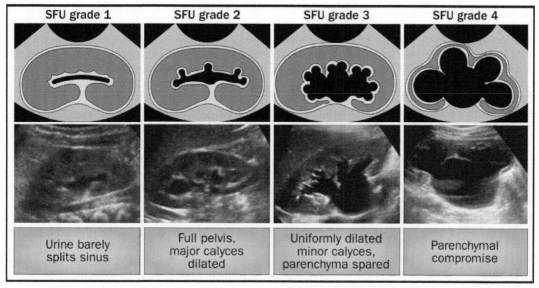

Fig. 1. The SFU grading system uses a 5-point grading system (0–4) to grade UTD and is based on US imaging. The system is scored on the degree of dilatation of collecting system and parenchymal integrity. Grade 0 is normal and not pictured. Grade 1: urine barely splits the renal sinus. Grade 2: urine fills pelvis and major calyces dilated. Grade 3: SFU grade 2 plus dilatation of minor calyces, normal parenchyma. Grade 4: SFU grade 3 plus parenchyma compromise. (*From* Timberlake MD, Herndon CDA. Mild to moderate postnatal hydronephrosis—grading systems and management. Nat Rev Urol 2013;10(11):649–56; with permission.)

- Grade IV: gross dilatation of the renal pelvis and calyces, parenchymal atrophy seen as cortical thinning

Urinary Tract Dilatation Classification System

In an effort to promote uniformity and consistency for both prenatal and postnatal grading of UTD, a new system was developed and captured within the multidisciplinary consensus statement on UTD. It combines both the objective and subjective parameters of the APD and SFU systems. The UTD classification expanded the grading system to analyze findings not only within the kidney but also within the ureter and lower urinary tract. The system applies to UTD that presents prenatally or postnatally. The UTD grading system was proposed by a multispecialty team that included maternal fetal medicine, pediatric radiology, pediatric urology, and pediatric nephrology. The UTD system is based on 6 categories of US findings: (1) APRPD; (2) calyceal dilatation; (3) renal parenchymal thickness; (4) renal parenchymal appearance; (5) bladder abnormalities; and (6) ureteral abnormalities.[2]

The consensus document called for standardization of technique inclusive of parameters that are measured as well as reporting nomenclature. For imaging technique, prenatal images should be obtained with the spine in the 6 o'clock or 12 o'clock position. Postnatally, the mid region of the kidney marked by the hilar structures should be used in the transverse plan to measure the APD. Serial imaging should be obtained in a similar position to the previous study, and either supine or prone position should be used. In terms of the APD measurement, it should be the maximal distance within the confines of the renal parenchyma, and avoid measuring the largest APD that may rest outside of the renal parenchyma, as commonly seen with an extrarenal dilated renal pelvis. These parameters are used to assign a level of risk. There are 2 antenatal and 3 postnatal categories of risk: A1 (low risk) or A2–3 (intermediate/high risk) for antenatal UTD; and P1 (low), P2 (intermediate), P3 (high risk) for postnatal UTD.[2]

In the UTD A1 group, APD measuring 4 to 7 mm at less than 28 weeks and 7 to less than 10 mm at greater than or equal to 28 weeks and the absence of peripheral calyceal involvement is considered low risk for postnatal urologic disorder. The UTD A2 to A3 group is considered to be at increased risk for postnatal urologic disorder based on APD greater than or equal to 7 mm at less than 16 to 27 weeks and greater than or equal to 10 mm at greater than or equal to 28 weeks. The increased risk group (A2–3) is also associated with any of the following findings: peripheral calyceal dilatation, abnormal parenchymal thickness or appearance, visibly dilated ureter, abnormal bladder, or the presence of unexplained oligohydramnios.[2] The UTD classification system was simplified to allow conversion from existing grading systems to the UTD system. For example, when converting the SFU to UTD system, SFU grade I to II would be equivalent to UTD P1, SFU grade III to UTD P2, and SFU grade IV to UTD P3. The postnatal evaluation and management recommendations are based on the risk stratification. Several studies have shown consistency for both the SFU and UTD for inter-rater and intrarater reliability aside from the SFU for moderate degrees of dilatation, which was slightly superior.[12] Equally, the UTD classification system was as effective as the SFU at predicting resolution of UTD for both low-grade and high-grade disease.[13]

Prenatal imaging and management

Ultrasonography In the United States, ultrasonography is the primary means of fetal imaging and routine screening US is typically performed during the second trimester ($\sim$20 weeks). On average, 2 US scans are obtained in a low-risk pregnancy and 4 scans in high-risk pregnancy.[14] Up to 3% of all pregnancies involve urinary tract anomalies and most prenatally diagnosed UTD is transient or physiologic; however, significant disease may be detected, and studies have shown that the degree of UTD correlates with an increased risk of urologic disorder.[15] The renal pelvis APD is considered normal when the measured value is less than 4 mm at less than 28 weeks' GA, less than 7 mm at greater than 28 weeks GA, and less than 10 mm in the postnatal period.[3] Of note, the APD threshold of less than 10 mm was only recently described with the intent to decrease the large number of additional evaluative studies for patients with a strong likelihood of having a nonpathologic condition. When prenatal UTD is detected, a complete fetal survey should be performed; level III fetal US and additional parameters should aid in guiding further need for evaluation and may aid in determining potential cause of UTD.

Prenatally 2 risk stratifications exist (A1 UTD and A2–3 UTD) based in part on the degree of APD that is indexed with GA and the degree of calyceal dilatation (**Fig. 2**). In the UTD A1 group, APD that measures 4 to 7 mm at less than 28 weeks' GA and 7 to greater than or equal to 10 mm at greater than or equal to 28 weeks' GA with only central calyceal involvement, when present, is considered low risk for postnatal urologic disorder (**Fig. 3**). The UTD A2 to A3 group is considered to be at increased risk for postnatal urologic disorder based on APD greater than or equal to 7 mm at less than 28 weeks' GA and greater than or equal to 10 mm at greater than or equal to 28 weeks' GA

(**Fig. 4**). The A2 to A3 increased risk group is also associated with any of the following US findings: peripheral calyceal dilatation, abnormal parenchyma thickness or appearance, visibly dilated ureter, abnormal bladder, or the presence of unexplained oligohydramnios.[16]

MRI MRI does not use ionizing radiation and is a noninvasive procedure that may be a valuable adjunct when fetal US is indeterminate. It allows for in utero characterization of anatomic details of fetal genitourinary tract abnormalities that may aid in prenatal consultation. Although US is the reference standard for fetal imaging, the assessment may be limited by factors such as amniotic fluid volume, fetal position, maternal body habitus, maternal bowel gas, and/or pelvic bony structures.[17,18] Kajbafzadeh and colleagues[19] showed that fetal MRI accurately diagnoses fetal UTD while providing additional information regarding different forms of urinary tract obstruction ranging from ureteropelvic junction (UPJ) obstruction to posterior urethral valve (PUV).

Management overview

When UTD is detected during the second trimester, a complete fetal survey US scan should be obtained. Most cases of fetal UTD are clinically insignificant; however, parental concerns still exist. These concerns may play a role in the abundance of overtesting that traditionally has driven up health care cost associated with prenatal care without showing an improvement in postnatal outcome.[20] The primary goal of prenatal care for urologic disease is to identify the patients who can be safely observed with an appropriate degree of certainty that will dictate the timing of subsequent prenatal imaging. Intervention is rarely needed and should be reserved for select cases in which pulmonary compromise is suspected.[21]

Up to 88% of prenatal patients with UTD show resolution in the prenatal or early neonatal period, which has led to increased expectant management.[22] When UTD is detected, the optimal timing of subsequent imaging depends on the GA at initial diagnosis and the severity of UTD. The risk level should dictate the timing and frequency of subsequent imaging. When UTD A1 is diagnosed before 32 weeks of gestation, an additional prenatal US scan should be obtained at greater than or equal to 32 weeks of gestation. If resolution of UTD is seen at greater than or equal to 32 weeks in the presence of normal parenchyma, bladder, and ureters, no further prenatal or postnatal imaging is necessary. Persistent UTD A1 or UTD A2 to A3 warrants postnatal evaluation. In low-risk fetuses (UTD A1), the first postnatal US scan should be

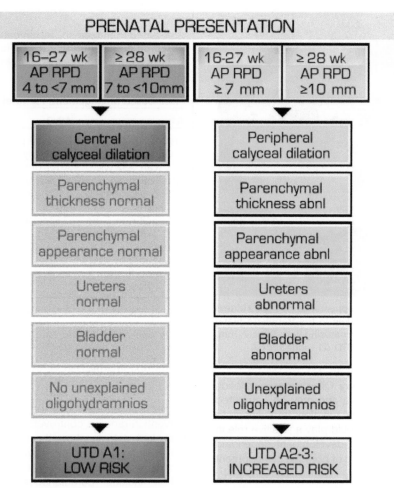

Fig. 2. Prenatal UTD risk stratification: UTD A1 (low risk) and UTD A2–3 (increased risk). The classification is based on the presence of the most concerning feature shown on US, regardless of the APRPD measurement. (*From* Nguyen HT, Benson CB, Bromley B. Multidisciplinary consensus on the classification of prenatal and postnatal urinary tract dilation (UTD classification system). J Pediatr Urol 2014;10(6):982–98; with permission.)

obtained at greater than 48 hours of age. In the increased risk group (UTD A2–3), repeat US is recommended within 4 to 6 weeks of the initial diagnosis of UTD. The recommendations regarding timing of subsequent interval assessment varies based on presence of severe unilateral UTD, bilateral UTD, and suspected bladder outlet obstruction and requires more frequent US evaluation[3,16] (**Table 2**).

If there is concern for significant risk of long-term renal impairment or possible need for surgical intervention, a prenatal consultation with a pediatric urologist and/or nephrologist is recommended. A repeat US scan after birth is recommended after 48 hours of life but before 1 month; however, the clinician should perform follow-up sooner in patients with suspected obstructive uropathy, such as PUV (suggested by thickened bladder wall

with persistent dilatation of the posterior urethra) or for bilateral conditions.[23] It is important to educate the parents on the ultrasonography findings, the possible cause, the potential significance, and the possible steps involved if the fetus will require further prenatal management. The finding of severe bilateral UTD of the kidneys, ureter, and bladder with/without the presence of the so-called keyhole sign and decreased amniotic fluid indicates lower urinary tract obstruction (LUTO). The exact cause is difficult to discern but most commonly includes PUV, urethral atresia, or prune-belly syndrome. These conditions can be differentiated from other conditions that result in severe dilatation of the entire urinary system, such as megacystis-microcolon-intestinal hypoperistalsis syndrome, which may maintain normal amniotic fluid.

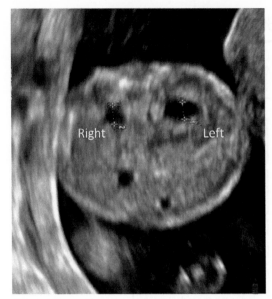

Fig. 3. Ultrasonography appearance of fetal kidneys at 20 weeks' gestation taken in the transverse plane shows bilateral APRPD measuring less than 7 mm, which is consistent with UTD A1 range for GA.

Fetal intervention/surgery Oligohydramnios leads to pulmonary hypoplasia and may be correlated with poor postnatal renal function. Intervention to restore amniotic fluid could play a positive role in pulmonary and/or renal development depending on the degree and timing of both the development

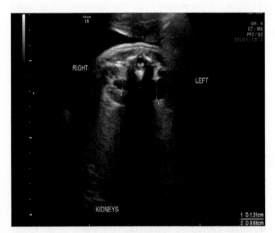

Fig. 4. US appearance of UTD A2–3: ultrasonography appearance of fetal kidneys at 37 weeks' gestation taken in the transverse plane shows an APRPD measurement taken with the spine at the 12 o'clock position with the calipers placed at the widest part of the intrarenal fluid collection. The right APRPD measures less than 7 mm, which is within the normal range. The left APRPD measures greater than 7 mm, which is within UTD A2–A3 range for GA.

Table 2
Risk-based management recommendations based on prenatal urinary tract dilatation risk stratification of urinary tract dilatation A1 and A2–3

Risk-Based Management, Prenatal Diagnosis	
A1	**A2–3**
Prenatal period: One additional US scan ≥32 wk	Prenatal period: Initially in 4–6 wk[a]
After birth: Two additional US scans: 1. >48 h to 1 mo 2. 1–6 mo later	After birth: US scan at >48 h to 1 mo of age[a]
Other: Aneuploidy risk modification if indicated	Other: Specialist consultation; eg, nephrology, urology

[a] Certain situations (eg, PUV, bilateral severe hydronephrosis) may require more expedient follow-up.

From Nguyen HT, Benson CB, Bromley B. Multidisciplinary consensus on the classification of prenatal and postnatal urinary tract dilation (UTD classification system). J Pediatr Urol 2014;10(6):982–98; with permission.

and relief of bladder outlet obstruction. Prenatal intervention remains controversial because of the insufficient data to show the potential benefits, such as long-term patient survival and improvement of renal outcome.[24–27] Methods of fetal intervention include percutaneous fetal shunting (vesicoamniotic shunts [VASs]) and fetal endoscopy (fetoscopy). Fetal intervention has been isolated to very select cases of suspected bladder outlet obstruction (primarily caused by PUV) associated with oligohydramnios between 18 and 24 weeks' GA and evidence of preserved renal function on serial fetal urine biochemistry profiles. The assessment of renal function is based on analysis of urine biomarkers such as urine sodium, chloride, calcium, osmolarity, and beta-2-microglobulin obtained via serial fetal bladder aspirations.[28,29]

A multicenter, prospective randomized trial, Percutaneous Shunting in Lower Urinary Tract Obstruction (PLUTO), was designed to determine the efficacy of vesicoamniotic shunting to improve survival and renal outcome compared with conservative management. However, the study was terminated because of poor enrollment and thus was underpowered. The study cohort included only pregnancies in which it was not clear whether intervention was appropriate. The study suggested shunting may improve perinatal survival but was unclear on the impact of renal function, with only 2 of 16 showing normal renal function.[30] Complications were common and occurred in 44% of the shunted group, similar to previous reports in the literature.[31]

Fetal cystoscopy offers the potential advantage of providing benefits similar to VAS placement without the dependence of maintaining a functional device throughout pregnancy. In addition, it allows for bladder cycling and direct visualization of the cause for LUTO, thereby facilitating the correct diagnosis and treatment when possible.[29,32,33] Complications associated with fetal cystoscopic therapy are similar to VAS with an additional risk of cutaneous or rectal fistula reported in 10% of those undergoing ablation.[34] The procedure is performed in an antegrade manner with a neodymium-doped yttrium aluminum garnet (Nd:Yag) laser, which puts the surgeon at an anatomic disadvantage compared with retrograde.

In a large multicenter comparative analysis, a total of 111 consecutive patients with fetal LUTO were retrospectively reviewed and fetal interventions were performed in 50 (34 fetal cystoscopy, 16 VAS). A clear survival advantage was shown with any intervention with a negligible difference between VAS and fetal cystoscopy. There was evidence of potential benefit in improving renal function when comparing fetal cystoscopy with VAS, with an adjusted relative risk ratio (ARR) of 1.73 (95% confidence interval [CI], 0.97–3.08; $P = .06$). When comparing those with postnatal confirmation of PUV, fetal cystoscopy further improved renal function, with an ARR of 2.66 (95% CI, 1.25–5.70; $P = .01$) that was not seen with VAS.[29]

These procedures remain controversial because of limited information on the long-term improvement in outcomes, potential risk to mother and fetus, and high complication rates. After extensive parental counseling regarding the risks and benefits, odds of neonatal survival, and renal outcome, in utero intervention should be discussed with and performed under the guidance and expertise of a specialist at a high-volume center with significant experience in these procedures.

Postnatal evaluation and management

The postnatal evaluation and management of prenatal UTD has become more conservative over the last decade. Following the publication of the multidisciplinary consensus statement on UTD and several other studies, the continuous evolution of management strategies has shifted away from aggressive screening toward a more conservative postnatal management approach of these infants. This approach has been coupled with a concerted effort to minimize the indiscriminate use of prophylactic antibiotics (PAs). The goal is to identify the infants with significant urologic disease while avoiding unnecessary testing, invasive procedures, and radiation in patients with transient, physiologic UTD. A more practical screening approach is directed at detecting those at highest risk of urinary tract infection (UTI) and renal detrioration.[21,35–38] Common imaging modalities used in postnatal evaluation of UTD include renal/bladder US, voiding cystourethrography (VCUG), diuretic renal scintigraphy, and magnetic resonance urography (MRU). The postnatal evaluation and treatment recommendations developed by the consensus statement were based on a risk stratification system.[2]

Imaging

Renal/bladder ultrasonography The postnatal evaluation of a neonate with a history of prenatal UTD begins with US. US is a paramount first step in formulating the risk stratification process. The first postnatal US scan should be delayed for at least 48 hours after birth. This delay allows for the resolution of the initial postnatal oliguric state, which occurs secondary to intravascular depletion and would underestimate the degree of UTD.[39,40] The study should evaluate the entire urinary tract, including the bladder and ureters, for the presence of dilatation and adhere to the principals outlined in the multidisciplinary consensus document.[2] US imaging provides an almost universally available modality to both evaluate and monitor UTD without the risk of radiation exposure. Also, serial imaging permits longitudinal follow-up and may obviate diuretic renal scintigrapy.[41] By comparing the degree of UTD identified on the prenatal US scan with the postnatal US scan, UTD is classified as resolved, stable, improving, or worsening. Of note, based on SFU hydronephrosis registry data, 25% of the infants with evidence of UTD resolution on postnatal imaging may still have significant urologic disease such as VUR, and up to 28% of patients may have recurrence of UTD or present later with UPJ obstruction.[42–44]

Voiding cystourethrography VCUG is an imaging modality used to evaluate the bladder and aids in the diagnosis of disorder involving the lower urinary tract, such as VUR, PUV, or ureterocele. The decision to perform lower urinary tract imaging to screen infants with prenatal UTD has shifted toward a more conservative approach over the last decade. The risk of developing urologic disease (eg, UTI), as opposed to the possibility of identifying VUR, should be the basis for recommending VCUG.[45] Historical data show an overall VUR incidence rate of up to 20% when patients with UTD are uniformly screened.[21,46] It is recognized that the degree of prenatal UTD does not correlate with the presence or severity of VUR.[15,47]

A more selective approach directing the use of lower urinary tract imaging toward those with an increased risk of UTI (high-grade VUR, women, intact foreskin, and ureteral dilatation) is recommended. The timing of the study should be based on the severity of UTD. Almost all patients screened with initial postnatal US may be discharged, and subsequent lower urinary tract imaging may be performed electively as an outpatient. In patients for whom there is concern of possible bladder outlet obstruction, the study should be performed before discharge. PAs should be used in patients who are considered high risk for UTI (UTD P2 or P3). The benefit of identifying asymptomatic VUR in the neonatal period remains unclear, but extrapolated data from older children with VUR undergoing active surveillance seem to show that it may be benign and may not increase risk of UTI.[48,49]

Recently, a standardization of technique white paper was endorsed by American Academy of Pediatrics, which serves to optimize the procedure and should allow more consistent studies to be performed. Pediatric urologists and other pediatric physicians are encouraged to ensure that their institutions follow the protocol.[50] The protocol recommends minimizing radiation while obtaining high-quality images by observing the "as low as (is) reasonably achievable" (ALARA) and Image Gently guidelines.[51,52] The procedure involves insertion of a nonballoon catheter into the bladder and instillation of contrast material into the bladder. Then, fluoroscopic images are obtained, including a scout KUB (kidneys, ureters, and urinary bladder) film, bladder filling, and voiding phases. This procedure may be repeated because several groups have shown an increased reliability to detect VUR with cyclic filling.[53,54] The procedure is usually well tolerated by infants.

Renal scintigraphy Renal scintigraphy is used in infants with persistent UTD to identify obstruction and evaluate the differential renal function. Radionucleotide studies are inferior in showing anatomic detail compared with other modalities such as US, MRI, or computed tomography. These studies are usually deferred until at least 6 weeks of age to allow the renal function to mature. The so-called well-tempered renogram involves administration of a diuretic and is measured in 2 phases (cortical imaging and tubular imaging phase) and is a well-established and adopted protocol.[55] The diuretic renogram is an invasive procedure and should follow the standardized protocol, including the placement of an urethral catheter, intravenous hydration, a small dose of radiation, patient positioning, and monitoring the region of interest.[16] However, the degree of radiation exposure is related to the severity of obstruction.[56] At present, the agent of choice is Tc-mercaptoacetyltriglycine (MAG3), and it is best suited to evaluate drainage of the kidney because it is bound primarily by plasma proteins and cleared by renal tubular secretion.[16] The major roles of MAG3 scan are identification of clinically relevant obstruction and split differential renal function in infants with a history of prenatal UTD and persistent postnatal UTD.[16] The approach to prenatally detected UTD has trended toward a more conservative management involving appropriately timed renal US studies and selective use of radionuclide scans in infants with persistent postnatal UTD P2 or P3 (similar to SFU grade III and IV dilatation). The main disadvantage of interpretation involves patients with severe UTD because of associated extreme variability in individual anatomy. False-positive results may occur with a large collecting system that does not afford appropriate time for the capacious system to fill before diuretic administration. Recently, formal upright imaging as a subsequent step with measurements of the percentage drainage was noted to be more predictive of surgical management in patients with indeterminate drainage with less variability.[57]

Magnetic resonance urography MRU is recognized as a valuable adjunct and is increasingly used in the evaluation of UTD. It provides better anatomic detail to localize the abnormality, calculates differential function, and allows an assessment of drainage.[58,59] The detailed information obtained can assist in operative planning. There is a superior correlation reported with MRU compared with the current standard evaluation of UTD using US, VCUG, and renal scintigraphy.[60] The cost, need for sedation, use of gadolinium contrast, and lack of availability at all centers are some of the disadvantages limiting the widespread use of MRU. One specific issue is the need for prone positioning. It may be less than ideal positioning for a neonate under anesthesia within the confines of an MRI machine with limited accessibility. As the technology advances, it will likely play a larger role when evaluating patients with obstruction.

URINARY TRACT INFECTION/ANTIBIOTIC PROPHYLAXIS

Recently, the efficacy of PAs to prevent UTI in patients with prenatal UTD has been challenged. A critical evaluation of the literature characterizing associated risk factors for UTI includes a combination of retrospective and more recently prospective registry data, including 1 multicenter report.[21,35,38,61] The overall incidence of UTI ranges from 9% to 19%.[38,61,62] The general consensus of factors that increase risk of UTI include female gender, intact foreskin, and higher-grade UTD (ie, SFU grade III and grade IV). Other factors associated with increased risk of UTI, such as ureteral dilatation and VUR, have been identified in some studies but not validated in others.[62,63] In terms of VUR, it should be noted that a meaningful evidence-based risk assessment is not practical because of the lack of uniform screening for VUR and use of PAs in patients with prenatal UTD.

Several studies have addressed the utility of PAs or lack thereof to affect UTIs. A systematic review of the literature supported the ability of PAs to prevent UTIs in high-grade UTD but not low-grade UTD. The risk reduction was about 50%, with 14.6% developing UTI on PAs and 28.9% off PAs. However, other single-center studies have shown discrepancies, noting a lack of benefit, indifferent results, or a clear benefit for isolated grades that show postnatal VUR.[37,64,65] Controversy exists between the 2 prospective registry reports by Braga and Zee.[35,38] The Braga group showed a UTI incidence of 14.6% on PAs and 28.9% without PAs.[35] The American multicenter registry did not validate these results and showed a lack of benefit for PAs for both low-grade and high-grade UTD. It did show that 89% of UTIs occurred within the first year of life.[38] However, the American registry included lower grades of UTD and less identified VUR because of less screening with VCUG. Also, it showed no reported harm secondary to prophylaxis. Therefore, those at risk regardless of the presence of VUR should be managed for the first year on PAs.

RISK STRATIFICATION BASED ON URINARY TRACT DILATATION CLASSIFICATION

The postnatal evaluation of UTD should be tailored toward the overall risk of urologic disorder. The variables affecting this risk include degree of prenatal UTD, gender, and the presence of lower UTD. The primary goal should be identifying those with clinically significant disease while avoiding unnecessary testing in infants with transient, physiologic UTD. The natural history of postnatal UTD is not clearly defined, thus making it increasingly difficult to differentiate the patients with significant disease from those with transient, insignificant dilatation. Note that a concerted effort was made

with the recommendations from the consensus document to redefine normalcy for UTD by affording an APD up to 9 mm, which should lead to less testing in the low-risk population.

The goal of the UTD classification system is to create a more uniform approach that can seamlessly be applied to both the prenatal and the postnatal UTD populations and used universally by all providers. This classification system is based on postnatal risk stratification, with the management recommendations specifying the timing and type of imaging modality as well as a recommendation toward the use of antibiotic prophylaxis (**Fig. 5**).

The recommendations given here apply to isolated unilateral UTD. In cases of bilateral UTD, possible bladder outlet obstruction, or presence of multiorgan disease, expert consultation by pediatric urology and/or pediatric nephrology is recommended (**Table 3**).

P1 (LOW-RISK) URINARY TRACT DILATATION

Most patients with persistent postnatal dilatation have UTD P1, and recent studies suggest that the use of PAs is not beneficial because of the low risk of infants developing a UTI.[38,61] The low risk affects the need for lower urinary tract imaging as well, despite the fact that VUR may be present in up to 20% of this group.[21,46] Parents and providers should be aware that the lack of screening does not equate to the absence of disease. Any child with fever and signs of UTI should be screened for VUR after an appropriate course of antibiotics.

The interval of postnatal US should be based on the probability of disease progression. Data from the SFU registry suggest patients with low-grade UTD rarely progress to higher grades and resolution is seen in almost all cases within 48 months of life.[66] Subsequent follow-up imaging should be obtained 3 to 6 months after the initial study. In patients with a normal initial postnatal US, it is recommended to repeat US within 3 to 6 months to ensure resolution has occurred (**Fig. 6**). When resolution of postnatal UTD is noted on further follow-up imaging, a follow-up US scan is recommended 1 year later to confirm the resolution. Following this confirmatory US, no further follow-up is warranted.

P2 (INTERMEDIATE-RISK) URINARY TRACT DILATATION

No uniform agreement exists regarding the use of PA, lower urinary tract imaging, or subsequent postnatal imaging for UTD P2 (**Fig. 7**). Survey data from pediatric urologists indicates that PA recommendations range from 24% to 46% based

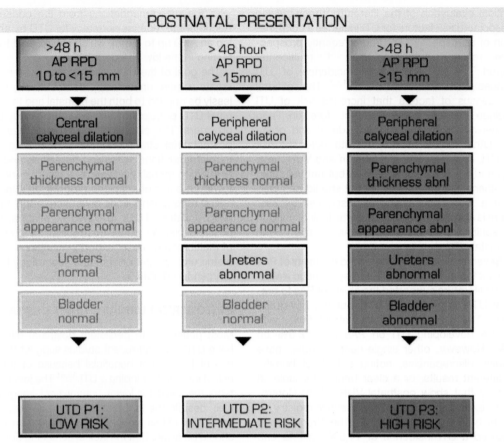

Fig. 5. Postnatal UTD risk stratification: UTD P1 (low risk), UTD P2 (intermediate risk), and UTD P3 (high risk). The risk stratification is based on the presence of the most concerning feature shown on US, regardless of the APRPD measurement. (*From* Nguyen HT, Benson CB, Bromley B. Multidisciplinary consensus on the classification of prenatal and postnatal urinary tract dilation (UTD classification system). J Pediatr Urol 2014;10(6):982–98; with permission.)

on gender and foreskins status, whereas 78% recommend lower urinary tract imaging and 58% recommend renal scintigraphy to assess the function and drainage in the presence of UTD.[67] At present, the recommendations regarding PA, VCUG, and renal scintigraphy are left to the discretion of physicians. There exists a clear need for further research to study this population.

Table 3
Risk-based management recommendations based on urinary tract dilatation risk stratification of postnatal urinary tract dilatation P1, P2, and P3

Risk-based Management, Postnatal Diagnosis		
P1	**P2**	**P3**
Follow-up US:	Follow-up US:	Follow-up US:
3 to 6 mo	1 to 3 mo	1 mo
VCUG:	VCUG:	VCUG:
Not recommended	Discretion of clinician	Recommended
Antibiotics:	Antibiotics:	Antibiotics:
Not recommended	Discretion of clinician	Recommended
Functional scan:	Functional scan:	Functional scan:
Not recommended	Discretion of clinician	Discretion of clinician

From Nguyen HT, Benson CB, Bromley B. Multidisciplinary consensus on the classification of prenatal and postnatal urinary tract dilation (UTD classification system). J Pediatr Urol 2014;10(6):982–98; with permission.

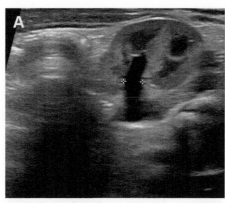
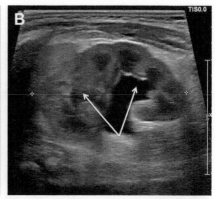

Fig. 6. Postnatal US appearance of UTD P1. (*A*) Imaging in the transverse plane shows APRPD less than 10 mm. (*B*) Imaging in the sagittal plane shows central calyceal dilatation (*arrows*) without peripheral dilatation with normal renal parenchyma.

P3 (HIGH-RISK) URINARY TRACT DILATATION

The use of PA, lower urinary tract imaging, and renal scintigraphy is highly recommended by pediatric urologists in patients with high-risk P3 UTD[67] (**Fig. 8**). Postnatally, repeat US imaging is recommended at intervals of 4 to 6 weeks to assess for possible disease progression.[68] This imaging can be combined with VCUG if the patient was not evaluated after delivery before discharge. In situations in which no visible improvement or disease progression is evident, a well-tempered renal scan should be obtained.

SEVERE BILATERAL PRENATAL URINARY TRACT DILATATION

Severe bilateral prenatal UTD is suggestive of LUTO and may indicate the presence of PUV, prune-belly syndrome, bilateral VUR, bilateral UPJ or ureterovesical junction obstruction, or any combination of these findings. Infants, who are diagnosed with severe bilateral prenatal UTD,

should undergo prompt evaluation after birth with US and VCUG because of the increased likelihood of significant disease. The VCUG may aid in identification of PUV or bilateral VUR. PUV is the most important diagnosis to rule out in boys with bilateral UTD, because it may be associated with an impairment of renal function. In girls, the most common cause is an obstructing ectopic ureterocele. After birth, it is important to promptly decompress the bladder, initiate antibiotic prophylaxis, and correct obstruction with the appropriate intervention.

TRANSIENT/PHYSIOLOGIC URINARY TRACT DILATATION

Transient dilatation is the most common urinary tract abnormality found during the prenatal evaluation, diagnosed in up to 70% of patients.[16] This condition is benign, usually resolves during the third trimester or soon after birth, and does not represent significant disorder.[66,69] Multiple studies

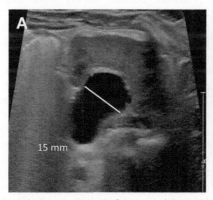
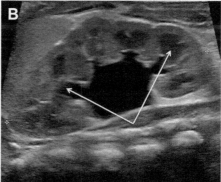

Fig. 7. Postnatal US appearance of UTD P2. (*A*) Transverse plane imaging shows APRPD greater than or equal to 15 mm (*white line*). (*B*) Imaging in the sagittal plane shows peripheral and central calyceal dilatation (*arrows*) with normal renal parenchyma.

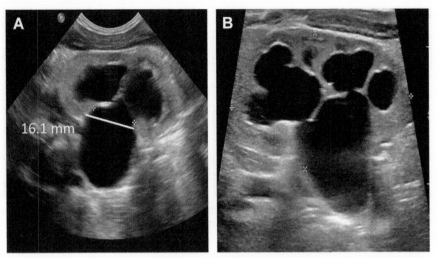

Fig. 8. Postnatal US appearance of UTD P3. (*A*) Transverse plane imaging shows APRPD greater than or equal to 15 mm (*white line*). Of note, the APRPD should be measured within confines of the renal parenchyma. (*B*) Sagittal plane imaging shows parenchymal thinning with peripheral and central calyceal dilatation.

have shown similar findings of mild to moderate prenatal UTD resolving or remaining mild/stable on subsequent postnatal imaging.[70,71] The SFU hydronephrosis registry study indicated that most infants show transient UTD and most resolve within 2 to 4 years of life depending on the grade of UTD.[66] This finding is important because parents and providers commonly have questions for their primary care physicians related to the expected timing of resolution.

URETEROPELVIC JUNCTION OBSTRUCTION

UPJ obstruction represents the most common pathologic urologic condition associated with UTD.[15] UPJ obstruction increases in frequency with increasing severity of UTD.[15] Most patients with UPJ obstruction can be monitored clinically without the need for operative management; however, separating benign from clinically relevant disorder continues to be an area of concern. The patients without the need for operative intervention may be followed with longitudinal imaging. Serial US imaging may help clinicians assess for evidence of disease progression.[72] Multiple studies have shown thresholds of dilatation (APRD, SFU, or UTD) that are predictive of, or correlate with, the need for surgical correction of UPJ obstruction.[6,7,12,73]

Dhillon[6] of Great Ormond Street conducted the benchmark study based on unilateral UTD (APD>15 mm) and differential renal function greater than 40%. In this prospective randomized trial, patients were randomly allocated to either observation or surgery for UPJ obstruction. Less than 20% of the patients in the conservative group

required surgical intervention for deterioration in renal function or increasing hydronephrosis. Of the conservative group, 33% remained stable on follow-up and 47% resolved or improved to mild dilatation. Of those who underwent surgical intervention, the APD measurements ranged from 20 to 40 mm.

Operative correction of UPJ obstruction is uniformly successful and recently has moved toward a minimally invasive approach.[74–77] A retrospective study of a single surgeon followed the transition of a practice from open to laparoscopic approach and noted the learning curve should be fairly flat after 15 cases, thus allowing for a successful transition in most busy practices within 6 months to a year.[77] The reoperative rate is 3% for all modalities, with open technique showing lowest cost and minimally invasive surgery providing less pain and improved cosmesis.

Practice pattern survey data suggest that 2 years of age seems to be a threshold at which minimally invasive surgery (MIS) including robotics is recommended by most pediatric urologist for UPJ obstruction. The survey data also suggest that open pyeloplasty is the preferred procedure in patients less than 6 months of age. There was also a trend toward MIS among the more recently fellowship-trained pediatric urologists[67] (**Fig. 9**). Recently, neonatal robotics has been proved to be effective with a specific premium placed on port placement and techniques to maximize working space by minimizing depth of port placement.[78] It is common practice to follow these patients with serial US after pyeloplasty is performed unless signs of obstruction persist.[67]

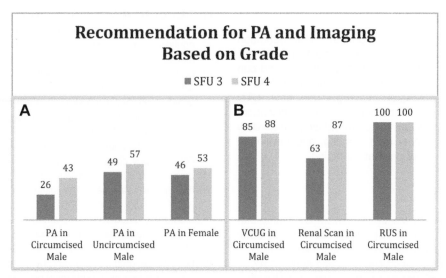

Fig. 9. (*A*) The percentage of respondents who recommend administering PAs to a 1-mo-old with unilateral UTD associated with the variables of circumcision status, gender, and grade of UTD. (*B*) The percentage of respondents who obtain VCUG, renal scan, and/or renal ultrasonography (RUS) for evaluation of a 1-mo-old circumcised boy with unilateral UTD. (*Data from* Jackson JN, Zee RS, Martin AN. A practice pattern assessment of members of the Society of Pediatric Urology for evaluation and treatment of urinary tract dilation. J Pediatr Urol 2017;13(6):602–7.)

VESICOURETERAL REFLUX

VUR is the third most common urologic condition presenting as prenatal UTD.[16] It is most common in boys and is typically bilateral and high grade. Of note, a disproportionate number of these patients resolve or can be managed nonoperatively. Multiple studies have noted a poor correlation between the degree of UTD and the presence of VUR.[15,79] The importance of diagnosing VUR in neonates with prenatally detected UTD remains a topic of debate; however, most agree that the selective use of lower urinary tract imaging to detect those at greatest risk of UTI is appropriate. Physicians should have an informed discussion with the family reviewing the risks and benefits of screening for VUR and use of antibiotics in this population.

MULTICYSTIC DYSPLASTIC KIDNEY

Multicystic dysplastic kidney is a congenital form of cystic kidney disease with the diagnostic findings of multiple large noncommunicating cysts, minimal to absent renal parenchyma, and absence of central large cysts. This disease is not progressive and is expected to involute early after birth. When detected on prenatal US, postnatal renal US is recommended to confirm the presence and quality of cysts. VCUG should be considered because the prevalence of VUR is as high as 20% based on some studies.[80] Radionuclide

imaging with dimercaptosuccinic acid (DMSA) historically has been recommended to confirm the absence of function; however, recent data suggest that it may not be necessary.[80] At present, the use of antibiotics is not recommended, because multicystic dysplastic kidney is not associated with an increased risk of UTI.

POSTERIOR URETHRAL VALVES/BLADDER OUTLET OBSTRUCTION

PUV is an important diagnosis to be made on prenatal US in boys with UTD. A prenatal US scan with bilateral UTD, thickened bladder wall with dilated posterior urethra, and in severe cases dysplastic renal parenchyma indicates PUV. The specific postnatal treatment of this entity is not covered in this article aside from recommending a prompt postnatal evaluation with bladder decompression. It is strongly recommended that all patients with suspected bladder outlet obstruction participate in prenatal counseling, which should involve maternal fetal medicine, pediatric urology, pediatric nephrology, and neonatology. Families should be made aware of the indication and limitations of prenatal intervention as well as the natural history of the disease. In addition to the timing interval of subsequent imaging, a thorough plan of delivery should be developed, including hospital location and contingency planning in case preterm labor occurs.

SUMMARY

UTD is the most common pathologic condition identified prenatally. However, most of these patients are at low risk for urologic disease and can be followed safely without the need for PAs or extensive postnatal imaging. The new UTD grading system incorporates risk stratification, which may dictate recommendations regarding PAs, lower urinary tract imaging, and the timing and frequency of postnatal imaging.

REFERENCES

1. Hamilton BE, Martin JA, Ventura SJ. Births: preliminary data for 2012. Natl Vital Stat Rep 2013; 62(3):1–20. Available at: http://www.ncbi.nlm.nih.gov/pubmed/24321416. Accessed April 7, 2017.

2. Nguyen HT, Benson CB, Bromley B, et al. Multidisciplinary consensus on the classification of prenatal and postnatal urinary tract dilation (UTD classification system). J Pediatr Urol 2014;10(6):992–8.

3. Zanetta VC, Rosman BM, Bromley B, et al. Variations in management of mild prenatal hydronephrosis among maternal-fetal medicine obstetricians, and pediatric urologists and radiologists. J Urol 2012; 188(5):1935–9.

4. Odibo AO, Marchiano D, Quinones JN, et al. Mild pyelectasis: evaluating the relationship between gestational age and renal pelvic anterior-posterior diameter. Prenat Diagn 2003;23(10):824–7.

5. Chitty LS, Altman DG. Charts of fetal size: kidney and renal pelvis measurements. Prenat Diagn 2003;23(11):891–7.

6. Dhillon HK. Prenatally diagnosed hydronephrosis: the Great Ormond Street experience. BJU Int 1998;81(S2):39–44.

7. Coplen DE, Austin PF, Yan Y, et al. The magnitude of fetal renal pelvic dilatation can identify obstructive postnatal hydronephrosis, and direct postnatal evaluation and management. J Urol 2006;176(2):724–7.

8. Shamshirsaz AA, Ravangard SF, Egan JF, et al. Fetal hydronephrosis as a predictor of neonatal urologic outcomes. J Ultrasound Med 2012;31(6):947–54. Available at: http://www.ncbi.nlm.nih.gov/pubmed/22644692. Accessed April 7, 2017.

9. Fernbach SK, Maizels M, Conway JJ. Ultrasound grading of hydronephrosis: introduction to the system used by the Society for Fetal Urology. Pediatr Radiol 1993;23(6):478–80. Available at: http://www.ncbi.nlm.nih.gov/pubmed/8255658. Accessed April 9, 2017.

10. Marks A, Maizels M, Mickelson J, et al. Effectiveness of the computer enhanced visual learning method in teaching the society for fetal urology hydronephrosis grading system for urology trainees. J Pediatr Urol 2011;7(2):113–7.

11. Erickson BA, Maizels M, Shore RM, et al. Newborn Society of Fetal Urology grade 3 hydronephrosis is equivalent to preserved percentage differential function. J Pediatr Urol 2007;3(5):382–6.

12. Braga LH, McGrath M, Farrokhyar F, et al. Associations of initial Society for Fetal Urology grades and urinary tract dilatation risk groups with clinical outcomes in patients with isolated prenatal hydronephrosis. J Urol 2017;197(3):831–7.

13. Braga LH, McGrath M, Farrokhyar F, et al. Society for Fetal Urology classification vs urinary tract dilation grading system for prognostication in prenatal hydronephrosis: a time to resolution analysis. J Urol 2017. https://doi.org/10.1016/j.juro.2017.11.077.

14. Siddique J, Lauderdale DS, VanderWeele TJ, et al. Trends in prenatal ultrasound use in the United States. Med Care 2009;47(11):1129–35.

15. Lee RS, Cendron M, Kinnamon DD, et al. Antenatal hydronephrosis as a predictor of postnatal outcome: a meta-analysis. Pediatrics 2006;118(2):586–93.

16. Nguyen HT, Herndon CDA, Cooper C, et al. The Society for Fetal Urology consensus statement on the evaluation and management of antenatal hydronephrosis. J Pediatr Urol 2010;6(3):212–31.

17. Hayashi S, Sago H, Kashima K, et al. Prenatal diagnosis of fetal hydrometrocolpos secondary to a cloacal anomaly by magnetic resonance imaging. Ultrasound Obstet Gynecol 2005;26(5):577–9.

18. Huisman TAGM, van der Hoef M, Willi UV, et al. Pre- and postnatal imaging of a girl with a cloacal variant. Pediatr Radiol 2006;36(9):991–6.

19. Kajbafzadeh A-M, Payabvash S, Sadeghi Z, et al. Comparison of magnetic resonance urography with ultrasound studies in detection of fetal urogenital anomalies. J Pediatr Urol 2008;4(1):32–9.

20. Clayton DB, Brock JW. Prenatal ultrasonography: implications for pediatric urology. J Pediatr Urol 2011;7(2):118–25.

21. Herndon CD, McKenna PH, Kolon TF, et al. A multicenter outcomes analysis of patients with neonatal reflux presenting with prenatal hydronephrosis. J Urol 1999;162(3 Pt 2):1203–8. Available at: http://www.ncbi.nlm.nih.gov/pubmed/10458467. Accessed April 16, 2017.

22. Sairam S, Al-Habib A, Sasson S, et al. Natural history of fetal hydronephrosis diagnosed on mid-trimester ultrasound. Ultrasound Obstet Gynecol 2001;17(3):191–6.

23. Psooy K, Pike J. Investigation and management of antenatally detected hydronephrosis. Can Urol Assoc J 2009;3(1):69–72. Available at: http://www.ncbi.nlm.nih.gov/pubmed/19293983. Accessed April 7, 2017.

24. Biard J-M, Johnson MP, Carr MC, et al. Long-term outcomes in children treated by prenatal vesicoamniotic shunting for lower urinary tract obstruction. Obstet Gynecol 2005;106(3):503–8.

25. Morris RK, Malin GL, Khan KS, et al. Systematic review of the effectiveness of antenatal intervention for the treatment of congenital lower urinary tract obstruction. BJOG 2010;117(4):382–90.

26. Freedman AL, Johnson MP, Smith CA, et al. Long-term outcome in children after antenatal intervention for obstructive uropathies. Lancet 1999;354(9176): 374–7.

27. Nassr AA, Shazly SAM, Abdelmagied AM, et al. Effectiveness of vesico-amniotic shunt in fetuses with congenital lower urinary tract obstruction: an updated systematic review and meta-analysis. Ultrasound Obstet Gynecol 2016. https://doi.org/10.1002/uog.15988.

28. Johnson MP, Corsi P, Bradfield W, et al. Sequential urinalysis improves evaluation of fetal renal function in obstructive uropathy. Am J Obstet Gynecol 1995; 173(1):59–65. Available at: http://www.ncbi.nlm.nih.gov/pubmed/7631728. Accessed March 3, 2018.

29. Ruano R, Sananes N, Sangi-Haghpeykar H, et al. Fetal intervention for severe lower urinary tract obstruction: a multicenter case-control study comparing fetal cystoscopy with vesicoamniotic shunting. Ultrasound Obstet Gynecol 2015;45(4): 452–8.

30. Morris RK, Malin GL, Quinlan-Jones E, et al. Percutaneous vesicoamniotic shunting versus conservative management for fetal lower urinary tract obstruction (PLUTO): a randomised trial. Lancet 2013;382(9903):1496–506.

31. Elder JS, Duckett JW, Snyder HM. Intervention for fetal obstructive uropathy: has it been effective? Lancet 1987;2(8566):1007–10. Available at: http://www.ncbi.nlm.nih.gov/pubmed/2889913. Accessed March 29, 2018.

32. Quintero RA, Johnson MP, Romero R, et al. In-utero percutaneous cystoscopy in the management of fetal lower obstructive uropathy. Lancet 1995; 346(8974):537–40. Available at: http://www.ncbi.nlm.nih.gov/pubmed/7658779. Accessed March 28, 2018.

33. Morris RK, Ruano R, Kilby MD. Effectiveness of fetal cystoscopy as a diagnostic and therapeutic intervention for lower urinary tract obstruction: a systematic review. Ultrasound Obstet Gynecol 2011;37(6): 629–37.

34. Sananes N, Cruz-Martinez R, Favre R, et al. Two-year outcomes after diagnostic and therapeutic fetal cystoscopy for lower urinary tract obstruction. Prenat Diagn 2016;36(4):297–303.

35. Braga LH, Mijovic H, Farrokhyar F, et al. Antibiotic prophylaxis for urinary tract infections in antenatal hydronephrosis. Pediatrics 2013;131(1):e251–61.

36. Zareba P, Lorenzo AJ, Braga LH. Risk factors for febrile urinary tract infection in infants with prenatal hydronephrosis: comprehensive single center analysis. J Urol 2014;191(5 Suppl):1614–8.

37. Alconcher L, Tombesi M. Mild antenatal hydronephrosis: management controversies. Pediatr Nephrol 2004;19(7):819–20.

38. Zee RS, Herbst KW, Kim C, et al. Urinary tract infections in children with prenatal hydronephrosis: a risk assessment from the Society for Fetal Urology Hydronephrosis Registry. J Pediatr Urol 2016;12(4): 261.e1-7.

39. Dejter SW, Gibbons MD. The fate of infant kidneys with fetal hydronephrosis but initially normal postnatal sonography. J Urol 1989;142(2 Pt 2):661–2 [discussion 667–8]. Available at: http://www.ncbi.nlm.nih.gov/pubmed/2664232. Accessed April 10, 2017.

40. Laing FC, Burke VD, Wing VW, et al. Postpartum evaluation of fetal hydronephrosis: optimal timing for follow-up sonography. Radiology 1984;152(2):423–4.

41. Herndon CDA. Editorial comment. J Urol 2015; 193(2):642.

42. Herndon CD, McKenna PH, Kolon TF, et al. A multicenter outcomes analysis of patients with neonatal reflux presenting with prenatal hydronephrosis. J Urol 1999;162(3 Pt 2):1203–8. Available at: http://www.ncbi.nlm.nih.gov/pubmed/10458467. Accessed April 9, 2017.

43. Aksu N, Yavaşcan Ő, Kangın M, et al. Postnatal management of infants with antenatally detected hydronephrosis. Pediatr Nephrol 2005;20(9):1253–9.

44. Gatti JM, Broecker BH, Scherz HC, et al. Antenatal hydronephrosis with postnatal resolution: how long are postnatal studies warranted? Urology 2001; 57(6):1178. Available at: http://www.ncbi.nlm.nih.gov/pubmed/11377338. Accessed April 9, 2017.

45. Zee RS, Herndon CDA. Prenatal diagnosis of congenital anomalies of the kidney and urinary tract. In: Barakat AJ, Rushton HG, editors. Congenital anomalies of the kidney and urinary tract. Cham (Switzerland): Springer International Publishing; 2016. p. 265–86.

46. Ismaili K, Avni FE, Hall M, Brussels Free University Perinatal Nephrology (BFUPN) Study Group. Results of systematic voiding cystourethrography in infants with antenatally diagnosed renal pelvis dilation. J Pediatr 2002;141(1):21–4.

47. Phan V, Traubici J, Hershenfield B, et al. Vesicoureteral reflux in infants with isolated antenatal hydronephrosis. Pediatr Nephrol 2003;18(12):1224–8.

48. Cooper CS, Chung BI, Kirsch AJ, et al. The outcome of stopping prophylactic antibiotics in older children with vesicoureteral reflux. J Urol 2000;163(1):269–73.

49. Kitchens DM, Herndon A, Joseph DB. Outcome after discontinuing prophylactic antibiotics in children with persistent vesicoureteral reflux. J Urol 2010; 184(4):1594–7.

50. Frimberger D, Mercado-Deane M-G, Section on Urology, Section on Radiology. Establishing a standard protocol for the voiding cystourethrography. Pediatrics 2016;138(5) [pii:e20162590].

51. NRC: Glossary – ALARA. Available at: https://www.nrc.gov/reading-rm/basic-ref/glossary/alara.html. Accessed March 30, 2018.

52. Pediatric Radiology & Imaging | Radiation safety – image gently. Available at: http://www.imagegently.org/. Accessed March 30, 2018.

53. Alexander SE, Arlen AM, Storm DW, et al. Bladder volume at onset of vesicoureteral reflux is an independent risk factor for breakthrough febrile urinary tract infection. J Urol 2015;193(4):1342–6.

54. Papadopoulou F, Efremidis SC, Economou A, et al. Cyclic voiding cystourethrography: is vesicoureteral reflux missed with standard voiding cystourethrography? Eur Radiol 2002;12(3):666–70.

55. Conway JJ, Maizels M. The "well tempered" diuretic renogram: a standard method to examine the asymptomatic neonate with hydronephrosis or hydroureteronephrosis. A report from combined meetings of The Society for Fetal Urology and members of The Pediatric Nuclear Medicine Council–The Society of Nuclear Medicine. J Nucl Med 1992;33(11):2047–51. Available at: http://www.ncbi.nlm.nih.gov/pubmed/1432172. Accessed April 15, 2017.

56. Stratton KL, Pope JC, Adams MC, et al. Implications of ionizing radiation in the pediatric urology patient. J Urol 2010;183(6):2137–42.

57. Sussman RD, Blum ES, Sprague BM, et al. Prediction of clinical outcomes in prenatal hydronephrosis: importance of gravity assisted drainage. J Urol 2017;197(3):838–44.

58. Jones RA, Perez-Brayfield MR, Kirsch AJ, et al. Renal transit time with MR urography in children. Radiology 2004;233(1):41–50.

59. McMann LP, Kirsch AJ, Scherz HC, et al. Magnetic resonance urography in the evaluation of prenatally diagnosed hydronephrosis and renal dysgenesis. J Urol 2006;176(4 Pt 2):1786–92.

60. Perez-Brayfield MR, Kirsch AJ, Jones RA, et al. A prospective study comparing ultrasound, nuclear scintigraphy and dynamic contrast enhanced magnetic resonance imaging in the evaluation of hydronephrosis. J Urol 2003;170(4 Pt 1):1330–4.

61. Braga LH, Farrokhyar F, D'Cruz J, et al. Risk factors for febrile urinary tract infection in children with prenatal hydronephrosis: a prospective study. J Urol 2015;193(5):1766–71.

62. Merguerian PA, Herz D, McQuiston L, et al. Variation among pediatric urologists and across 2 continents in antibiotic prophylaxis and evaluation for prenatally detected hydronephrosis: a survey of American and European pediatric urologists. J Urol 2010;184(4 Suppl):1710–5.

63. Braga LH, Pemberton J, Heaman J, et al. Pilot randomized, placebo controlled trial to investigate the effect of antibiotic prophylaxis on the rate of urinary tract infection in infants with prenatal hydronephrosis. J Urol 2014;191(5 Suppl):1501–7.

64. Coelho GM, Bouzada MCF, Pereira AK, et al. Outcome of isolated antenatal hydronephrosis: a prospective cohort study. Pediatr Nephrol 2007;22(10):1727–34.

65. Estrada CR, Peters CA, Retik AB, et al. Vesicoureteral reflux and urinary tract infection in children with a history of prenatal hydronephrosis—Should voiding cystourethrography be performed in cases of postnatally persistent grade II hydronephrosis? J Urol 2009;181(2):801–7.

66. Zee RS, Herndon CDA, Cooper CS, et al. Time to resolution: a prospective evaluation from the Society for Fetal Urology hydronephrosis registry. J Pediatr Urol 2017;12(17). https://doi.org/10.1016/j.jpurol.2016.12.012.

67. Jackson JN, Zee RS, Martin AN, et al. A practice pattern assessment of members of the Society of Pediatric Urology for evaluation and treatment of urinary tract dilation. J Pediatr Urol 2017;13(6):602–7. Available at: http://spuonline.org/abstracts/2016/MP13.cgi. Accessed April 15, 2017.

68. Herndon CDA. Fetal urology. J Pediatr Urol 2012;8(2). https://doi.org/10.1016/j.jpurol.2012.01.001.

69. Mandell J, Kinard HW, Mittelstaedt CA, et al. Prenatal diagnosis of unilateral hydronephrosis with early postnatal reconstruction. J Urol 1984;132(2):303–7. Available at: http://www.ncbi.nlm.nih.gov/pubmed/6737582. Accessed April 9, 2017.

70. Maayan-Metzger A, Lotan D, Jacobson J, et al. The yield of early postnatal ultrasound scan in neonates with documented antenatal hydronephrosis. Am J Perinatol 2011;28(8):613–8.

71. Barbosa JABA, Chow JS, Benson CB, et al. Postnatal longitudinal evaluation of children diagnosed with prenatal hydronephrosis: insights in natural history and referral pattern. Prenat Diagn 2012;32(13):1242–9.

72. Herndon CD, DeCambre M, McKenna PH. Changing concepts concerning the management of vesicoureteral reflux. J Urol 2001;166(4):1439–43. Available at: http://www.ncbi.nlm.nih.gov/pubmed/11547107. Accessed April 10, 2017.

73. Ross SS, Kardos S, Krill A, et al. Observation of infants with SFU grades 3–4 hydronephrosis: worsening drainage with serial diuresis renography indicates surgical intervention and helps prevent loss of renal function. J Pediatr Urol 2011;7(3):266–71.

74. Cain MP, Rink RC, Thomas AC, et al. Symptomatic ureteropelvic junction obstruction in children in the era of prenatal sonography-is there a higher incidence of crossing vessels? Urology 2001;57(2):338–41. Available at: http://www.ncbi.nlm.nih.gov/pubmed/11182349. Accessed April 12, 2017.

75. Sweeney DD, Ost MC, Schneck FX, et al. Laparoscopic pyeloplasty for ureteropelvic junction obstruction in children. J Laparoendosc Adv Surg Tech A 2011;21(3):261–5.

76. Minnillo BJ, Cruz JAS, Sayao RH, et al. Long-term experience and outcomes of robotic assisted laparoscopic pyeloplasty in children and young adults. J Urol 2011;185(4):1455–60.

77. Herndon CDA, Herbst K, Smith C. The transition from open to laparoscopic pediatric pyeloplasty: a single-surgeon experience. J Pediatr Urol 2013; 9(4):409–14.

78. Avery DI, Herbst KW, Lendvay TS, et al. Robot-assisted laparoscopic pyeloplasty: multi-institutional experience in infants. J Pediatr Urol 2015;11(3): 139.e1-5.

79. Herndon CD, Ferrer FA, Freedman A, et al. Consensus on the prenatal management of antenatally detected urological abnormalities. J Urol 2000;164(3 Pt 2):1052–6. Available at: http://www. ncbi.nlm.nih.gov/pubmed/10958739. Accessed April 12, 2017.

80. Calaway AC, Whittam B, Szymanski KM, et al. Multicystic dysplastic kidney: is an initial voiding cystourethrogram necessary? Can J Urol 2014; 21(5):7510–4. Available at: http://www.ncbi.nlm. nih.gov/pubmed/25347379. Accessed April 9, 2017.

Surgery of Anomalies of Gonadal and Genital Development in the "Post-Truth Era"

Daniela B. Gorduza, MD, FEAPU[a,b],
Charmian A. Quigley, MBBS[c],
Anthony A. Caldamone, MD, MMS, FAAP, FACS[d],
Pierre D.E. Mouriquand, MD, FRCS(Eng), FEAPU[a,b,*]

KEYWORDS

- Atypical gonadal/genital development • Disorders of sex development • AGD • AGD surgery

KEY POINTS

- Management of anomalies of gonadal and genital development (AGD) is highly complex and controversial, with diverse and often conflicting arguments for and against early surgical intervention.
- We chose the term "AGD" to avoid the confusion and discomfort associated with previous terminologies.
- Surgery primarily entails management of anomalies of the gonads, genital tubercle (masculinization or feminization), urethra, vagina, and perineum.
- Proponents of early surgery point out surgeons' greater experience with early (vs late) surgery. The more favorable genital anatomy in infants, the greater magnitude and potential for morbidity of genital surgery in adolescent and adult individuals and the limited psychological awareness of infants, support early surgery.
- Opponents of early surgery believe that affected individuals have a right to be involved in decisions regarding nonurgent, particularly irreversible interventions, that there is a significant risk of altering genital sensitivity, and that early surgery removes the child's right to an open future.

INTRODUCTION

Few subjects in pediatric urology have moved so rapidly during the past 3 decades as the management of the anomalies of gonadal and genital development (AGD). Changes in the terminology, the understanding of genetics and anatomy, the rationale for surgery, the outcome evaluation, and the psychological and societal contexts of AGD have driven all parties involved in care of individuals with AGD and their families toward major ongoing reflections. These changes have been triggered by patients, advocacy associations, and other groups who have voiced their defiance against lack of societal acceptance of genital variations and against some aspects of medical and surgical management. In the "post-truth era,"[1] opinions and emotions may oust facts and foster confusion. The difficulty is increased by the limits and pitfalls of

Disclosure Statement: The authors have nothing to disclose.
[a] Department of Paediatric Urology, Université Claude-Bernard, Hospices Civils de Lyon, Lyon, France; [b] Service d'Urologie Pédiatrique, Hôpital Mère-Enfant, 59, Boulevard Pinel, Bron 69500, France; [c] Sydney Children's Hospital, Randwick, New South Wales, Australia; [d] Division of Urology, Hasbro Children's Hospital, Warren Alpert School of Medicine, Brown University, 2 Dudley Street, Providence, RI 02905, USA
* Corresponding author. Service d'Urologie Pédiatrique, Hôpital Mère-Enfant, 59, Boulevard Pinel, Bron 69500, France.
E-mail address: pierre.mouriquand@chu-lyon.fr

Urol Clin N Am 45 (2018) 659–669
https://doi.org/10.1016/j.ucl.2018.06.012

"evidence-based medicine,"[2] a methodology that may be incompatible with some ethical considerations, leaving "experience-based medicine" as the only tool to forge current attitudes.

WHO ARE WE TALKING ABOUT?

We are talking about individuals with atypical gonadal or genital development identified either before birth, when the ultrasound scan of the genital area does not match the karyotype; or more frequently at birth or in the perinatal period, when the external genital appearance is unexpected, with atypical features affecting the genital tubercle, the genital folds, the urethral meatus, or the vaginal opening. Presentation during childhood may occur when a young girl undergoes surgery for what appears to be a simple inguinal hernia and testicles are found (complete androgen insensitivity syndrome [CAIS]) or a boy is found to have Mullerian structures during an unrelated surgical procedure; or at adolescence when an individual living as female shows unexpected signs of virilization (eg, clitoral enlargement, deepening of the voice, unusual body hair growth) or when an individual living as male shows signs of feminization (eg, breast development, female body habitus).

The terminology used to describe conditions affecting gonadal and genital development has long been confusing, controversial, and in some cases hurtful to affected individuals. The 2005 consensus conference organized by the Pediatric Endocrine Society (North America) and the European Society for Pediatric Endocrinology in Chicago introduced a nomenclature based primarily on the chromosomal profile, and although not entirely satisfactory, helped to foster consistent classification of these conditions.[3,4] However, the umbrella term, "disorders of sex development" ("DSD") was problematic for many people, particularly affected individuals and their families.[5]

The 3 primary categories under the 2006 terminology were "sex chromosome DSD," representing conditions associated with variations in the number of X or Y chromosomes in some or all of the body's cells (eg, 45,X; 47,XXY or chromosomal mosaicisms [45,X/46,XY; 46,XX/46,XY]); "46,XY DSD," affecting gonadal/genital development in 46,XY individuals: and "46,XX DSD," affecting gonadal/genital development in 46,XX individuals.

The conditions differ from each other etiologically and to some extent anatomically and clinically, and some of the current controversy is related to the tendency to group together very distinct conditions. In fact, the "DSD" terminology in many ways increased the confusion and distress. Some believe that unusual genital anatomy should not be considered an abnormality or "disorder,"[6] and, therefore, should not be managed as a medical condition unless medical consequences are likely to arise (eg, persistent incontinence, urinary tract infection, pain). To soften the impact of the term, some medical, ethical and support organizations redefined the "D" of the acronym to represent "differences" of sex development (eg, Androgen Insensitivity Syndrome–Differences of Sex Development Support Group, USA; American Academy of Pediatrics; Council of Europe; Swiss Ethics Commission; German Ethics Council).[7–16] The term "sex" in the "DSD" acronym added further confusion, as it may overlap in the minds of some people with a common English term for sexual relations. Furthermore, the term "sex" amalgamates brain imprinting ("brain sex" or "personal identity") with genital anatomy, which are separate issues, as evidenced by the discordance between gender identity and genital anatomy in transgender individuals. Although there has been continued debate on these semantic issues, we chose the term "anomalies of gonadal/genital development (AGD)" to outline the 2018 surgical approach of these very distinct conditions and address many current questions and controversies regarding each of them.[17]

THE 5 SUBTYPES OF ANOMALIES OF GONADAL AND GENITAL DEVELOPMENT

1. 46,XX AGD is mainly represented by girls with congenital adrenal hyperplasia (CAH), in which the cleavage between the lower part of the urinary tract and the genital tract (partitioning of the cloacal cavity at approximately 6 weeks of gestation) failed due to androgen excess. In 95% of cases, CAH is caused by deficiency of the enzyme 21 hydroxylase, due to mutations in the CYP21A gene.[18] Although fetal ovarian function is normal, this adrenal enzyme deficiency leads to androgen-mediated development of external and internal genitalia,[19,20] including augmented genital tubercle (GT[a]), fusion of the genital folds, and confluence between the vaginal

---

[a]The term "genital tubercle" (GT) is used throughout this article to refer to any structure derived from the embryonic genital tubercle: penis in typical male development, clitoris in typical female development, and variations of these structures in atypical genital development.

cavity and the posterior wall of the urethra. The external features are similar to those of a 46,XY child with hypospadias and nonpalpable testes. There is usually no gender issue in this group, except in the case of late diagnosis and markedly masculinized genitalia. Surgical management issues for this group mostly focus on the rationale and arguments for and against genital surgery, its timing, and long-term outcome evaluation.

Much less common forms of 46,XX AGD include 46,XX testicular AGD or 46,XX ovotesticular AGD, in which aberrant expression of testis-determining genes results in all or part of the gonads of a 46,XX fetus developing as testes. The development of reproductive and genital structures reflects the amount and function of testicular versus ovarian tissue in the gonads. Ovotesticular AGD is discussed further in subtype 4 in this list.

2. 46,XY AGD is a more heterogeneous group that includes 3 main classes: conditions affecting gonadal development (eg, dysgenetic gonads due to SRY deficiency, SF1 deficiency, or other genetic anomalies); conditions causing insufficient synthesis of testicular hormones by otherwise healthy gonads (eg, deficiency of androgens, due to conditions such as 17β hydroxysteroid dehydrogenase [17βHSD2] deficiency or deficiency of anti-Mullerian hormone [AMH]); conditions caused by reduced target tissue responses to hormones (5α reductase deficiency, partial or complete androgen insensitivity, AMH resistance). However, many patients with 46,XY AGD have no genetic or endocrine condition identifiable using currently available standard diagnostic techniques.

The typical clinical findings include underdevelopment of the GT (hypospadias and/or small penis), undescended and/or incompletely developed gonads, and possible persistence of Mullerian structures. Gender-of-rearing issues in 46,XY AGD are most often associated with conditions in which external genital development is intermediate between typical male and typical female. Management questions include timing and nature of surgical and hormonal treatment, and long-term evaluation. The risks and benefits of retaining versus removing the gonads may be considered for some patients, particularly those with gonadal dysgenesis, for whom there may be an increased risk of gonadal tumors.

3. Individuals with chromosomal mosaicism or chimerism also represent a genetically and clinically heterogeneous group.[21,22] Two primary forms are associated with AGD: 45,X/46,XY (formerly known as "mixed gonadal dysgenesis") and 46,XX/46,XY mosaicism or chimerism, which differ in terms of gonadal development, function, and malignancy potential, as well as clinical features. Because of the monosomic 45,X cell line, gonads of 45,X/46,XY individuals may have areas of atrophy/dysgenesis, whereas the presence of the Y-containing cell line renders these gonads at risk for gonadal tumor. In contrast, 46,XX/46,XY gonads contain 2 complete cell lines (ie, both have the usual complement of 2 sex chromosomes) and, therefore, the gonads are not dysgenetic and have no increase in risk of malignancy. However, in both conditions, the gonads may contain areas of both testicular development and ovarian development ("ovotestes"), with correspondingly variable hormone production; therefore, genital and reproductive development spans the spectrum from typical female to typical male. The genitalia may be asymmetric, with a palpable gonad on one side situated in a scrotum or labial fold and a nonpalpable gonad on the other side (often located in the abdomen), associated with a labia majora and inguinal hernia on that side. In 45,X/46,XY mosaicism the nonpalpable gonad is often underdeveloped or nondifferentiated (eg, streak gonad) and the GT is underdeveloped. Gender of rearing, rationale, timing and type of surgery, and tumor risks are the main surgical issues in these patients. In addition, due to the presence of the 45,X cell line, individuals with 45,X/46,XY mosaicism may have clinical features of Turner syndrome.[23]

4. Ovotesticular AGD is another complex group of conditions, in which the gonads contain ovarian and testicular elements, resulting in hormonal and genital/reproductive development that generally reflects the function of the different portions of the gonads. Most individuals with this very rare condition have 46,XX karyotype, with the testicular portion of the gonads developing as a result of aberrant expression of testis-determining genes. Most of the management issues overlap with those of children with 46,XX/46,XY mosaicism and, like this group, the risk of gonadal malignancy is low.[24]

5. The heterogeneous category of "Other" AGD includes patients with 46,XY and 46,XX cloacal exstrophy who have incompletely developed GT, those with 46,XY aphallia and some complex cloacal anomalies.[25] The potential genital, reproductive, urologic, and psychological consequences of these conditions raise similar questions to other groups, in addition to issues of intestinal function.

WHAT DOES SURGERY ENTAIL?
Aims of Surgery

In listing the following aims of surgery, it is acknowledged that not all of these goals are considered appropriate by, or relevant for, all patients, caregivers, or health care providers[26]:

- Reduce urologic hazards related to genitourinary anomalies (urinary tract infections with upper urinary tract and renal involvement, urinary incontinence)
- Reduce the risk of gonadal cancers in those patients with substantially increased risk
- Avoid virilization at puberty in 46,XY individuals living as girls whose testes have androgen-producing capacity and whose tissues have androgen responsiveness (eg, those with 17βHSD deficiency; 5α-reductase deficiency; some with partial androgen insensitivity syndrome [AIS])
- Avoid breast development in individuals living as boys (eg, ovotesticular AGD and some with partial AIS)
- Refashion, create, restore a genital anatomy more concordant with gender of rearing that will facilitate future penetrative intercourse (whether living as male or female), if desired
- Preserve erogenous sensitivity of genital tissues
- Facilitate future reproduction (as a male or female individual) when possible
- Avoid fluid or blood retention in vaginal or uterine cavities
- Help foster development of "personal" and "social" identities by providing anatomy concordant with gender of living
- Reduce risk of stigmatization related to atypical anatomy
- Respond to parents' wishes for their child

The Genital Tubercle

The GT appearance can be extremely variable from fully masculinized to fully feminized, hypospadias and small penis being the most common features in 46,XY groups and enlargement of the clitoris with incomplete vaginal opening being typical in 46,XX groups.

Three primary modes of surgery are used for anomalies of the GT: reduction (feminization), construction (masculinization), and replacement.

A. Reduction (feminization) of the GT involves the removal of part of the corpora cavernosa after a careful sparing dissection of the neurovascular bundles that surround the corpora.[27] Understanding the anatomy of the nerves and vessels leading to the glans and clitoris has changed the surgery of reduction of the GT.[28] Preserving the sensitivity of the clitoris is a major challenge and its evaluation remains quite subjective, making analysis of literature on this subject problematic. Most, if not all, procedures reducing the length of the GT are irreversible, although some surgeons have reported techniques in which corpora are left hidden in the vulvar region.[29] There is no published report claiming that these hidden corpora can later be unburied and refashioned as a penis. The irreversibility of these procedures and the potential damage to clitoral sensitivity restrict these operations to those individuals with significantly enlarged clitoris, especially if symptomatic. There is ongoing controversy regarding whether such surgery should be performed only with the full consent of the affected individual, with complete disclosure of the potential consequences as well as unknowns, both of intervention and nonintervention.

B. Masculinization of the GT follows the 3 major steps of hypospadias surgery, which include the following:

1. The degloving of the GT to determine the level of division of the corpus spongiosum, which is the best criterion to define the severity of hypospadias, the degree of hypoplasia of the ventral tissues, and the subsequent ventral curvature. This first step allows the choice of the most appropriate technique of urethroplasty and the possible straightening of the GT.

2. The repair or construction of the deficient urethra. Many techniques of urethroplasty have been reported.[30] They can be distinguished as belonging to 4 primary categories:

   a. Techniques solely using ventral tissues (eg, Thiersch-Duplay, tubularized incised-plate, Mathieu), which raise some concerns on a long-term basis, as the tissues distal to the division of the corpus spongiosum are hypoplastic and may not grow at the same pace as the rest of the GT.[31]

   b. Techniques combining ventral and dorsal tissues (eg, onlay island flap urethroplasty) are used more often than ventral tissue–only procedures in severe (midshaft or proximal) hypospadias and generally have good long-term outcomes, as the dorsal tissues have normal growth potential. In perineal hypospadias, a large mobilization of the dorsal, lateral, and ventral penile tissues with their blood supply (Koyanagi-Hayashi procedures) permits construction of a full-length penile urethra. Complications related to the amount and nature of skin tissue used in this procedure are quite common,[32] and may require urethral revisions. Staged procedures may be used in this population as well.

   c. Techniques using free skin or buccal grafts (eg, Cloutier Bracka) have their place in either proximal hypospadias or in cases of redo surgery. Revisions are quite common, as these procedures require a graft and commonly a second or third operation to complete the process.

   d. For distal hypospadias, a full mobilization of the penile urethra down to the peno-scrotal junction (Beck-Koff procedure)[33] is an elegant way to remove the ventral dysplastic tissues and to avoid a proper urethroplasty. The selection of patients for this method is important to avoid meatal and distal stenosis (short urethroplasty [<2 cm], distal urethra surrounded by spongiosum tissue).

3. Fashioning of the meatus, the glans, and the skin shaft cover. Follow-up of long-term results (until adulthood) of these procedures is mandatory to assess outcomes and identify complications.[34] Five groups of complications may affect these surgeries, in the following order of frequency: (1) inadequate cosmesis; (2) healing complications (urethral fistulae and urethral dehiscence), these 2 groups are probably the most common troubles following hypospadias surgery; (3) urethral flow complications (stenosis, urethrocele), which are more complicated to repair and often require a redo-urethroplasty; (4) persistent or new penile curvature and anomalies that may come to light with the growth of the GT; and (5) sexual or functional complications. The latter have been poorly evaluated but are likely to be significant in the adolescent and adult populations.

C. Replacement surgery is technically highly complex and is undertaken infrequently. Aphallia, extremely underdeveloped GT, or desire for gender change from female to male may lead to request for penile creation (phalloplasty). This request typically arises at adolescence or later, although this surgery has occasionally been performed during childhood.[35] Phalloplasties are extremely complex, multistaged, challenging procedures that should be performed only in rare specialized centers.[35–37]

The Vaginal Cavity

In girls with CAH, the vaginal cavity opens into the posterior wall of a normally formed urethra. This embryologic situation is different from the urogenital sinus, which is a distinct entity in which the nonseparation between the urinary and the genital compartments leads to a single, joint vesicovaginal cavity. The surgical challenge is to separate the vaginal cavity from the urethra and to bring its opening down to the pelvic floor. In most cases, a perineal approach allows the connection of the vagina, either using a "top-down" approach in which the urethra is mobilized up to the confluence or a "down-top" approach involving the mobilization of the mucosa sitting under the GT (ie, urethral plate), which is split into 2 vertical strips to fashion a mucosal introitus. Both techniques can be combined. In rare cases, the confluence is too high to allow a safe connection to the pelvic floor. In this situation, the classical option is the "anterior sagittal transrectal approach" (ASTRA). A less invasive approach is the laparoscopic pull-through of the vagina combined with a perineal approach.[38]

The principles of vaginal surgery remain the same in 45,X/46,XY patients raised as girls, although the vaginal cavity is more narrow, more tubular and rigid, increasing the technical challenges.

In girls with CAIS, the distal third of the vagina is usually patent and can be enlarged by natural dilatation that occurs with sexual intercourse later in life. However, the vagina is typically shorter than usual, and in rare cases exists only as a perineal dimple (this is also the case in girls with Mayer-Rokitansky-Kuster-Hauser syndrome). In these latter situations, the shortened or vestigial vagina usually can be dilated by the patient herself using a series of graduated cylindrical rods ("bougies")[39,40] or small vibrators.[41] However, the dilated vagina will resume its small size unless dilatation is continued, so should be undertaken only by girls/women who are preparing for intercourse, which will help to maintain the dilated state. Vaginal dilatation should not be performed in children at any time before they have attained the cognitive capacity to understand, consent to, and self-direct the procedure.

Discussions to define the timing of any vaginal surgery must be undertaken on a case-by-case basis with the affected child and family.[42] Those against early (prepubertal) genitoplasty believe that an individual should be given the opportunity to participate in the decision to refashion her genital anatomy, that a child does not need a vagina, that early vaginoplasty/genitoplasty may require revision at puberty, and that because of its potential detrimental effects on neurocognitive function, anesthesia should be avoided in infants unless required for protection of life or health.[43] Those who support early genitoplasty believe that genital tissues are more suitable for surgical intervention in infancy due to the brief increase in sex hormone production during the first few months of life (the so-called "minipuberty" of infancy). They also support the idea of undertaking surgery of both the GT and the vagina at the same time, as the tissues located under the GT are used to create a mucosal introitus. The distance between the perineal floor and the urethra-vaginal confluence is greater in older children, which implies a more extensive dissection of the genital region. It is also believed by supporters of early surgery that separation of the vagina from the urethra is more complicated in older children, who are believed to be at greater risk of bleeding and infection than infants. Psychological impact of late versus early surgery needs to be evaluated, as well as the potential consequences of growing up with atypical genitalia versus the alternative of discovering in childhood or adolescence that one's genitals had been surgically altered in infancy.

The Gonads

Depending on the clinical circumstances, testes can be partially or totally removed (orchidectomy), brought down (orchidopexy), or simply monitored with regular clinical examination, ultrasound scans, MRI, and, rarely, biopsies. The main reason to perform an early orchidectomy is the risk of tumor, particularly in 2 AGD groups: 46,XY gonadal dysgenesis and 45,X/46,XY mosaicism.[24,44] In addition, undescended but otherwise normally developed testes are at greater risk, compared with scrotal testes, for development of seminoma in young adulthood and should be monitored carefully.[45–48]

Testes that have acceptable risk of tumor are typically kept in place until the patient is fully informed and able to decide their fate for himself or herself. Teenage girls and women with CAIS are increasingly choosing to retain their testes into adulthood[49] on the basis of their preference for the natural hormones produced by the testes rather than synthetic hormones provided as hormone replacement therapy following orchidectomy.[50] Testosterone produced by the testes undergoes aromatization to estradiol, which induces and maintains feminization (breast development, female body habitus). Testicular hormone secretion in both CAIS and partial AIS may also contribute to bone health[51] and possibly libido.[52] Preservation of germ cells harvested from the prepubertal testis (eg, by cryopreservation), is a hypothetical possibility whose application using assisted reproductive technologies for individuals with AGD and healthy testes is beginning to be explored.[53]

Prepubertal orchidectomy may be considered in children with AGD living as girls who have substantial risk of virilization (eg, 45,X/46,XY AGD, ovotestis, 17βHSD deficiency, 5α-reductase deficiency, some with partial AIS), although alternative hormonal treatments to block pubertal hormone secretion are available to allow irreversible decisions to be deferred.

In ovotesticular AGD,[54] the ovarian part of an ovotestis can be removed to avoid breast development in individuals raised as boys; again, hormonal medications to prevent the feminizing effects of aromatization of testosterone to estradiol may be an alternative to surgery, particularly as gender outcomes in this group are variable and unpredictable.

Mullerian Structures

Mullerian remnants, such as fallopian tubes, utricular cavity, or vestigial uterus, are usually left in place if asymptomatic. When associated with hernia, or if they cause dysuria, cyclic pain, stone formation, or infections they can be removed either laparoscopically or with open surgery. Malignancy has rarely been reported in these tissues.[48]

The Perineum

In feminization procedures, the creation of labia minora using the skin of the shaft of the GT and the repositioning of the genital folds allows the fashioning of a vulva in most cases. For boys, surgery for penoscrotal transposition or bifid scrotum may be necessary to give a masculine appearance to the perineum. Although AGD surgery has been considered by some to be nonessentially "cosmetic surgery," the cosmetic aspect of the genitalia and the related risk of stigma may be important issues for some patients. Those who favor delayed surgery believe that because such procedures are not essential for physical health and well-being, they can be deferred until the individual can participate in decision making.

Breasts

Breasts can be either removed (bilateral mastectomy if unwanted), or enhanced (hormones; prosthesis) at or after puberty.

TIMING OF SURGERY

The timing of genital surgery has been a topic of major discussion and no consensus has been achieved. Arguments are presented as follows both against and in favor of early genital surgery.[26,55–57]

Against Early Surgery

- The nonconsultation of the affected individual until a hypothetical age of understanding her or his body and the choices available for the future.
- The inability of the young patient to understand the potential risks and benefits of the procedures, to be involved in shared decision making, and to provide informed consent for himself or herself (Human Rights Watch 2017).
- The withdrawal of the child's right to an open future.[58]
- The irreversibility of the procedures accompanied by the chance that the affected individual may choose in later life to live in a gender other than the one he or she was assumed to be or assigned in infancy.
- The feedback from some adult patients who received surgery during childhood.[59]
- The disappointing outcomes of some prior AGD surgery.
- The fact that the vagina is functionally unnecessary in a child.
- The risk of altering clitoral and vaginal sensitivity.
- The rejection by some of societal standards of "normality" and a binary or dichotomous society, with the belief that genital development instead represents a spectrum.
- The belief by some parents that their child should not be subject to surgery unless medically necessary and until the child's gender is clearly established.

In Favor of Early Surgery

- The pressure from parents to give their child a genital appearance consistent with their expectations for gender of rearing.
- The unevaluated consequences of living with atypical genitalia (potential for stigmatization).
- The magnitude and potential physical morbidity of late surgery.
- The paucity of data concerning the outcome of late surgery.
- The experience of surgeons with early AGD surgery in dedicated centers and lack of experience of AGD surgery at a later age.
- The possibly reduced psychological impact of AGD surgery performed in infants and the potential psychological impact of AGD surgery

during adolescence, which is known to be a difficult period for many individuals.
- The feedback from some adult patients who received surgery during childhood.

PATIENT, PARENT, AND EXPERT VIEWPOINTS

The views of patients and parents are as diverse as the conditions they represent and the cultural, societal, and religious frameworks in which they live. In the first few years of life children do not typically voice judgments about their own or others' appearances, and are, therefore, represented by their parents. Whereas some families feel that children should be given the opportunity to experience the bodies with which they were born, and to make their own decisions when old enough to express their gender identity and understand the consequences, others feel strongly that everything possible should be done to protect their child from the potential challenges of life with genitalia that do not fulfill societal expectations.

In the 1990s, a small but strong group of adult patients who experienced surgical treatment in childhood began a movement against genital surgery. They argued that alterations made to their genital and reproductive tissues without their consent had caused irreversible harm, and pushed for changes in the legal framework surrounding such surgeries. As a consequence, performance of surgery altering the genitalia and/or the gonads is restricted in some jurisdictions and may require legal approval to determine whether it is "medically necessary" (eg, Chile, Australia, Kenya, Malta).

Expert viewpoints have been published with increasing frequency in the 2000s and 2010s, from ethicists, governmental and nongovernmental agencies (eg, Australian Human Rights Commission, Council of Europe, United Nations, Swiss Ethics Commission, German Ethics Council, Human Rights Watch), patient support organizations (eg, Advocates for Informed Choice, InterACT), expert panels (eg, US Surgeon General, June 2017; North American Society and Adolescent Gynecology 2017), and legal entities. A number of key focal points are described in the following sections.

Consent for Irreversible Interventions

Advocacy groups believe that individuals have the right to bodily autonomy and reproductive integrity, and, therefore, that no irreversible procedures should be performed without the understanding and consent of the individual unless required to prevent medically significant consequences. The 2017 decision by the Court of South Carolina,

United States, to award compensation to a child who underwent feminizing genital and gonadal surgery at 16 months of age and subsequently self-identified as a boy highlights the scrutiny to which such procedures are subjected.[60] Overall, physicians working with families of children with AGD should be aware of the trend for legal and human rights organizations to increasingly emphasize preserving patient autonomy.[61]

The age at which a child is capable of contributing to informed decision making regarding his or her care cannot be rigorously defined, and will vary based on individual developmental maturity, in addition to familial, social, and cultural factors. However, the basic principle is that the views of the child regarding any nonurgent interventions, particularly those that are irreversible, should be sought and given full consideration. In the context of AGD, a key concern is that gender identity may be unclear or fluid in these children until mid or late childhood, so ethical principles would favor leaving all options open for the child's future (ie, protecting "the right to an open future"). To address this issue, one small pilot study assessed the feasibility of deferring genital surgery in CAH until adolescence, finding no psychological problems in girls with intact genitalia up to age 8, and spontaneous reduction in clitoral length by more than 50%.[62] The investigators propose further study to determine long-term outcomes of this strategy.

Parental Role

The role of the parents in the care of, and advocacy for, children with AGD is critical and must be fully acknowledged. However, the legal rights of parents are controversial and will vary by jurisdiction. According to ethicist Claudia Wiesemann, "The right to represent the child and to decide on its behalf is normally accorded to the parents as legal guardians. However, their role in DSD management is contested."[9]

Depending on approaches to care, communication, and counseling, some parents may face prolonged and recurrent shock, anxiety, and grief in adjusting to the diagnosis of a child with AGD.[8] Some researchers have likened the parental experience in context of the diagnosis of CAH (a condition that in addition to genital anomalies, includes potentially life-threatening hormonal deficiencies) to a form of posttraumatic stress disorder.[63] Others have highlighted the importance of counseling and peer support in mitigating that stress.[64] The overarching responsibility of parent(s) is to ensure that they are fully informed about the long-term as well as short-term risks, benefits, knowns, and unknowns of the choices they are making on behalf of their child. Furthermore, they have the critical obligation to make choices that preserve, as far as possible, the child's options for the future.

Counseling and Peer Support

Recognizing that AGD may result in significant stress and psychological challenges, advocacy organizations believe that psychological counseling and support should be offered to all affected individuals and families living with various forms of AGD.[65] Many published guidelines and position papers in the past 10 years have proposed that the care of children and families living with AGD should be provided by multidisciplinary (or preferably *inter*disciplinary, implying collaborative teamwork across disciplines) teams comprising both medical and nonmedical personnel. The inclusion of psychological support in such teams is critical, and the 2006 Chicago guidelines advised "Psychosocial care provided by mental health staff with expertise in DSD should be an integral part of management to promote positive adaptation."[3] The 2016 updated guidelines expanded on this concept, stating "Advocates and clinicians recommend team and communication skills training for health professionals to advance well-being. However, formalized training programs are lacking."[66,67] With the inherent difficulty of implementing consistent structured training across geographies and among diverse institutions the European Society for Pediatric Endocrinology provides an online training course for "DSD."[68] In addition, all individuals involved in care of families living with AGD, including psychologists, social workers, and other health care providers, should be encouraged to communicate with and learn from affected families who can share their life experiences. Whenever possible, attendance at a patient support group meeting can provide a wealth of insight and personal experience from which health professionals can learn.

Follow-up of Long-Term Outcomes

Echoing the guidance by various professional societies, patient advocacy organizations believe that long-term outcome data on surgical and nonsurgical management of individuals with AGD is profoundly deficient, and this gap must be addressed.

REFERENCES

1. Available at: https://en.oxforddictionaries.com/definition/post-truth.
2. Davidoff F, Haynes RB, Sackett DL, et al. Evidence-based medicine. Br Med J 1995;310:1085–6.

3. Hughes IA, Houk C, Ahmed SF, et al, Lawson Wilkins Pediatric Endocrine Society/European Society for Paediatric Endocrinology Consensus Group. Consensus statement on management of intersex disorders. J Pediatr Urol 2006;2(3):148–62.

4. Lee PA, Houk CP, Ahmed SF, et al, International Consensus Conference on Intersex Organized by the Lawson Wilkins Pediatric Endocrine Society and the European Society for Paediatric Endocrinology. Consensus statement on management of intersex disorders. International consensus conference on intersex. Pediatrics 2006;118(2):e488–500.

5. Johnson EK, Rosoklija I, Finlayson C, et al. Attitudes towards "disorders of sex development" nomenclature among affected individuals. J Pediatr Urol 2017;13:608.

6. Lin-Su K, Lekarev O, Poppas DP, et al. Congenital adrenal hyperplasia patient perception of "disorders of sex development" nomenclature. Int J Pediatr Endocrinol 2015;2015(1):9.

7. Gillam LH, Hewitt JK, Warne GL. Ethical principles for the management of infants with disorders of sex development. Horm Res Paediatr 2010;74:412–8.

8. Karkazis K, Rossi WC. Ethics for the pediatrician: disorders of sex development: optimizing care. Pediatr Rev 2010;31:e82–5.

9. Wiesemann C, Ude-Koeller S, Sinnecker GHG, et al. Ethical principles and recommendations for the medical management of differences of sex development (DSD)/intersex in children and adolescents. Eur J Pediatr 2010;169:671–9.

10. Council of Europe Commissioner for Human Rights. Human rights and Intersex People. 2015.

11. Council of Europe, Parliamentary Assembly (PACE), resolution 1952 (2013) final version of children's rights to physical integrity, 1 October 2013, para 7.5.3.

12. European Union Agency for Fundamental Rights. The Fundamental Rights Situation of Intersex People: FRA Focus. 2015.

13. German Ethic Council 2013. Intersexuality (Opinion). Available at: http://ethikrat.org:files:$/opinion-intersexuality.pdf.

14. Swiss National Advisory Committee on Biomedical Ethics. On the Management of Differences of Sex Development: Ethical Issues Relating to Intersexuality. Opinion number 20/2012. Berne, November, 2012.

15. United Nations Convention on the Right of the Child. Committee on the Right of the Child (CRC/C/CHE/CO/2-4). 2015.

16. United Nations General Assembly, Human rights Council. Discrimination and Violence against Individuals Based on their Sexual Orientation and Gender Identity. A/HRC/29/23. 2015.

17. Mouriquand P. Commentary to "attitudes towards 'disorders of sex development' nomenclature among affected". J Pediatr Urol 2017;13:610.

18. Speiser PW, Azziz R, Baskin LS, et al, Endocrine Society. Congenital adrenal hyperplasia due to steroid 21-hydroxylase deficiency: an Endocrine Society clinical practice guideline. J Clin Endocrinol Metab 2010;95:4133.

19. Prader A. Genital findings in the female pseudohermaphroditism of the congenital adrenogenital syndrome; morphology, frequency, development and heredity of the different genital forms. Helv Paediatr Acta 1954;9(3):231–48.

20. Gorduza D, Tardy-Guidollet V, Robert E, et al. Late prenatal dexamethasone and phenotype variations in 46,XX CAH: concerns about current protocols and benefits for surgical procedures. J Pediatr Urol 2014;10(5):941–7.

21. Martinerie L, Morel Y, Gay C-L, et al. Impaired puberty, fertility, and final stature in 45,X/46,XY mixed gonadal dysgenetic patients raised as boys. Eur J Endocrinol 2012;166(4):687–94.

22. Lindhardt Johansen M, Hagen CP, Raipert-De Meyts E, et al. 45,X/46,XY mosaicism: phenotypic characteristics, growth, and reproductive function– a retrospective longitudinal study. J Clin Endocrinol Metab 2012;97:1540.

23. Gravholt CH, Andersen NH, Conway GS, et al, International Turner Syndrome Consensus Group. Clinical practice guidelines for the care of girls and women with Turner syndrome: proceedings from the 2016 Cincinnati International Turner Syndrome Meeting. Eur J Endocrinol 2017;177:G1–70.

24. Cools M, Drop SLS, Wolffenbuttel KP, et al. Germ cell tumors in the intersex gonad: old paths, new directions, moving frontiers. Endocr Rev 2006;27:468–84.

25. Mouriquand P. Congenital disorders of the bladder and the urethra. In: Whitfield HN, Henry WF, Kirby RS, et al, editors. Textbook of genitourinary surgery – volume 1 – second edition. London: Black well Science Publishers; 1998. p. 205–44.

26. Mouriquand PD, Gorduza DB, Gay CL, et al. Surgery in disorders of sex development (DSD) with a gender issue: if (why), when, and how? J Pediatr Urol 2016;12:139.

27. Vidal I, Gorduza DB, Haraux E, et al. Surgical options in disorders of sex development (DSD) with ambiguous genitalia. Best Pract Res Clin Endocrinol Metab 2010;24:311.

28. Kaefer M, Rink RC. Treatment of the enlarged clitoris. Front Pediatr 2017;28(5):125.

29. Pippi Salle JL, Braga LP, Macedo N, et al. Corporeal sparing dismembered clitoroplasty: an alternative technique for feminizing genito-plasty. J Urol 2007;178:1796.

30. Djordjevik M. In: Djordjevik, editor. Hypospadias surgery challenges and limits. 2014.

31. Grosos C, Bensaid R, Gorduza DB, et al. Is it safe to solely use ventral penile tissues in hypospadias repair? Long-term outcomes of 578 Duplay

urethroplasties performed in a single institution over a period of 14 years. J Pediatr Urol 2014;10:1232–7.

32. Catti M, Lottmann H, Babloyan S, et al. Original Koyanagi urethroplasty versus modified Hayashi technique: outcome in 57 patients. J Pediatr Urol 2009;5:300.

33. Thiry S, Gorduza D, Mouriquand P. Urethral advancement in hypospadias with a distal division of the corpus spongiosum: outcome in 158 cases. J Pediatr Urol 2014;10:451.

34. Mouriquand PDE, Gorduza DB, Noché M-E, et al. Long-term outcome of hypospadias surgery: current dilemmas. Curr Opin Urol 2011;21(6):465–9.

35. De Castro R, Rondon A, Barroso U, et al. Phalloplasty and urethroplasty in a boy with penile agenesis. J Pediatr Urol 2013;9(1):108.e1-2.

36. Callens N, De Cuypere G, T'Sjoen G, et al. Sexual quality of life after total phalloplasty in men with penile deficiency: an exploratory study. World J Urol 2015;33(1):137–43.

37. Terrier JÉ, Courtois F, Ruffion A, et al. Surgical outcomes and patients' satisfaction with suprapubic phalloplasty. J Sex Med 2014;11(1):288–98.

38. Birraux J, Mouafo FT, Dahoun S, et al. Laparoscopic-assisted vaginal pull-through: a new approach for congenital adrenal hyperplasia patients with high urogenital sinus. Afr J Paediatr Surg 2015;12:177.

39. Frank R. The formation of an artificial vagina without operation. Am J Org 1938;1053–5.

40. Gargollo PC, Cannon GM Jr, Diamond DA, et al. Should progressive perineal dilation be considered first line therapy for vaginal agenesis? J Urol 2009; 182:1882.

41. Available at: https://www.acog.org/Clinical-Guidance-and-Publications/Committee-Opinions/Committee-on-Adolescent-Health-Care/Mullerian-Agenesis-Diagnosis-Management-and-Treatment.

42. Wolffenbuttel KP, Crouch NS. Timing of feminising surgery in disorders of sex development. Endocr Dev 2014;27:210.

43. Andropoulos DB, Greene MF. Anesthesia and developing brains—Implications of the FDA warning. N Engl J Med 2017;376:905–7.

44. Cools M, Looijenga LHJ, Wolffenbuttel KP, et al. Managing the risk of germ cell tumourigenesis in disorders of sex development patients. Endocr Dev 2014;27:185–96.

45. Hoei-Hansen CE, Rajpert-De Meyts E, Daugaard G, et al. Carcinoma in situ testis, the progenitor of testicular germ cell tumours: a clinical review. Ann Oncol 2005;16:863.

46. Ghazarian AA, Trabert B, Devesa SS, et al. Recent trends in the incidence of testicular germ cell tumors in the United States. Andrology 2015;3:13–8.

47. Pettersson A, Richiardi L, Nordenskjold A, et al. Age at surgery for undescended testis and risk of testicular cancer. N Engl J Med 2007;356(18):1835–41.

48. Picard JY, Cate RL, Racine C, et al. The persistent Müllerian Duct Syndrome: an update based upon a personal experience of 157 cases. Sex Dev 2017;11(3):109.

49. Nakhal RS, Hall-Craggs M, Freeman A, et al. Evaluation of retained testes in adolescent girls and women with complete androgen insensitivity syndrome. Radiology 2013;268:153.

50. Deans R, Creighton SM, Liao LM, et al. Timing of gonadectomy in adult women with complete androgen insensitivity syndrome (CAIS): patient preferences and clinical evidence. Clin Endocrinol (Oxf) 2012; 76:894–8.

51. Marcus R, Leary D, Schneider DL, et al. The contribution of testosterone to skeletal development and maintenance: lessons from the androgen insensitivity syndrome. J Clin Endocrinol Metab 2000;85:1032.

52. Ko JKY, King TFG, Williams L, et al. Hormone replacement treatment choices in complete androgen insensitivity syndrome: an audit of an adult clinic. Endocr Connect 2017;6:375.

53. Finlayson C, Fritsch MK, Johnson EK, et al. Presence of germ cells in disorders of sex development: implications for fertility potential and preservation. J Urol 2018.

54. Verkauskas G, Jaubert F, Lortat-Jacob S, et al. The long-term followup of 33 cases of true hermaphroditism: a 40-year experience with conservative gonadal surgery. J Urol 2007;177:726–31.

55. Creighton S, Chernausek SD, Romao R, et al. Timing and nature of reconstructive surgery for disorders of sex development—introduction. J Pediatr Urol 2012; 8(6):602.

56. Cools M, Simmonds M, Elford S, et al. Response to the Council of Europe Human Rights Commissioner's Issue Paper on Human Rights and Intersex People. Eur Urol 2016;70(3):407.

57. Springer A, Baskin LS. Timing of hypospadias repair in patients with disorders of sex development. Endocr Dev 2014;27:197–202.

58. Kon AA. Ethical issues in decision-making for infants with disorders of sex development. Horm Metab Res 2015;47:340–3.

59. Kohler B, Kleinemeier E, Lux A, et al, DSD Network Working Group. Satisfaction with genital surgery and sexual life of adults with XY disorders of sex development: results from the German clinical evaluation study. J Clin Endocrinol Metab 2012;97: 577–88.

60. Available at: https://www.buzzfeed.com/azeenghorayshi/intersex-surgery-lawsuit-settles?utm_term=.ca9xp775MK#.ad45lyyw1r.

61. Hunter D, Pierscionek BK. Children, Gillick competency and consent for involvement in research. J Med Ethics 2007;33:659.

62. Bougnères P, Bouvattier C, Cartigny M, et al. Deferring surgical treatment of ambiguous genitalia into

adolescence in girls with 21-hydroxylase deficiency: a feasibility study. Int J Pediatr Endocrinol 2017;2017:3.

63. Pasterski V, Mastroyannopoulou K, Wright D, et al. Predictors of posttraumatic stress in parents of children diagnosed with a disorder of sex development. Arch Sex Behav 2014;43:369.

64. Streuli JC, Vayena E, Cavicchia-Balmer Y, et al. Shaping parents: impact of contrasting professional counseling on parents' decision making for children with disorders of sex development. J Sex Med 2013; 10:1953.

65. Bennecke E, Werner-Rosen K, Thyen U, et al. Subjective need for psychological support (PsySupp) in parents of children and adolescents with disorders of sex development (DSD). Eur J Pediatr 2015;174:1287–97.

66. Liao LM, Green H, Creighton SM, et al. 'Service users' experiences of obtaining and giving information about disorders of sex development. Br J Obstet Gynaecol 2010;117:193.

67. Lee PA, Nordenström A, Houk CP, et al, Global DSD Update Consortium. Global disorders of sex development update since 2006: perceptions, approach and care [review]. Horm Res Paediatr 2016;85(3): 158–80 [Erratum appears in Horm Res Paediatr 2016;85(3):180].

68. Available at: https://www.eurospe.org/education/e-learning/.

Statement of Ownership, Management, and Circulation
UNITED STATES POSTAL SERVICE ® (All Periodicals Publications Except Requester Publications)

1. Publication Title	2. Publication Number	3. Filing Date
UROLOGIC CLINICS OF NORTH AMERICA	000 – 711	9/18/2018

4. Issue Frequency	5. Number of Issues Published Annually	6. Annual Subscription Price
FEB, MAY, AUG, NOV	4	$374.00

7. Complete Mailing Address of Known Office of Publication (Not printer) (Street, city, county, state, and ZIP+4®)

ELSEVIER INC.
230 Park Avenue, Suite 800
New York, NY 10169

Contact Person
STEPHEN R. BUSHING

Telephone (Include area code)
215-239-3688

8. Complete Mailing Address of Headquarters or General Business Office of Publisher (Not printer)

ELSEVIER INC.
230 Park Avenue, Suite 800
New York, NY 10169

9. Full Names and Complete Mailing Addresses of Publisher, Editor, and Managing Editor (Do not leave blank)

Publisher (Name and complete mailing address)

TAYLOR E BALL, ELSEVIER INC.
1600 JOHN F KENNEDY BLVD. SUITE 1800
PHILADELPHIA, PA 19103-2899

Editor (Name and complete mailing address)

KERRY HOLLAND, ELSEVIER INC.
1600 JOHN F KENNEDY BLVD. SUITE 1800
PHILADELPHIA, PA 19103-2899

Managing Editor (Name and complete mailing address)

PATRICK MANLEY, ELSEVIER INC.
1600 JOHN F KENNEDY BLVD. SUITE 1800
PHILADELPHIA, PA 19103-2899

10. Owner (Do not leave blank. If the publication is owned by a corporation, give the name and address of the corporation immediately followed by the names and addresses of all stockholders owning or holding 1 percent or more of the total amount of stock. If not owned by a corporation, give the names and addresses of the individual owners. If owned by a partnership or other unincorporated firm, give its name and address as well as those of each individual owner. If the publication is published by a nonprofit organization, give its name and address.)

Full Name	Complete Mailing Address
WHOLLY OWNED SUBSIDIARY OF REED/ELSEVIER, US HOLDINGS	1600 JOHN F KENNEDY BLVD. SUITE 1800 PHILADELPHIA, PA 19103-2899

11. Known Bondholders, Mortgagees, and Other Security Holders Owning or Holding 1 Percent or More of Total Amount of Bonds, Mortgages, or Other Securities. If none, check box ▶ ☐ None

Full Name	Complete Mailing Address
N/A	

12. Tax Status (For completion by nonprofit organizations authorized to mail at nonprofit rates) (Check one)
The purpose, function, and nonprofit status of this organization and the exempt status for federal income tax purposes:
☒ Has Not Changed During Preceding 12 Months
☐ Has Changed During Preceding 12 Months (Publisher must submit explanation of change with this statement)

PS Form 3526, July 2014 [Page 1 of 4 (see instructions page 4)] PSN: 7530-01-000-9931 PRIVACY NOTICE: See our privacy policy on www.usps.com.

---

13. Publication Title	14. Issue Date for Circulation Data Below
UROLOGIC CLINICS OF NORTH AMERICA	MAY 2018

15. Extent and Nature of Circulation			Average No. Copies Each Issue During Preceding 12 Months	No. Copies of Single Issue Published Nearest to Filing Date
a. Total Number of Copies (Net press run)			231	431
b. Paid Circulation (By Mail and Outside the Mail)	(1)	Mailed Outside-County Paid Subscriptions Stated on PS Form 3541 (include paid distribution above nominal rate, advertiser's proof copies, and exchange copies)	110	201
	(2)	Mailed In-County Paid Subscriptions Stated on PS Form 3541 (include paid distribution above nominal rate, advertiser's proof copies, and exchange copies)	0	0
	(3)	Paid Distribution Outside the Mails Including Sales Through Dealers and Carriers, Street Vendors, Counter Sales, and Other Paid Distribution Outside USPS®	77	132
	(4)	Paid Distribution by Other Classes of Mail Through the USPS (e.g. First-Class Mail®)	0	0
c. Total Paid Distribution (Sum of 15b (1), (2), (3), and (4))		▶	187	333
d. Free or Nominal Rate Distribution (By Mail and Outside the Mail)	(1)	Free or Nominal Rate Outside-County Copies included on PS Form 3541	35	78
	(2)	Free or Nominal Rate In-County Copies Included on PS Form 3541	0	0
	(3)	Free or Nominal Rate Copies Mailed at Other Classes Through the USPS (e.g. First-Class Mail)	0	0
	(4)	Free or Nominal Rate Distribution Outside the Mail (Carriers or other means)	0	0
e. Total Free or Nominal Rate Distribution (Sum of 15d (1), (2), (3) and (4))		▶	35	78
f. Total Distribution (Sum of 15c and 15e)		▶	222	411
g. Copies not Distributed (See instructions to Publishers #4 (page #3))		▶	9	20
h. Total (Sum of 15f and g)		▶	231	431
i. Percent Paid (15c divided by 15f times 100)			84.23%	81.02%

* If you are claiming electronic copies, go to line 16 on page 3. If you are not claiming electronic copies, skip to line 17 on page 3.

16. Electronic Copy Circulation		Average No. Copies Each Issue During Preceding 12 Months	No. Copies of Single Issue Published Nearest to Filing Date
a. Paid Electronic Copies	▶	0	0
b. Total Paid Print Copies (Line 15c) + Paid Electronic Copies (Line 16a)	▶	187	333
c. Total Print Distribution (Line 15f) + Paid Electronic Copies (Line 16a)	▶	222	411
d. Percent Paid (Both Print & Electronic Copies) (16b divided by 16c × 100)	▶	84.23%	81.02%

☒ I certify that 50% of all my distributed copies (electronic and print) are paid above a nominal price.

17. Publication of Statement of Ownership
☒ If the publication is a general publication, publication of this statement is required. Will be printed
in the NOVEMBER 2018 issue of this publication. ☐ Publication not required.

18. Signature and Title of Editor, Publisher, Business Manager, or Owner

STEPHEN R. BUSHING - INVENTORY DISTRIBUTION CONTROL MANAGER

Date 9/18/2018

I certify that all information furnished on this form is true and complete. I understand that anyone who furnishes false or misleading information on this form or who omits material or information requested on the form may be subject to criminal sanctions (including fines and imprisonment) and/or civil sanctions (including civil penalties).

PS Form 3526, July 2014 (Page 2 of 4) PRIVACY NOTICE: See our privacy policy on www.usps.com.

Moving?

Make sure your subscription moves with you!

To notify us of your new address, find your **Clinics Account Number** (located on your mailing label above your name), and contact customer service at:

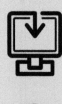

Email: journalscustomerservice-usa@elsevier.com

800-654-2452 (subscribers in the U.S. & Canada)
314-447-8871 (subscribers outside of the U.S. & Canada)

Fax number: 314-447-8029

Elsevier Health Sciences Division
Subscription Customer Service
3251 Riverport Lane
Maryland Heights, MO 63043

*To ensure uninterrupted delivery of your subscription, please notify us at least 4 weeks in advance of move.

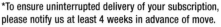
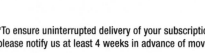